The PEDIATRIC PAIN HANDBOOK

Jayant K. Deshpande, MD, FAAP
Associate Professor of Pediatrics and Anesthesiology, Director, Division of Pediatric Critical Care and Anesthesia, Vanderbilt Children's Hospital, Nashville, Tennessee

Joseph D. Tobias, MD
Director, Pediatric Critical Care, The University of Missouri, Columbia, Missouri

Medical Illustrations by
Paul Gross and Dominic Doyle,
Department of Biomedical Communications,
Vanderbilt University Medical Center

with 33 illustrations

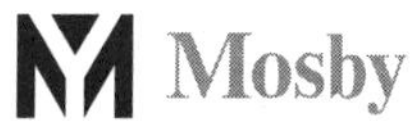

St. Louis Baltimore Boston Carlsbad Chicago Naples New York
Philadelphia Portland London Madrid Mexico City Singapore
Sydney Tokyo Toronto Wiesbaden

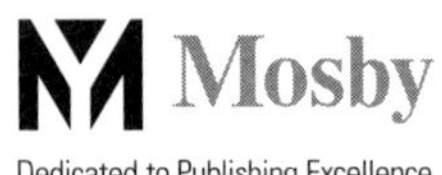

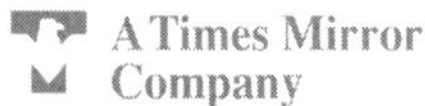

Senior Editor: *Laurel Craven*
Developmental Editor: *Sandra Clark Brown*
Project Manager: *Dana Peick*
Production Editor: *Jeffrey Patterson*
Manufacturing Supervisor: *Tony McAllister*
Book Designer: *Amy Buxton*

Printed in the United States of America
Composition by Top Graphics
Printing/binding by Malloy

Mosby–Year Book, Inc.
11830 Westline Industrial Drive
St. Louis, MO 63146

International Standard Book Number ISBN 0-8151-2431-7

96 97 98 99 00 / 9 8 7 6 5 4 3 2 1

This book is provided as an educational service from Astra USA, Inc.

Astra USA products, such as EMLA Cream (lidocaine 2.5% and prilocaine 2.5%) are mentioned. Astra advocates the use of its products within approved labeling, as specified in the full prescribing information for its products. The opinions expressed in this book are not necessarily those of Astra, USA.

PLEASE NOTE THE FOLLOWING:

- Ch. 1, pgs. 33-34: Regarding EMLA

(A) EMLA Cream should not be used in infants under the age of one month or in those rare patients with congenital or idiopathic methemoglobinemia or in infants under the age of twelve months who are receiving treatment with methemoglobin-inducing agents

- Ch. 3, pgs. 81-112 and Ch. 4, pgs. 113-156: Regarding Local Anesthetics

(B) Please consult the full prescribing information for a local anesthetic prior to its use

- Ch. 5, pg. 183: Regarding EMLA

(C) EMLA Cream is indicated as a topical anesthetic for use on **normal intact skin** for local analgesia. The insertion site for a chest tube is not considered to be normal intact skin and EMLA should not be used.

- Ch. 6, pg. 201 and pg. 212: Regarding EMLA

SEE NOTE (A) ABOVE; EMLA should not be used in infants under the age of 1 month. ***EMLA is not approved for use prior to circumcision.***

- Ch. 8, pgs. 298-299: Regarding EMLA

SEE NOTE (A) ABOVE: EMLA should not be used in infants under the age of 1 month.

CONTRIBUTORS

Kanwal J.S. Anand, MBBS, PhD, FAAP
Assistant Professor of Pediatrics, Anesthesia, and Psychiatry, Associate Investigator, Stress Neurobiology Laboratory, Division of Critical Care Medicine, Eggleston's Children's Hospital at Emory University, Atlanta, Georgia

Christi Capers, PharmD
Pediatric Clinical Pharmacist, Vanderbilt Children's Hospital, Nashville, Tennessee

Jayant K. Deshpande, MD, FAAP
Associate Professor of Pediatrics and Anesthesiology, Director, Division of Pediatric Critical Care and Anesthesia, Vanderbilt Children's Hospital, Nashville, Tennessee

David F. Gregory, DPh
Pediatric Pharmacy Coordinator, Vanderbilt Children's Hospital, Nashville, Tennessee

Shannon L. Hersey, MD
Assistant Professor of Anesthesiology and Pediatrics, Division of Pediatric Critical Care and Anesthesia, Vanderbilt Children's Hospital, Nashville, Tennessee

Sandra V. Lowe, MD
Assistant Professor of Anesthesiology and Pediatrics, Division of Pediatric Critical Care and Anesthesia, Vanderbilt Children's Hospital, Nashville, Tennessee

Brenda C. McClain, MD
Assistant Professor of Anesthesiology and Pediatrics, Division of Pediatric Clinical Care and Anesthesia, Director, Pediatric Pain Clinic, Vanderbilt Children's Hospital, Nashville, Tennessee

Gail E. Rasmussen, MD
Assistant Professor of Anesthesiology and Pediatrics, Division of Critical Care and Anesthesia, Vanderbilt Children's Hospital, Nashville, Tennessee

Berklee Robins, MD
Assistant Professor of Anesthesiology and Pediatrics, Division of Pediatric Critical Care and Anesthesia, Vanderbilt Children's Hospital, Nashville, Tennessee

Joseph D. Tobias, MD
Director, Pediatric Critical Care, The University of Missouri, Columbia, Missouri; Formerly Associate Professor of Anesthesiology and Pediatrics, Associate Director, Division of Pediatric Critical Care and Anesthesia, Director, Pediatric Pain Medicine Service, Vanderbilt Children's Hospital, Nashville, Tennessee

To our young patients and their families
and
To My Parents (JDT)
For My Sons Neel and Shyam (JKD)

FOREWORD

"Suffer the little children to come unto me and forbid them not." . . . Mark 10:14

Pain is an important component, and at times the only component, of most disease processes in man. Healthcare professionals approached pain management in a very simplistic fashion until recent times when it became clear that this approach was woefully inadequate and unsatisfactory. The pioneering efforts of the late John Bonica and others highlighted the need to approach pain management in a different light, and in recent times it has become clear that new approaches to pain management had to be implemented. For the past twenty years this new direction has resulted in a proliferation of many pain clinics all over the world, especially in the United States. This new direction has highlighted the need to differentiate between acute pain management and chronic pain management and has, as a consequence, brought tremendous pain relief and satisfaction to healthcare providers and patients alike. While most of these innovations have been taking place, pain management in children has been largely ignored until approximately seven years ago when serious attempts were made to effectively address pediatric pain management. The prime objective and, in fact, the major accomplishment of this text, *The Pediatric Pain Handbook,* has been to provide a clear, logical, concise, practical, and authoritative approach to the management of pain in children.

Most surgical procedures in patients are associated with pain; infants and children are no exception. The perioperative pain associated with those procedures has been largely ignored in the past. The commencement of an intravenous line, the insertion of a catheter, the changing of dressings, the performance of lumbar puncture, and many other similar procedures, though relatively minor from an adult standpoint, are associated with significant pain in children. The emotional, physiological, and psychological consequences of unmanaged pain associated with these perioperative procedures can have significant implications for the child, both in the short and long terms. Thus, effective perioperative pain management is important for the well being of the infant and child. Drs. Deshpande and Tobias and their colleagues have produced an outstanding text which may be useful to all healthcare professionals who treat infants and children.

The text corrects the long-standing and deep-rooted myth that infants in particular and children in general do not suffer pain or at least do not suffer as much pain as adults. In an attempt to correct that myth, they have reviewed the basic anatomy and physiology of neonates and children and have discussed the various pharmacological issues relevant to infants and children. The manner in which this task was accomplished has been very meaningful and comprehensive; further, they have provided a review of the current approaches to pain management in infants and children.

The chapter on Postoperative Pain Management by Dr. Tobias is thorough and complete. Dr. Tobias is eminently qualified to review that subject and is an acknowledged expert in pediatric pain management. He shares his experience in a very erudite and informative fashion and his contributions to this book are truly noteworthy. His chapter provides good information not only for the practical management of pediatric patients but also for the candidate preparing for different certifying examinations. There are very few reliable sources of information regarding nerve blocks in infants and children. This handbook provides such a source and does so with special emphasis on the differences between adults and the pediatric population, while paying particular attention to the dosing schedules of pediatric patients.

There are a number of disease processes and pain syndromes associated with the pediatric patient population. These syndromes and their respective manifestations are unique as far as their presentation is concerned. Further, their management requires an adequate understanding of the individual disease pathogeneses so as to implement effective therapy. Dr. McClain and colleagues have done an outstanding job in outlining those syndromes and diseases and have presented a clear review of the therapeutic approaches to pain management in these pediatric patients. Their contributions will be very useful to the practicing pediatric pain physician and other healthcare professionals who manage pediatric patients with pain.

Time spent as an adult patient in the Intensive Care Unit is usually associated with multiple diagnostic testing, administration of painful procedures, and implementation of therapeutic modalities that may usually be associated with pain. These issues are even more critical in the pediatric patient, who is removed from his or her natural environment and also from the love and care of parents. In this uncomfortable environment and with the constant background noises continually present (human and equipment-related noises), the bright lights and the ambient activity renders the child more apprehensive and thus more prone to perceive relatively innocuous stimuli as painful and painful stimuli as horrendous. In that environment, it is important to have well-planned procedures for the provision of sedation in the Intensive Care Unit and also of sedation for the administration of special procedures including cardiac catheterization, CT scan, MRI, and various interventional radiologic procedures. These issues have been eloquently addressed in an accessible form and should be very useful to all healthcare professionals caring for the pediatric patient in the Intensive Care Unit and beyond.

All in all, Dr. Deshpande and colleagues should be congratulated for putting together such a comprehensive text and doing so in a scholarly, efficient, and concise manner that should be useful not only to the pain specialist but to all healthcare professionals caring for pediatric patients in pain.

Winston C.V. Parris, MD, FACPM
Professor of Anesthesiology,
Director, Pain Control Center,
Vanderbilt University Hospital,
Nashville, Tennessee

FOREWORD

It has been said that we are born into a painful world. Indeed, there are few among us who exit the delivery room or nursery without some assault on our bodies, be it in the form of a heel-stick or perhaps a circumcision. Later on come infrequent, but nonetheless uncomfortable, minor surgical procedures or invasive diagnostic techniques that require both pain relief and sedation. Each of these circumstances presents a challenge to those who give care to infants and children. For the average practitioner, the challenge is not an easy one, for it requires a fair amount of knowledge about a variety of issues. What are the indications for pain relief and sedation? Which medication or procedure, if any, should be chosen? What is the correct dosage for a particular pain medication or sedative? Does the dosage vary with age or with weight? What are the drug interactions? What are the drug synergies? . . . and on and on. The sheer number of questions posed all too frequently results in a therapeutic paralysis, or at least lethargy, about doing anything, which is hardly in the best interest of children. Perhaps this is what Euripides was referring to when he said, "only time cancels young pain."

This book goes a long way to fill the void most have about pain management and sedation for the young. Drs. Tobias and Deshpande have assembled a group of expert contributors who effectively demystify the process of pain relief and sedation in the pediatric age group. While not every aspect of this work will be relevant to all practitioners, there is something here for each of us.

Read on and see how infants, children, and adolescents can be made comfortable when comfort is truly needed.

James A. Stockman III, MD
President,
The American Board of Pediatrics, Inc.,
Chapel Hill, North Carolina

PREFACE

The relief of pain and anxiety in children has been ignored by healthcare professionals for many years, possibly because of the perceived high risk of cardiorespiratory compromise. Over the last decade practitioners have realized that pain and anxiety may have profound, deleterious effects on children. This realization, coupled with humanitarian concerns, mandates that we search for safe and effective means to provide sedation and pain control. This handbook is not meant to be an exhaustive review of the literature, since there is a limited number of clinical studies on the subject. Instead, our goal is to summarize our clinical experience and outline methods, which we have found effective to sedate children for procedures, and to prevent and treat pain. We hope this handbook provides practical guidelines that the practitioner can use when caring for children undergoing invasive procedures or suffering from acute pain.

Acknowledgments

We would like to thank the nurses and residents of the Vanderbilt Children's Hospital whose quest to improve the quality of hospital life for their patients pointed out the need for this handbook. We also need to express our thanks to Tonda Rice, Judy Ledgerwood, and Brenda Gray for their secretarial support of this project.

Jayant K. Deshpande and Joseph D. Tobias

CONTENTS

1 Basic Aspects of Acute Pediatric Pain and Sedation, 1
Jayant K. Deshpande
Kanwal J.S. Anand

2 Postoperative Pain Management, 49
Joseph D. Tobias

3 Epidural and Spinal Anesthesia and Analgesia, 81
Gail E. Rasmussen

4 Regional Nerve Blocks and Interpleural Analgesia, 113
Joseph D. Tobias

5 The Management of Pain Associated With Medical Illnesses, 157
Brenda C. McClain
Gail E. Rasmussen
Berklee Robins

6 Neonatal Pain Management, 197
Brenda C. McClain
Kanwal J.S. Anand

7 Sedation in the Pediatric Intensive Care Unit, 235
Joseph D. Tobias

8 Sedation for Imaging and Invasive Procedures, 263
Sandra Lowe
Shannon Hersey

Appendixes I-IV, 319

Index, 365

The PEDIATRIC PAIN HANDBOOK

1

BASIC ASPECTS OF ACUTE PEDIATRIC PAIN AND SEDATION

Jayant K. Deshpande
Kanwal J.S. Anand

NEUROANATOMY AND NEUROPHYSIOLOGY OF THE DEVELOPING PAIN SYSTEM
- NEUROBIOLOGY OF THE PAIN SYSTEM
- DORSAL HORN OF THE SPINAL CORD
- GATE-CONTROL THEORY OF PAIN
- SUPRASPINAL CENTERS
- EVIDENCE FOR INCREASED SENSITIVITY TO PAIN IN NEONATES

PHARMACOLOGIC AGENTS
- NONSTEROIDAL ANTIINFLAMMATORY DRUGS
- OPIOIDS AND ANALOGS
- OPIOID ANTAGONISTS
- INTRAVENOUS ANESTHETIC AGENTS (SEDATIVES AND HYPNOTICS)
  - Ketamine
  - Etomidate
  - Propofol
  - Barbiturates
  - Benzodiazepines
  - Benzodiazepine antagonist
  - Chloral hydrate
- LOCAL ANESTHETIC AGENTS
  - Eutetic mixture of local anesthetics
- PSYCHOTROPIC AGENTS
  - Antidepressants
  - Antihistamines

Phenothiazines
Neuromuscular blocking agents
Succinylcholine
Pancuronium
d-Tubocurarine
Vecuronium
Atracurium
Doxacurium
Mivacurium
Rocuronium
Inhalational anesthetic agents
SAFETY CONSIDERATIONS
Patient assessment
Monitoring
Personnel
Fasting guidelines

Sedation and pain management have been on the back burner of medical education for many years. In particular, the care of a child undergoing a painful procedure or one that requires the child to be quiet and still for any period of time has received little attention. Most practitioners resort to physical restraint of the child and tolerate the anxiety, discomfort, and crying that the child exhibits during the procedure. Alternatively, many children are sedated for painful procedures (e.g., suturing of lacerations) with the "pedi cocktail." This mixture of Demerol, Phenergan, and Thorazine (DPT) combines a varying dosage of each of the medications to achieve a quiet and cooperative child. However, the significant risk to the patient of using such a combination was essentially ignored until recently. Children were often left to "sleep off the medication" for hours without ascertaining that they had normal protective airway reflexes or that they were hemodynamically stable. The morbidity that occurred with this technique, including airway obstruction and apnea, was either overlooked or underplayed.

Over the last 10 years it has become clear that a more rational approach is necessary to care for the child who needs sedation or pain management. Many investigators have worked to clarify the understanding of the mechanisms of pain and anxiety, as well as the pharmacology of sedative agents in infants and children. Other authors have advanced the knowledge concerning techniques available to provide analgesia and sedation under various circumstances. It is beyond the scope of this handbook to present an extensive review of the available information. This handbook is designed to provide a basic understanding of and a practical approach to the management of sedation and acute pain in infants and children. It presents brief discussions on mechanisms of pain in children and the basic pharmacology of the commonly used drugs, and it emphasizes pragmatic approaches to some common clinical situations.

The basic premise in this book is that infants and children perceive pain and suffer because of it. To treat a child inappropriately for his or her pain, or to fail to sedate a child when required, is inhumane. Recent information supports the fact that infants and children perceive pain, and such experiences may have long-term residual effects if their pain is inadequately treated. Furthermore, because of improved knowledge of the pharmacology and pharmacokinetics of the medications available and an ability to provide appropriate monitoring and cardiopulmonary support to an infant or child, the patient can be safely sedated, and his or her pain can be alleviated in nearly all types of clinical situations.

This chapter focuses on the general aspects of managing sedation and treating acute pain in infants and children. The first section is a review of the developmental neuroanatomy of pain. The second part is a brief overview of the pharmacologic armamentarium available to treat patients. The final section of this chapter addresses the basic safety considerations that must be kept in mind when undertaking sedation or treatment of acute pain in children.

NEUROANATOMY AND NEUROPHYSIOLOGY OF THE DEVELOPING PAIN SYSTEM

Neurobiology of the Pain System

The pain system develops during the second and third trimesters of human gestation, with additional maturation changes occurring during the first two years of postnatal life[1,2,3] (Fig. 1-1). Thereafter, the perception of pain changes very little, although major changes occur in the emotional aspects of painful experiences, the interpretations of the meaning of pain, and the repertoire of behavioral and cognitive expressions of pain.

Traditionally, the pain system was thought to be underdeveloped in the neonate and older infant. Because neonates, or nonverbal infants, are not capable of describing the subjective phenomenon of pain, it was concluded that these age groups are also incapable of pain perception. These widespread notions led to the clinical practices of providing either minimal or no anesthesia during surgery and no analgesia for invasive procedures or after

---

FIG 1-1.

Graphical representation of the mature pain system. *A,* A-δ fibers; *C,* C-fibers; *DRG,* dorsal root ganglion; *DH,* dorsal horn of the spinal cord; *SR,* spinoreticular tract; *SM,* spinomesencephalic tract; *ST,* lateral spinothalamic tract; *NP,* nucleus proprius; *RF,* medullary and pontine reticular formation; *PAG,* periaqueductal gray matter; *VPL,* ventroposterolateral nucleus of the thalamus; *VPM,* ventroposteromedial nucleus of the thalamus; *CN,* central and intralaminary nuclei of the thalamus; *OB,* olfactory bulb; *F,* fornix; *MB,* mammillary bodies; *AB,* amygdaloid body (central nucleus of the amygdala); *H,* hippocampus; *CG,* cingulate gyrus; *PCG,* postcentral gyrus; *V & Vm,* sensory and motor roots of the trigeminal nerve; *MN,* motor nucleus of the trigeminal nerve; *PSN,* principal sensory nucleus of the trigeminal nerve; *SSN,* spinal sensory nucleus of the trigeminal nerve; *TL,* trigeminal lemniscus; *VII,* facial nerve; *IX,* glossopharyngeal nerve; *X,* vagus nerve. Numbers in the cerebral cortex indicate the cortical fields of Broadmann.

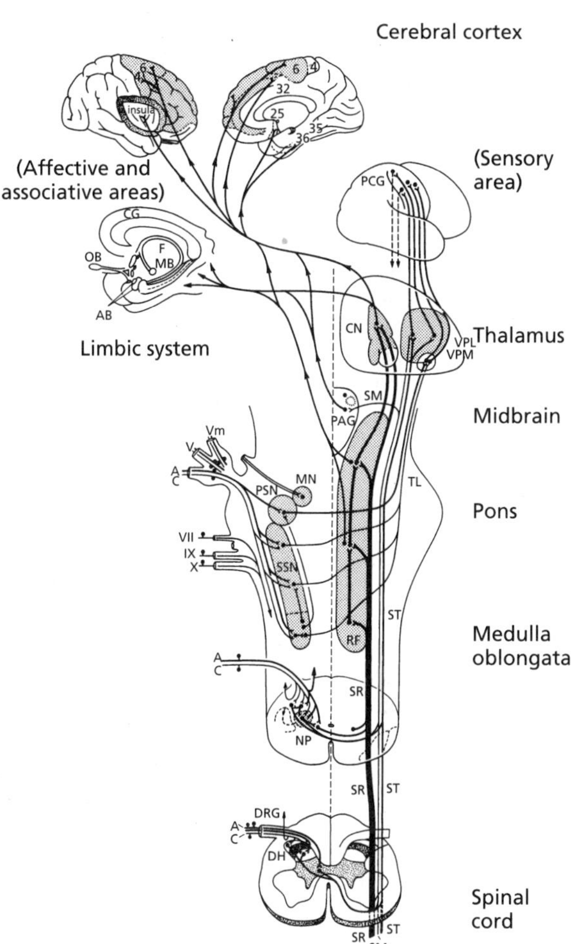
Cerebral cortex
(Affective and associative areas)
(Sensory area)
insula
6
4
32
25
35
36
PCG
CG
F
MB
OB
AB
Limbic system
CN
Thalamus
VPL
VPM
SM
PAG
Midbrain
Vm
V
A
C
MN
PSN
TL
Pons
VII
IX
X
SSN
ST
RF
Medulla oblongata
SR
NP
SR
ST
DRG
DH
Spinal cord
SR
SM
ST

surgery. These practices were commonly practiced in newborns, particularly premature neonates. Recommendations for analgesia or sedation during intensive care were also made without considering the developmental neurobiology of pain mechanisms or the physiologic and behavioral responses to pain and stress in neonates and small infants.

Pain-related pathways may be traced from sensory receptors in the skin to the cerebral cortex. The development of each of these components provides a framework to study the development of the pain system. For the sake of clarity, a description of the pain system is arbitrarily divided in Table 1-1.

Histologic studies show that the density of nociceptive nerve endings in newborn skin is similar to that of adult skin. Microneurographic investigations show that the neurophysiologic properties of the earliest nociceptors are also similar to those of adult skin. Rapidly-adapting pressure receptors are the first to appear during fetal life, followed by the development of slowly-adapting pressure receptors, rapidly-adapting mechanoceptors, and occasional muscle afferents. The depolarization responses of these receptors to mechanical injury, chemical irritants, and inflammatory mediators are similar to those of adult receptors before they establish synaptic connections with neurons in the dorsal horn. Signal transduction mechanisms via linkage to G-protein complexes appear to mature rapidly in these early receptors.

Fetal sensory receptors are located on or close to the skin surface soon after development and gradually become subepidermal with the development of the stratum corneum. Studies in the 1940s note reflexes to cutaneous sensory stimulation from the perioral area of the human fetus in the seventh week of gestation; from the rest of the face, palms of the hands, and the soles of the feet by the eleventh week; from the trunk and proximal parts of the arms and legs by the fifteenth week; and from all cutaneous and mucous surfaces by the twentieth week. The development of sensory reflexes was somatotopically preceded by synaptogenesis between afferent fibers and sensory neurons in the dorsal horn of the spinal cord. Thicker, myelinated fibers are the first to grow into the de-

TABLE 1-1. Anatomy of the Pain System

Anatomical Location	Components	Biological Function
The peripheral pain system	High-threshold mechanoceptors, free nerve endings, polymodal nociceptors, C-fibers, silent C-fibers, A-δ fibers, ?lymphocytes	Registering the initial noxious stimulus, local pain reactions (vasomotor, inf'ammatory), conduction to the central nervous system
Dorsal horn of the spinal cord	Dorsal root ganglion cells, substantia gelatinosa, inhibitory interneurons, lamina V neurons, projection neurons, descending inhibitory fibers, ascending pain tracts	Integration of pain and other sensory stimuli, sensory hyperexcitability or windup phenomenon, gate-control mechanisms/modulation of pain, chronic pain mechanisms (e.g., neuropathic pain, causalgia, etc.)
Supraspinal centers	Raphe magnus, periaqueductal grey, reticular activating system, locus coeruleus, inferior olivary nucleus, paraventricular nucleus & other hypothalamic centers, thalamic nuclei, limbic system (amygdala, hippocampus), cingulate gyrus, postcentral gyrus, some frontal and parietooccipital areas	Integration and processing of painful information, localization and identification of pain characteristics, emotional reactions, matching with memories of pain, cognitive interpretation, arousal and attention, modulation of pain perception, stimulation of systemic responses to pain (cardiovascular, hormonal, immune, etc.)

veloping spinal cord and form connections with deeper layers of the dorsal horn, with collaterals to neurons in the substantia gelatinosa. With the ingrowth of C-fibers and synaptogenesis with superficial dorsal horn neurons, these collaterals undergo developmental degeneration. Nociceptive stimuli in fetal life (and in micropremature neonates) are therefore conducted by myelinated A-β and A-δ fibers until the maturation of C-fiber connections.

Dorsal Horn of the Spinal Cord

Development of the dorsal horn begins with the closure of the neural canal in the first trimester of pregnancy. Sequential electron microscopic and immunocytochemical studies during the second trimester demonstrate that the development of the various neuronal cell types in the dorsal horn, together with their laminar arrangement, interneuronal connections, and the expression of their specific neurotransmitters and receptors, begins before 13 weeks of gestation and is completed by 30 to 32 weeks. Initially, the receptive fields of dorsal horn neurons are very large with an extensive overlap between the receptive fields of adjacent neurons. As maturation occurs, the receptive fields of individual dorsal horn cells progressively decrease and can be more precisely defined.

The transmission of nociceptive impulses through the dorsal horn of the spinal cord is mediated via the release of excitatory neurotransmitters, such as substance P, glutamate, calcitonin-gene-related peptide (CGRP), vasoactive intestinal polypeptide (VIP), neuropeptide Y, and somatostatin. Modulation of this nociceptive transmission occurs primarily by the release of met-enkephalin from local interneurons, as well as norepinephrine, dopamine, and serotonin from descending inhibitory axons. These descending inhibitory axons originate in supraspinal centers and terminate at all levels of the spinal cord and brainstem. Of the nociceptive neurotransmitters, substance P, CGRP, and somatostatin are expressed in the dorsal horn of 8- to 10-week-old human fetuses, whereas glutamate, VIP, and neuropeptide Y appear at about 12 to 16 weeks of human gestation. Modulation of incoming noxious or nonnoxious sensory stimuli in extremely premature infants may occur by the local release of met-enkephalin, which is first expressed at 12 to

16 weeks of gestation, although this mechanism is unlikely to be effective in diminishing the transmission of intense painful stimuli. In the latter half of the third trimester, as the descending inhibitory control from supraspinal centers develops and matures, inhibition of incoming sensory stimuli occurs with the release of dopamine and norepinephrine. These neurotransmitters are first expressed at 34 to 38 weeks of human gestation followed by the appearance of serotonin in the postneonatal period.

Gate Control Theory of Pain

The result of the activity of these different neuronal subgroups is responsible for controlling the context-dependence of the behavioral responses to pain, such as the effects of the child's attention, the degree of arousal and behavioral state, and the presence of other incoming afferent impulses at the time that the noxious stimulus occurs. Selective modulation or enhancement of painful stimuli occurs at various levels in the central nervous system (CNS) and forms the physiologic basis for the gate-control theory of pain. Other neurobehavioral phenomena that are dependent on these mechanisms include habituation to nonnoxious stimuli, hypersensitivity, muscle contracture, resting joint positions that occur after severe injury or inflammation, the summation of noxious stimuli with close anatomical proximity, and other common clinical manifestations of pain.

Pain was previously described as a process in which specific nociceptive receptors are stimulated and produce standard responses within dorsal horn neurons in the spinal cord, with well-defined patterns of conduction to the brainstem, thalamus, and other subcortical centers. Such concepts of the pain system and other simple explanations of pain mechanisms were abandoned since accumulating clinical and experimental evidence described the phenomenon of pain as a remarkable adaptive neuronal and neurochemical process. Within neuronal networks at various levels of the CNS the elements may increase or decrease in number. Such adaptive processes were noted to be dependent on the characteristics of the noxious stimulus, the context in which it is applied, the behavioral state at the time of application, and various other factors, all of which produce significant alterations in the form or degree of pain experienced. Within this framework proposed by Wall and Melzack in 1965, the experience of pain was likened to a "need state," which elicited a complex neuronal response with regulatory outflows at various levels of the CNS, produced in order to modulate the intensity of pain, respond to it, or adapt to it.

Traditional classifications of nociceptive neurons were also challenged by these novel concepts. Since there are no fixed relationships between excitation of peripheral fibers and sensory or behavioral outcome, or between the input and output of individual dorsal horn neurons, it was proposed the input-output schemes within the pain system are context-dependent. For example, strong or repeated nociceptive stimuli were thought to trigger widespread increases of neural excitability within the spinal cord, with changes in the sensitivity of dorsal horn neurons and expansion of their cutaneous receptive fields.

Supraspinal Centers

It is now known that the integration of afferent signals occurs in multiple time frames at each level of sensory processing through both excitatory and inhibitory input and is interwoven with efferent output from higher centers, which may accentuate or modify the cascade of neurochemical events triggered by nociception. This elaborate system provides a plasticity characteristic of the nervous system, and may form the basis for memory and learning from nociceptive experiences. It also produces variable responses to the multiplicity of nociceptive experiences within the environment, responses which may initiate or influence widespread processes such as awareness, cardiovascular activation, respiratory adaptation, hormonal stimulation, metabolic alterations, changes in immune function, and a host of other bodily functions. These widespread responses within the CNS are coordinated by neuronal networks, which are particularly dense loci for the processing, transmission, and integration of painful stimuli, collectively labeled as the supraspinal centers for pain.

Conduction of nociceptive impulses to the supraspinal centers occurs via the spinothalamic, spinoreticular, and spinomesencephalic tracts located mainly in the anterolateral and lateral white matter of the spinal cord. Lack of myelination in these nerve tracts was proposed as an index of immaturity in the neonatal CNS and was used to support the argument that neonates cannot feel pain. This argument was widely supported despite the common knowledge that incomplete myelination does not imply lack of function but merely imposes a slower conduction velocity in the central nerve tracts of neonates. In addition, any slowing in the central conduction velocity would be completely offset by the shorter interneuronal distances traveled by the impulse. Quantitative neuroanatomical data from the Collaborative Perinatal Project show that nociceptive nerve tracts to the brain stem and thalamus are completely myelinated by 30 weeks of human gestation, and the thalamocortical pain fibers are myelinated by 37 weeks. The timing of the thalamocortical connection is of crucial importance for cortical perception, since most sensory pathways to the neocortex have synapses in the thalamus. In the primate fetus, thalamic neurons produce axons that arrive in the cerebrum before midgestation. These fibers wait just below the neocortex until migration and dendritic arborization of cortical neurons are complete and finally establish synaptic connections at 20 to 24 weeks of gestation.

Functional maturity of the cerebral cortex is suggested by fetal and neonatal electroencephalographic (EEG) patterns and by the behavioral development of neonates. Intermittent EEG bursts in both cerebral hemispheres first seen at 20 weeks of gestation become sustained at 22 weeks and are bilaterally synchronous at 26 to 27 weeks of gestation. By 30 weeks the distinction between wakefulness and sleep can be made on the basis of EEG patterns. Cortical components of somatosensory, auditory, and visually evoked potentials have been recorded in preterm babies before 26 weeks of gestation. Several forms of behavior imply cortical function during fetal life. Well-defined periods of quiet sleep, active sleep, and wakefulness occur even in utero, beginning at 28 weeks of gestation. In addition to the specific behavioral responses to pain described below, neonates have various cognitive, coordinative, and associative capabilities in response to visual and auditory stimuli, attesting to the presence of cortical function. Several lines of evidence suggest that the complete nervous system is active during prenatal development and that detrimental or developmental changes in any part would affect the entire system. Thus, it is now well-established that even premature human newborns have the functional components of a pain system and are capable of pain perception. In fact, the development of a pain system suggests that the pain threshold may be decreased in preterm neonates compared with term neonates or older infants.

Evidence for Increased Sensitivity to Pain in Neonates

The cutaneous flexor reflex has a lower threshold in preterm neonates than in term neonates or adults.[4] Thresholds for the flexor withdrawal reflex are decreased (sensitized) after repeated stimulation or local tissue injury in preterm neonates. The prolonged hypersensitivity is abolished by topical analgesia if applied before injury. Sensitization of this reflex may result from immature segmental or descending inhibition in the spinal cord, the immaturity of other spinal or supraspinal mechanisms, or factors associated with intensive care (e.g., noise) and critical illness.

Neurotransmitter development in the dorsal horn of the spinal cord demonstrates the early and abundant expression of putative neurotransmitters mediating nociception (substance P, L-glutamate, VIP, CGRP) and increased somatosensory excitability in the premature spinal cord. In contrast, the neurotransmitters contained in descending inhibitory fibers from supraspinal centers (serotonin, norepinephrine, dopamine) are expressed postnatally, implying poorly developed gate-control mechanisms for pain in preterm neonates.

Opioid receptor labeling in the fetal brain stem demonstrates very high densities in multiple supraspinal centers associated with sensory perception. Theoretically, these inhibitory opioid receptors may protect developing neuronal systems from constant overstimulation, given the underdeveloped gate-control mechanisms in the dorsal horn of the spinal cord. Brain development in neonatal rats was significantly altered by exposure to naloxone but was relatively unaltered after treatment with exogenous opioids.

The magnitude of endocrine-metabolic and other stress responses to invasive procedures or surgical operations is much greater in neonates than in adults. Neonatal catecholamine and metabolic responses are 3 to 5 times those of adult patients undergoing similar types of surgery.

Pharmacokinetic studies of anesthetic drugs show that higher plasma concentrations are required to maintain effective surgical anesthesia in preterm neonates than in older age groups.

Further decreases in pain threshold (windup phenomenon) occur in preterm neonates after exposure to a painful stimulus or experience. During these prolonged periods of hypersensitivity, even nonnoxious stimuli (such as those produced by handling, physical examination, checking vital signs, etc.) are perceived as noxious stimuli, producing stress and stimulating the systemic physiologic stress responses. Although the assessment and treatment of acute painful stimuli have received greater attention in the past, it is likely that chronic noxious stimulation occurring as a result of this hypersensitivity may have substantially greater biologic and clinical importance in the management of preterm neonates.

PHARMACOLOGIC AGENTS

Nonsteroidal Antiinflammatory Drugs

There are several classes of drugs in the family known as nonsteroidal antiinflammatory drugs (NSAIDs) (Table 1-2). These agents exert their antiinflammatory effects by inhibiting prostaglandin synthesis at the level of cyclooxygenase, thereby blocking the production of prostaglandins that stimulates free nerve endings in the peripheral nervous system.[5,6] More recent evidence suggests that inhibition of central prostaglandin synthesis may also account for part of their analgesic actions. NSAIDs include the paraaminophenol derivatives (acetaminophen), propionic acid derivatives (ibuprofen, ketoprofen, and naproxen), indoles and

TABLE 1-2. Pediatric Dosage of Nonsteroidal Antiinflammatory Drugs for Acute Pain Management

	Single Dose (mg/kg) (PO)	Number of Daily Doses	Maximum Dose (mg/kg/day)
Acetaminophen	10-20	4-6	60-80
Aspirin	10-15	4-6	60
Diclofenac	1.0-2.0	3-4	?
Ibuprofen	10	3-4	40
Indomethacin	1	3	3
Ketoprofen	2.5	2	5
Naproxen	7	2	15
Piroxicam	0.4	1	?
Ketorolac	0.5	2-4	60

Modified from Schecter NL, Berde CB, Yaster M, editors: *Pain in infants, children, and adolescents,* Baltimore, 1993, Williams and Wilkins.
PO, Per os (by mouth).

pyrroles (indomethacin, tolmetin, and ketorolac), phenylacetic acid derivatives (diclofenac), oxicam (piroxicam) and salicylates (acetylsalicylic acid and choline magnesium trisalicylate). Because of its association to Reye's syndrome, acetylsalicylic acid should rarely be used for analgesia in children.

NSAIDs are weak organic acids that are rapidly and completely absorbed after oral administration. These products undergo metabolism via the cytochrome P-450 system of the liver and are excreted by the kidneys. Approximately 5% to 10% of the drug is excreted in the unmetabolized form. These drugs should be used with caution in patients with renal failure because their inhibition of renal prostaglandins can further decrease renal blood flow and the glomerular filtration rate (GFR). If used in high or toxic doses, NSAIDs may induce renal failure.

Clinical experience suggests that the risk of nephrotoxicity may be greater with certain NSAIDs, such as ketorolac; therefore, it is recommended to limit the use of such agents to 72 hours or less. Underlying renal disease, hypovolemia, and the concomitant administration of other nephrotoxic agents may increase the risk of renal insufficiency with NSAIDs.

Other side effects result from prostaglandin inhibition at sites distant from the area of inflammation. These include bronchoconstriction, gastric irritation, gastritis, vomiting, diarrhea, and elevation of serum liver enzymes. A significant and potentially dangerous side effect of NSAIDs is the inhibition of platelet function. This is particularly dangerous in patients at risk for significant postoperative bleeding (e.g., procedures involving the airway, such as tonsilloadenoidectomy) or patients with coagulation disorders. Acetaminophen or magnesium choline trisalicylate should be used in patients with qualitative or quantitative platelet disorders since neither agent alters platelet function.

Of the available medications, only acetaminophen, acetylsalicylic acid, tolmetin, naproxen, and ibuprofen are approved for pediatric use. Most practitioners have extensive experience with the use of acetaminophen to treat pain in children. The other agents are equally effective analgesics for relief of mild to moderate pain, and the selection of a particular drug is based on the preference and experience of the practitioner.

Ketorolac has recently been found to be effective in the treatment of acute pain in children.[7] Initial studies suggest that ketorolac may be as effective as opioids in treating postoperative pain. However, it should not be used as a replacement for opioids but as an adjunct to opioid analgesia. For example, in one study ketorolac administered intravenously (IV) just before the completion of the surgical procedure decreased the total morphine requirements and was associated with lower pain scores and a decreased incidence of adverse effects.[8] Ketorolac may also have a place in the treatment of inflammatory and musculoskeletal pain, such as that found in patients with a pleuritic type of pain or vasoocclusive crisis caused by sickle cell disease. A fixed-interval dosing of ketorolac (0.5 mg/kg to a maximum of 30 mg every 6 hrs) appears to be effective in decreasing total opioid requirements.

Opioids and Analogs

Opioids act as agonists at opioid receptors in the CNS and other tissues.[9] They exert their effects through specific receptors that are located throughout the CNS. Four major groups of receptors have been identified: mu, delta, kappa, and sigma (Table 1-3). The mu and delta receptors mediate analgesia, respiratory depression, euphoria, and physical dependence. Endogenous opioid-like substances, like enkephalins, are more potent delta agonists than mu agonists. Morphine, on the other hand, is 50 to 100 times more potent at the mu receptor than the delta. The kappa receptors are concentrated in the spinal cord and mediate spinal analgesia, miosis, and sedation. The sigma receptor is responsible for psychotomimetic effects, such as dysphoria and hallucinations, seen with some opioids.

Opioids may be classified according to their chemical structure as naturally occurring, semisynthetic, and synthetic. The naturally occurring opioids are derivatives of the poppy plant, *Papaver somni' ferum,* and include papaverine, thebaine, and morphine. Only morphine is used clinically in the United States. Chemical manipulation of the base compounds of morphine results in the semisynthetic agents. This group includes codeine, hydromorphone, oxycodone, and oxymorphone. Synthetic compounds resemble morphine chemically but are artificially manufactured. This group includes fentanyl, sufentanil, alfentanil, levorphanol, methadone, meperidine and pentazocine. From a clinical perspective, the major differences in opioids lie in their metabolites, cardiovascular effects, potency, and duration of ac-

TABLE 1-3. Opioid Receptors

Receptor	Drugs	Actions
Mu	Morphine Fentanyl Codeine Naloxone	Analgesia Respiratory depression Physical dependence
Delta	Enkephalin	Analgesia euphoria Respiratory depression Physical dependence
Kappa	Mixed agonist-antagonist	Spinal analgesia
Sigma	Phencyclidine Ketamine	Psychotomimetic effects Hallucinations, dysphoria

tion. The duration of action and potency of the various agents are outlined in Table 1-4.

Morphine is a naturally occurring opioid that has been widely used clinically for decades. As with all of the opioids, morphine undergoes hepatic metabolism. Liver N-demethylation and conjugation with glucuronide forms morphine-6-glucuronide (M6G), which is excreted in the urine. M6G possesses some analgesic and respiratory depressant properties and can accumulate in patients with renal insufficiency, leading to a prolonged effect of excessive respiratory depression. Age related differences in metabolism are also noted. The elimination half-life of morphine in the newborn is longer than in the older infant or child.

Meperidine is one tenth as potent as morphine but has a similar duration of action. Metabolism of the drug includes demethylation to normeperidine. This is subsequently conjugated with hepatic glucuronide and renally excreted. Normeperidine causes CNS excitation and can lead to seizures. As the compound is renally excreted accumulation may occur in the setting of renal failure.

The most recent additions to the opioid family are the synthetic agents fentanyl, sufentanil, and alfentanil. These agents are potent inhibitors of central sympathetic outflow and provide analgesia with relatively few hemodynamic consequences. Fentanyl is 80 to 100 times as potent as morphine. The primary problems associated with rapid administration of these drugs include bradycardia and chest wall rigidity. Chest wall rigidity may be avoided by slowly infusing fentanyl. When used with an anticholinergic agent such as atropine, the bradycardia associated with the fentanyl can be averted. At doses used for acute pain relief (1 to 4 μg), the hemodynamic effects of the agent are minimized. Neonatal clearance of fentanyl is comparable to that in the older child and adult. The premature infant, however, has a markedly decreased clearance of fentanyl. Plasma concentrations in infants and children are less than those achieved in adults with the same (μg/kg) dosage. The reasons for these differences may be attributed to the larger volume of distribution and the lower renal clearance in infants. Decreased clearance may also be seen in patients who have un-

TABLE 1-4. Commonly Used Mu-Agonist Drugs

Agonist	Equipotent IV Dose (mg/kg)	Duration (hrs)	Oral Bioavailability (%)	Comments
Morphine	0.1	3-4	20-40	Seizures in newborns and with patients at high doses Histamine release, vasodilation; therefore, avoid in asthmatics and patients with circulatory compromise
Meperidine	1.0	3-4	40-60	Ms contin®; 8 to 12 hour duration Catastrophic interactions with MAO inhibitors Tachycardia; negative inotrope Metabolite produces seizures; not recommended for chronic use
Methadone	0.1	6-24	70-100	Can be given IV even though the package insert says SQ or IM

Fentanyl	0.001	0.5-1		Bradycardia; minimal hemodynamic alterations Chest wall rigidity (>5 μg/kg rapid IV bolus). Treat with nalaxone or paralyze with succinylcholine or pancuronium
Codeine	1.2	3-4	40-70	Oral route only Prescribe with acetaminophen
Hydromorphone	0.015 to 0.02	3-4	40-60	Less itching and nausea than morphine Can be used with IV and epidural PCA
Oxycodone	0.15	3-4	50	One third less potent than morphine but with better bioavailability, it is often used when weaning from IV to oral medication

Modified from Schecter NL, Berde CB, Yaster M, editors: *Pain in infants, children, and adolescents,* Baltimore, 1993, Williams and Wilkins.

IV, Intravenous; *MAO,* monoamine oxidase; *SQ,* subcutaneous; *IM,* intramuscularly; *PCA,* patient-controlled analgesia.

dergone abdominal procedures because of an associated decrease in hepatic blood flow.

Fentanyl is now also available in a transmucosal preparation incorporated into a raspberry flavored lozenge (Fentanyl Oralet). Sedation results from the absorption of fentanyl across the buccal mucosa when the patient sucks on the lozenge. Analgesia and sedation generally occur in 10 to 15 minutes. If the lozenge is chewed and swallowed, only 5% to 10% is absorbed with limited, if any, effect. Three formulations of the Oralet are currently available: 200, 300, and 400 μg. The size that approximates the recommended dosage of 8 to 10 μg/kg should be used. Although this preparation has been used most frequently as a preoperative medication, it is also useful for treating acute pain and in the management of a child undergoing a painful procedure. Problems include a relatively high incidence of nausea, vomiting, and pruritus. Mild to moderate oxygen desaturation has also been noted with oral transmucosal fentanyl citrate (OTFC). Therefore the patient should be appropriately monitored regardless of the route of administration of sedative and analgesic agents.

Sufentanil is 10 times as potent as fentanyl. It is rarely indicated for acute pain relief or sedation in adults or children. The drug is a highly lipophilic compound that is rapidly distributed and taken up in all tissues. Metabolism of sufentanil occurs by o-demethylation and dealkylation. Sufentanil demonstrates higher protein binding compared with fentanyl and has a higher clearance rate. This results in a shorter elimination half-life and a shorter duration of action. Serum pH also affects protein binding of sufentanil. A pH of 7.0 increases protein binding by 28% compared with a normal pH of 7.4. Alkalosis to a pH of 7.8 will decrease protein binding by 28%. The hemodynamics of fentanyl and sufentanil appear to be similar.

The third of the synthetic opioids that is in common clinical use is alfentanil. Alfentanil is a fentanyl analog of lesser potency (one fifth to one third) and shorter duration of action than fentanyl. The drug is metabolized by N-dealkylation and glucuronidation. Similar to fentanyl and sufentanil, alfentanil is associated with hemodynamic stability. Like sufentanil, alfentanil is rarely used outside the operating room.

Codeine is an opioid that is commonly used to treat mild to moderate pain in children. This drug is available in both oral and parenteral forms. It exerts a respiratory depressant effect, causes sedation, and stimulates the chemoreceptor trigger zone to a similar degree as morphine and the other opioids when used in equipotent doses. Codeine also has potent antitussive properties. When ingested orally, the bioavailability is approximately 60%. Analgesia occurs by 20 minutes and peaks at 60 to 120 minutes. The plasma half-life is 2.5 to 3 hours. After nearly completed hepatic metabolism, the drug is excreted in the urine.

Codeine (0.5 to 1.0 mg/kg) is most often used orally in combination with acetaminophen (10 mg/kg) or salicylates. These drugs potentiate the analgesic effect, thereby reducing the dose of opioid required to produce the same degree of analgesia. Higher doses of codeine are associated with a dose-dependent increase in respiratory depression, delayed gastric emptying, nausea, vomiting, and constipation. The parenteral form of the drug produces significant pain when administered intramuscularly (IM) and has no advantage over morphine or other opioids. IV administration can be associated with significant histamine release and episodes of severe hypotension. For these reasons, parenteral codeine is not recommended in children.

Methadone is an excellent analgesic that is gaining popularity in the treatment of acute and chronic pain. The drug is available in oral and parenteral preparations. It is equipotent to morphine. The oral bioavailability of the agent approaches 80% to 90%. Methadone can exert analgesic effects for up to 12 to 36 hours after a single dose. It is metabolized slowly in the liver and has an elimination half-life that is the longest of any of the clinically available opioids (12 to 24 hours). The adverse effects of methadone are the same as those of other opioids and include respiratory depression and nausea. To treat acute pain, an initial dose of 0.1 to 0.2 mg/kg may be injected slowly IV; additional doses of 0.05 mg/kg may be given every 10 to 15 minutes until the desired effect is achieved. Subsequent doses (0.05 to 0.1 mg/kg) may be administered for pain by slow IV injection every 4 to 12 hours as needed. Berde has recommended the use of a "sliding scale" of methadone, by which small doses are administered IV over 20 minutes every 4 hours, in response to the patients rating of the degree of pain: 0.07 to 0.08 mg/kg for severe pain, 0.05 to 0.06 mg/kg for moderate pain, 0.03 mg/kg for little or no pain, and no drug is given if the child is somnolent.

Hydromorphone (Dilaudid) is a morphine derivative that is nearly 5 to 7 times more potent than the parent compound. It is available in oral and parenteral formulations. Like morphine, hydromorphone undergoes hepatic metabolism and has an elimination half-life of 3 to 4 hours. However, it has no active metabolites and is an appropriate alternative in patients with renal insufficiency. Analgesic effects may be seen within 5 minutes of an IV dose and 20 to 30 minutes of an oral dose. The duration of action is approximately 3 to 4 hours. As with other opioids, hydromorphone is associated with such side effects as respiratory depression, sedation, and nausea. However, clinical experience suggests that it may cause less histamine release and pruritis than morphine and may be an effective alternative in that setting.

Mixed opioid agonist-antagonists are also available for use as analgesic agents. These drugs exert a partial agonism at one opioid receptor subtype (kappa or delta) while acting as antagonists at another subtype (mu). Because of their mixed actions, these drugs may be associated with less respiratory depression. Although they are effective as analgesics, the agonist-antagonists have a "ceiling effect" that limits the maximum pain relief produced. The addition of a pure agonist (e.g., morphine) will not produce additional analgesia. Pentazocine (Talwin), butorphanol (Stadol), and nalbuphine (Nubain) are among the various agents available for oral and parenteral use. Each of these drugs can produce respiratory depression, sedation, and gastrointestinal symptoms similar to an equipotent dose of morphine. Agonist-antagonists have no advantage over properly dosed opioids because of their "ceiling effect" and the fact that these compounds reduce the effectiveness of additional doses of pure agonists (opioids) if additional analgesia is required. They should not be used in patients who are chronically receiving opioids, because the mu-antagonistic effects of these drugs can lead to acute withdrawal symptoms.

Opioid Antagonists

Opioid antagonists are used to counteract the side effects of opioids. The pure antagonists available are naloxone and nalmefene. These agents are competitive antagonists at all four of the opioid receptors. Recommended starting doses for naloxone are 1 to 4 μg/kg, titrated to achieve the desired effect. When administered in small incremental doses it may be possible to reverse the adverse effects (e.g., respiratory depression) without reversing the analgesia. The peak effect of IV administered naloxone occurs at 30 to 60 minutes with a duration of action of approximately 60 minutes. In patients who have been given opioids, reversal of the analgesic effects with large doses of naloxone may result in significant, adverse cardiovascular and neurologic effects. The reversal of opioid analgesia may produce a massive release of catecholamines resulting in ventricular irritability, increased mean arterial pressure, and increases in various cardiovascular parameters. If administered in the absence of opioids, naloxone has few hemodynamic consequences. In patients with compromised cardiovascular function who have received opioids for analgesia, naloxone should be used with extreme caution. If used to counteract significant respiratory depression associated with high dose opioids, naloxone can be titrated in small, incremental doses. However, it may be better to support the child's respiratory system until the effects of the opioid have subsided.

Intravenous Anesthetic Agents (Sedatives and Hypnotics)

IV anesthetics have emerged as pharmacologic mainstays of acute pain management and as important adjuncts for sedation. This group is composed of drugs from several classes of agents that exert their effects through a variety of mechanisms. This section briefly deals with agents that are commonly used for pain management and sedation.

KETAMINE

Ketamine is frequently used for infants and children undergoing painful procedures. It is a cyclohexamine derivative that produces a dissociative state. Ketamine blocks afferent impulses in the diencephalon and the associated cortical pathways. This agent may also exert an effect on the brain stem. The clinical effects of ketamine include analgesia of skin, muscle, and bone at lower doses (0.5 to 1 mg/kg). Higher doses (1 to 2 mg/kg) are associated with general anesthesia. The respiratory effects of this drug are minimal, and the gag reflex is preserved. Laryngeal irritability is also preserved or even slightly increased, and muscle tone is unaffected. Significant bronchorrhea may occur. The clinically effective doses of ketamine are higher in younger patients, particularly those under six months of age. This is probably due to the immaturity of the N-methyl-D-aspartate (NMDA) receptor to which ketamine binds. NMDA is an excitatory amine that may act on or modulate sigma opioid receptors. Ketamine may act as an antagonist at these NMDA sites.[10]

The anesthetic state produced by higher doses of ketamine is associated with minimal effects on respiration and blood pressure. In infants, the doses required for lack of movement may produce respiratory depression and apnea. In most cases, with doses commonly used for induction of anesthesia (1 to 2 mg/kg) and/or sedation, the hemodynamic and respiratory effects are minimal. Acute increases in pulmonary artery pressure have been seen in infants with congenital heart disease undergoing cardiac catheterization. However, the increase in pulmonary artery pressure is proportionate to that seen in systemic vascular resistance and mean arterial pressure. Therefore ketamine can usually be used safely in children with intracardiac shunts. The changes in pulmonary vascular resistance are further minimized with appropriate support of the airway and ventilation.

The etiology of the cardiorespiratory stimulation is not clear. Administration of ketamine is associated with elevated systemic catecholamines. The pressor effect of increased circulating epinephrine and norepinephrine may account for maintained or increased blood pressure, heart rate, and cardiac output.

Undesirable effects of ketamine in children include increased laryngeal irritability and bronchorrhea. Intracranial pressure may be increased after ketamine administration. Therefore the use of ketamine should be avoided in children at risk for intracranial hypertension. There are no documented reports of toxic effects of ketamine on the liver, kidneys, or other organ systems in older children and adults. This agent is associated with dysphoric reactions and hallucinations that can persist for several hours. The incidence of hallucinations is as high as 50% in adults but significantly lower in the younger age group. The psychotomimetic effects of ketamine can be reduced by pretreatment with benzodiazepines, such as midazolam (0.05 mg/kg IV).

Etomidate

Etomidate is an imidazole compound that is a potent, short-acting, sedative hypnotic that possesses no analgesic properties. It is almost completely metabolized through ester hydrolysis. The onset of action of etomidate is similar to that of the short-acting barbiturates. Etomidate produces less hemodynamic depression than the barbiturates. With doses of 0.2 to 0.3 mg/kg, which induce an anesthetic state, minimal depression of myocardial function is seen with little or no change in blood pressure. This is true for normal and hemodynamically compromised patients. The drug does produce a significant amount of pain and burning on injection and is also associated with myoclonic movements. The pain on injection can by minimized by pretreatment with IV lidocaine (10 to 20 mg). Myoclonic movements may be minimized by treatment with benzodiazepines, barbiturates, or opioids. Etomidate has one significant side effect which can produce significant morbidity and mortality—the suppression of adrenal steroidogenesis. Although this effect can be seen after a single dose, it is more likely to occur with higher doses and sustained administration. Therefore prolonged use of etomidate in children is not recommended. Etomidate is useful for sedating patients for cardioversion procedures where hemodynamic stability and a brief period of deep sedation are required. Like the barbiturates, it decreases the cerebral metabolic rate for oxygen and decreases cerebral blood flow (CBF) and intracranial pressure (ICP).

PROPOFOL

Propofol, an isopropylphenol derivative, is a short-acting, rapid onset, hypnotic agent that has no analgesic properties. The drug is rapidly redistributed and metabolized, accounting for its short duration of action. Because it is not water soluble, it is suspended in oil (10% soybean oil, 2.25% glycerol, and 1.2% egg phosphatide). Propofol undergoes nearly complete hepatic metabolism via conjugation with glucuronide and sulfate. It is associated with significant pain on injection, myoclonus, and, occasionally, anaphylaxis. Injection pain can be relieved by pretreatment with a small dose of IV lidocaine. Because of its extremely short duration of action and rapid metabolism, repeated doses or a continuous infusion (100 to 200 μg/kg/min) is usually used. In patients with normal cardiovascular function, the hemodynamic consequences of induction doses are minimal and include mild hypotension. However, significant hypotension and depression of cardiac function can be seen in patients with compromised function. Propofol has gained widespread popularity for accomplishing deep sedation or anesthesia in children undergoing cardiac catheterization or other procedures outside the operating room.

BARBITURATES

Barbiturates provide amnesia and sedation at low doses and induce anesthesia at higher doses.[6] They exhibit no analgesic properties. Four classes of agents (ultrashort-, short-, intermediate-, and long-acting) are distinguished by their onset of action and duration of the sedative effect. IV preparations are alkaline (pH 11) and can cause pain on injection. These are lipid-soluble agents with a large volume of distribution, which explains the short duration of action of an initial dose. All of the barbiturates undergo hepatic metabolism, and their duration of action can be prolonged in the presence of liver failure. Adverse effects of these medications include respiratory depression and apnea, coma, local vasculitis or thrombophlebitis, and, in some patients, excitation. Cardiovascular effects include peripheral vasodilation and decreased inotropy. Toxic doses of barbiturates (especially methohexital) may be associated with seizures. Barbiturates are contraindicated in patients with hypersensitivity reactions to them and in patients with acute intermittent porphyria. Thiopental and methohexital, two ultrashort-acting agents, and pentobarbital, an intermediate-acting agent, are commonly used for sedation of children.

Methohexital is administered per rectum (PR) (20 to 30 mg/kg) as a sedative for a painless procedure or as an anesthetic induction agent in children. Onset of action is 10 to 20 minutes after rectal administration. The sedative effect usually lasts up to 30 minutes. Thiopental, another ultrashort-acting barbiturate, is the most commonly used barbiturate for the IV induction of anesthesia. Doses for IV administration vary from 2 to 6 mg/kg with a duration of action of 3 to 5 minutes. Like all the barbiturates, thiopental has negative inotropic and vasodilator properties that can result in hypotension, especially in the setting of hypovolemia or underlying cardiovascular dysfunction. Rapid redistribution accounts for its short duration of action (5 to 10 minutes) after IV administration. It is a potent anticonvulsant and may be administered by continuous IV infusion to control refractory status epilepticus. It can also be administered PR (25 mg/kg) with a duration of action of approximately 90 minutes.

Pentobarbital is an intermediate-acting agent that remains a popular choice for pediatric sedation for nonpainful procedures, such as MR (magnetic resonance) scanning. The drug can be given IV (1 to 2 mg/kg) or IM (5 to 7 mg/kg). Because of pain on injection, IM administration is not recommended. The duration of action (45 to 60 minutes) after a single IV dose is considerably longer than with either methohexital or thiopental. The adverse effects of pentobarbital are similar to other barbiturates.

Benzodiazepines

The three most commonly used IV benzodiazepines in the United States are diazepam, midazolam, and lorazepam (Table 1-5). Of these, midazolam has become the most frequently used because of its water solubility and short duration of action. All of these agents produce a pleasant sedation or hypnosis with few respiratory or hemodynamic side effects when used alone in children. None of the benzodiazepines exhibit analgesic properties. Acting through the γ-aminobutyric acid (GABA) receptors in the amygdala of the limbic system and spinal neurons, the agents produce hypnosis, sedation, and amnesia. All of these agents are associated with cardiovascular stability with minimal effects on blood pressure, cardiac output, or heart rate at doses that produce sedation. Respiratory depression may occur after bolus doses or high doses of the agents. Metabolism of the three agents occurs primarily in the liver. Diazepam undergoes N-demethylation producing two active metabolites. Urinary excretion of the metabolites occurs in the oxidized and glucuronidated forms. Midazolam undergoes extensive hydroxylation and glucuronidation before excretion in the urine. Lorazepam also undergoes glucuronidation and urinary excretion.

These agents are most commonly used for premedication, for postoperative sedation, and as adjuncts for sedation during a variety

TABLE 1-5. Commonly Used Benzodiazepines (mg/kg)

Drug	Intravenous	Intra-muscular	Oral	Rectal	Intranasal
Diazepam	0.1-0.3		0.1-0.5	0.1-0.5	
Midazolam	0.02-0.03 (up to 0.15)	0.02-0.03	0.3-0.75	0.3-0.75	0.2-0.4
Lorazepam	0.05-0.1				

of procedures. They are effective when administered via a variety of routes: per os (PO) (midazolam, lorazepam, diazepam), intranasal (midazolam), PR (midazolam, lorazepam, diazepam), IV (midazolam, lorazepam, diazepam) and IM (midazolam, lorazepam). Dosing recommendations are listed in Table 1-5. Adverse effects of these drugs include respiratory depression and apnea, hypotension and decreased systemic vascular resistance, occasional nausea and vomiting, paradoxical excitation, and hallucinations.

Benzodiazepine Antagonist

Flumazenil is a competitive antagonist of benzodiazepines at the GABA receptor. It has recently been released for use in the United States. This agent has a very high affinity for GABA receptors with limited agonist effects. It can reverse, in a dose dependent manner, all of the effects produced by benzodiazepines. It is administered in doses of 8 to 15 μg/kg IV. This agent may need to be given every 30 to 60 minutes since the half-life in adults is relatively short. The precise pharmacology of flumazenil in children has not been defined. Use of flumazenil may be indicated in children who experience hypoventilation or oversedation because of benzodiazepine use. It should not be used in patients who are receiving chronic benzodiazepine therapy or who have toxic ingestion of other medications (e.g., tricyclic antidepressants). In these settings flumazenil can precipitate seizure activity.

Chloral Hydrate

Chloral hydrate is a sedative and hypnotic agent that is still commonly used in children. Only oral or rectal formulations are available, but it is well absorbed from the gastrointestinal tract. This drug undergoes metabolism in the liver to its active form, trichloroethanol, which has a half-life of 8 to 12 hours. Trichloroethanol is further metabolized (glucuronidated) before excretion in the urine. The onset of action occurs between 10 and 20 minutes after administration. Although it has no analgesic properties, it is a valuable and useful agent for brief, nonpainful procedures, such as computed tomography (CT) imaging. Adverse effects include unpleasant taste, nausea, epigastric pain, dizziness, ataxia, and malaise. Respiratory depression and apnea, decreased cardiac contractility, and hypotension are seen with high or repeated doses. If used repeatedly, tolerance and physical dependence may develop, and sudden discontinuation may lead to a severe withdrawal syndrome. Because of the possibility of accumulation of active metabolites, its use is not recommended in infants younger than 3 months of age or patients with hepatic dysfunction.

Local Anesthetic Agents

Two classes of local anesthetic agents are available for clinical use: esters (e.g., chloroprocaine) and amides (e.g., lidocaine or bupivacaine) (see Box 1-1).[9,11] These agents can be used for a variety of techniques, such as regional blocks (Table 1-6).

Esters undergo hydrolysis by plasma cholinesterase and amides undergo metabolism in the liver. The hepatic metabolism of amides poses a problem for the neonate. Because liver enzymes may be quickly saturated and are relatively immature, amides are less completely metabolized in the infant and young child, creating a potential hazard. The metabolism of ester anesthetics may be decreased because of a lower plasma pseudocholinesterase activity in infants. In newborns, serum proteins, such as alpha-1-acid glycoprotein, are found in lower levels than in adults. These pro-

BOX 1-1.
Commonly Used Local Anesthetics

Esters	Amides
Procaine	Ropivacaine
Tetracaine	Lidocainene
2-Chloroprocaine	Mepivacaine
	Bupivacaine
	Etidovaine
	Prilocaine

Modified from Cote CJ, Ryan JF, Todres ID et al, editors: *A practice of anesthesia for infants and children,* Philadelphia, 1993, WB Saunders.

TABLE 1-6. Use of Local Anesthetics to Produce Regional Anesthesia

Classification	Topical	Local Infiltration	Peripheral Nerve Block	Intravenous Regional (Bier) Block	Epidural Block	Spinal Block
Esters						
Procaine	No	Yes	Yes	No	No	No
2-Chloroprocaine	No	Yes	Yes	No	Yes	No
Tetracaine	Yes	No	No	No	No	Yes
Amides						
Lidocaine	Yes	Yes	Yes	Yes	Yes	Yes
Mepivacaine	No	Yes	Yes	No	Yes	No
Bupivacaine	No	Yes	Yes	No	Yes	Yes
Etidocaine	No	Yes	Yes	No	Yes	No
Prilocaine	No	Yes	Yes	Yes	No	No

Modified from Schecter NL, Berde CB, Yaster M, editors: *Pain in infants, children, and adolescents,* Baltimore, 1993, Williams and Wilkins.

teins are responsible for much of the protein binding of the local anesthetics. Therefore the free, or "nonbound," local anesthetic concentration is greater in the neonate than in the adult for the same dose. In turn, the potential for local anesthetic toxicity is greater in the neonate, particularly with repeated doses. For example, the hemodynamic effects of lidocaine are seen in early infancy at approximately half the dose used in adults. Thus, careful attention must be paid to the drug chosen, the total dose administered, the rate and the route of administration, and the use of vasoconstrictors. Table 1-7 outlines the maximum doses of some of the local anesthetics.

The highest systemic absorption (plasma concentration) of local anesthetics occurs with interpleural and intercostal nerve blocks. The rate of absorption is lower with other types of nerve blocks. These are, in descending order, caudal blocks, epidural blocks, brachial plexuses, and peripheral nerve blocks.

TABLE 1-7. Duration of Action, Maximum and Recommended Doses, and Commonly Used Local Anesthetics

Local Anesthetic	Maximum Dose (mg/kg)	Duration of Action (min)
Procaine	10	60-90
2-Chloroprocaine	20	30-60
Tetracaine	1.5	180-600
Lidocaine	5-7	90-200
Mepivacaine	7	120-240
Bupivacaine	3	180-600

Modified from Cote CJ, Ryan JF, Todres ID et al, editors: *A practice of anesthesia for infants and children*, Philadelphia, 1993, WB Saunders.

Epinephrine is often added to the local anesthetic injection as a vasoconstrictor. A vasoconstrictor is used to decrease systemic absorption and to prolong the block. The uptake of lidocaine, for instance, may be decreased by one half, resulting in a block of longer duration. The lower absorption, in turn, allows the use of a higher dose of lidocaine (3 to 7 mg/kg), producing a denser nerve block. In contrast, the use of epinephrine with bupivacaine does not result in a significant increase in the duration of the block, and it does not alter the total allowable dose. Vasoconstricting agents are contraindicated in nerve blocks at or near end-artery circulation (e.g., penis, digits, and ear).

Excessive doses of local anesthetics can cause significant systemic toxicity. The major adverse effects of these agents manifest in the cardiovascular system and the CNS. The earliest sign of local anesthetic toxicity may be tinnitus (ringing in the ears), a bad taste in the mouth, or circumoral paresthesias. Subsequently, the patient may experience dizziness, which can progress to visual and auditory difficulties. The patient may be more lethargic or comatose. CNS toxicity may proceed to slurred speech, myoclonus, and generalized tonic-clonic seizures. Before this, respiratory depression may be seen and may progress to respiratory arrest. Cardiovascular toxicity manifests as decreases in systemic blood pressure, direct myocardial depression, and arrhythmias. If unabated this may lead to cardiac arrest.

Bupivacaine toxicity may manifest as early, life-threatening, cardiac arrhythmias. Because bupivacaine is highly tissue bound, treatment of its toxicity is more difficult. Local anesthetic toxicity may be prevented by paying close attention to the following: the total dose, the site of administration, the route of administration, the rate of uptake, the rate of metabolism and excretion of the anesthetic, and the serum pH of the patient.

Local anesthetic toxicity must be diagnosed and managed quickly. The initial approach to treatment is the same for any child—the administration of the drug is stopped, followed by appropriate airway management and supplemental oxygen delivery. If seizures occur, IV diazepam, midazolam, or lorazepam may be appropriate. Alternately, thiopental IV is effective in terminating the seizure activity. Muscle relaxation may facilitate airway management and intubation if necessary.

The cardiovascular toxicity of local anesthetics is more difficult to treat, particularly with a bupivacaine overdose. In addition to airway management, the initial treatment should consist of IV fluid boluses (10 to 20 ml/kg) and the use of a peripheral vasoconstrictor, such as phenylephrine. Significant arrhythmias are often seen with bupivacaine toxicity and may require the use of bicarbonate IV to maintain normal to alkaline serum pH. This will decrease the amount of free drug and reduce the ongoing hemodynamic problems. Arrhythmias associated with bupivacaine toxicity may respond to IV bretylium, phenytoin, or magnesium. They are less likely to respond to lidocaine IV treatment. Bupivacaine toxicity can be severe and, if unresponsive to treatment, may result in patient death.

Eutetic Mixture of Local Anesthetics

A eutetic mixture of local anesthetics (EMLA) is a topical emulsion (cream) containing prilocaine and lidocaine. When applied to the desired area and covered with a biocclusive dressing for at least 60 minutes, the mixture produces excellent topical anesthesia. The systemic absorption of the local anesthetics is slow and the serum levels remain low, even in infants. Because of its long onset of action, EMLA has limited use in the acute setting. However, when a painful procedure can be planned (e.g., IV catheter placement, lumbar puncture, or venipuncture),[12] the cream is useful in minimizing the child's pain and related anxiety.

Psychotropic Agents

ANTIDEPRESSANTS

Psychotropic agents are often used to potentiate the analgesic effects of opioids. Numerous studies demonstrate that there can be a substantial emotional and behavioral aspect of a patient's perception of pain. Therefore medications that minimize the psychological reaction to the pain-producing situation are commonly used. There are several classes of drugs used as adjuncts, or "adjuvant medications." The use of these in conjunction with an appropriate dose of an opioid may reduce the total opioid dose required and improve the patient's response and satisfaction.

Antidepressants are commonly used in the treatment of chronic pain as adjuncts to opioid analgesia. They may be effective in patients who are clinically depressed. Their efficacy in the treatment of acute pain has not been demonstrated. Antidepressants block the reuptake of neurotransmitters in the brain. This action results in increased concentration of neurotransmitters (monoamines, norepinephrine, and serotonin) in the synapse that is thought to provide analgesia. In particular, the serotonergic medications (e.g., amitriptyline, fluoxetine, and fluvoximine) have gained a significant role in the management of chronic pain. Because they exert their effects via the CNS, improvement may not be evident for 5 to 7 days. Because of space limitations, only the medications in Table 1-8 are listed. The reader is referred to a textbook of pharmacology for more detailed discussions on these agents.

Antidepressants can have significant adverse side effects. At clinical doses these drugs produce anticholinergic effects (e.g., dry mouth, constipation, or blurred vision). Overt toxicity may occur with higher cumulative doses. These may result in deep sedation or coma, electrocardiograph changes (e.g., prolonged P-R intervals, prolonged QRS intervals, tachycardia, ventricular arrhyth-

TABLE 1-8. Psychotropic Adjuvant Analgesics

Drug	Starting Dose (mg) (Oral Administration)	Daily Dose
Tricyclic antidepressants		
Amitriptyline	10	3-5 mg/kg
Imipramine	10	3-5 mg/kg
Clomipramine	25	3-5 mg/kg
Nortriptyline	10	1-3 mg/kg
Doxepin	12.5	12.5-100 mg
Novel antidepressants		
Fluoxetine	10	10-20 mg
Phenothiazines		
Chlorpromazine	25	25-80 mg
Butyrophenones		
Haloperidol	0.25	0.25-2 mg
Antihistamines		
Hydroxyzine	25	25-100 mg
Diphenhydramine	25	25-100 mg

Modified from Heiligenstein E, Gerrity S: Psychotropics as adjuvant analgesics. In Schecter NL, Berde CB, Yaster M, editors: *Pain in infants, children, and adolescents,* Baltimore, 1992, Williams and Wilkins.

mias), and hypotension. Overdose with these agents requires hospitalization in the intensive care unit (ICU), alkalinization of the serum, and close monitoring for neurologic and hemodynamic compromise.

Antihistamines

Antihistamines have been demonstrated to be effective adjuncts to opioid analgesia in the treatment of pain. These drugs reduce histamine-induced responses in the autonomic nervous system and smooth muscles. The drugs also have some local anesthetic properties. When used in conjunction with opioids, the medications produce a higher satisfaction because of their analgesic and antiemetic properties. The two most commonly used drugs in this class are hydroxyzine (Vistaril, Atarax) and diphenhydramine (Benadryl) (0.25 to 0.5 mg/kg). Side effects of antihistamines include sedation, tremors, and gastrointestinal stress. An overdose may result in CNS excitation and seizures. The child may have a flushed appearance, a fever, and dilated pupils. If unabated, antihistamine toxicity can lead to cardiovascular failure and coma.

Phenothiazines

Phenothiazines and butyrophenones are categorized as the major tranquilizers and are generally used to treat psychiatric disturbances and severe nausea and for sedation. Of the many agents available, haloperidol is frequently chosen when less potent sedatives are ineffective. Haloperidol has a rapid onset of action with IV or IM injection, exerts minimal respiratory depression, and has no active metabolites. Adverse effects associated with the butyrophenones and phenothiazines include peripheral α-adrenergic blockade with hypotension, dystonia and extrapyramidal effects, and, in rare cases, neuroleptic malignant syndrome. Less common but more serious are the cardiac events, such as cardiac arrest and ventricular arrhythmias, including torsades de pointes, which may be seen with high doses. These drugs may also lower the seizure threshold.

Most commonly, pediatricians have used the phenothiazines in combination with other agents (e.g., DPT) for invasive procedures. This practice is no longer recommended since the combination may result in prolonged sedation and a risk of respiratory depression and apnea.

Neuromuscular Blocking Agents

Normal neuromuscular transmission includes the propagation of the impulse to the neuromuscular junction, depolarization of the neuron, and the release of acetylcholine into the synaptic cleft. Acetylcholine diffuses across the cleft and binds with specific receptors on the muscle cell. This binding leads to depolarization of the sarcolemma and subsequent muscle contraction. Neuromuscular blocking agents are used to interfere with this process and produce muscle paralysis.

Neuromuscular blocking agents (Table 1-9) are used in combination with sedative or anesthetic drugs to immobilize the patient during selected procedures. These drugs should never be used alone, since paralysis without proper sedation is inhumane and physiologically stressful for the child. Adequate airway support should be guaranteed, including endotracheal intubation and ventilatory support, when using neuromuscular blocking agents.

SUCCINYLCHOLINE

Succinylcholine is a depolarizing neuromuscular blocker. It binds to the acetylcholine receptors and produces depolarization of the sarcolemma. Unlike acetylcholine, succinylcholine is resistant to degradation by acetylcholinesterase; therefore, repolarization and susbequent muscle contractions cannot occur. The drug has a rapid onset (30 to 45 seconds) and a short duration (4 to 6 minutes) of action. It is metabolized by an enzyme in plasma (pseudocholinesterase). As a cholinergic agonist, the agent can produce transient bradycardia. It may also have negative inotropic effects, particularly in low doses. Bradyarrhythmias, nodal rhythms, and premature ventricular contractions (PVCs) may occur after succinylcholine administration. Because of its significant side effects, succinylcholine should be used only by experienced practitioners familiar with its pharmacology.

The remainder of the clinically used muscle relaxants are nondepolarizing agents. They competitively antagonize the effects of acetylcholine at the receptors. There are several agents in com-

TABLE 1-9. Neuromuscular Blocking Agents (mg/kg)

Drug	Intravenous	Intramuscular
Succinylcholine	1-2	4-5
Pancuronium	0.05-0.10	0.2-0.4
Atracurium	0.3-0.6	
Vecuronium	0.05-0.10	
Doxacurium	0.05	
Rocuronium	0.6-1.0	

mon clinical use. They differ in their metabolism, duration of action, and cardiovascular effects.

Pancuronium

Pancuronium has been a mainstay of neuromuscular blockade in children undergoing surgery. Pancuronium is a steroidal, nondepolarizing, neuromuscular blocker that produces a dose dependent increase in blockade. Pancuronium may also exert a β-adrenergic, mediated, positive, inotropic effect and has anticholinergic effects mediated through cardiac, muscarinic receptors which can produce tachycardia. In addition to the increased heart rate, the patient may experience increases in mean arterial pressure. Pancuronium is primarily (80%) dependent on renal excretion to terminate its effects.

d-Tubocurarine

d-Tubocurarine is a curare derivative that was one of the first agents introduced into clinical practice as a competitive neuromuscular blocker. It is dependent on both renal (60%) and hepatic (40%) elimination. The most profound effect on hemodynamics is a result of a large histamine release upon IV injection, which decreases the mean arterial blood pressure and increases the heart rate.

Vecuronium

Vecuronium is a steroidal muscle relaxant similar to pancuronium. Because of its duration of action (20 to 30 minutes), it is classified as an intermediate-acting agent. This agent is metabolized by the liver (70% to 80%). Hepatic metabolism results in active metabolites, including 3-hydroxy, 17-hydroxy, and 3, 17-dihydroxy vecuronium. The dihydroxy compound is a weak neuromuscular blocker with roughly half the potency of the parent compound. With the commonly used clinical doses, vecuronium has few cardiovascular effects. Vascular resistance is also minimally affected by clinically relevant doses of vecuronium but may be decreased with higher doses. In clinical use, the heart rate, mean arterial pressure, and cardiac output do not change after a dose of vecuronium.

Atracurium

Atracurium is an intermediate-acting, neuromuscular blocker metabolized by plasma esterases and spontaneous decomposition by Hoffmann degradation. Both of these reactions are pH and temperature sensitive. One of the metabolites, laudanosine, can cause seizures when present in high concentrations. However, to date, this metabolite has not been reported to cause clinical problems. Under usual clinical circumstances, ester hydrolysis is responsible for most of the breakdown of atracurium. The absence of pseudocholinesterase has no effect on atracurium metabolism. In normal patients an intubating dose of atracurium (0.6 mg/kg) has minimal effects on heart rate and blood pressure. Moderate degrees of histamine release and hypotension may also be seen with atracurium administration.

Doxacurium

Doxacurium is a new, nondepolarizing muscle relaxant that has recently been introduced into clinical use. The duration of action of doxacurium is similar to that of pancuronium. Unlike pancuronium, doxacurium has few cardiovascular effects. The effective dose of doxacurium in children is similar to that in adults; however, the duration of action in children may be shorter.

Mivacurium

Mivacurium is a new, short-acting, nondepolarizing, neuromuscular blocker. The unique feature of this agent is its metabolism by plasma cholinesterases. The drug has a recovery rate of 5 to 7 minutes (25% to 75% recovery). In children, the effective dose (ED_{95}) is 115 μg/kg. When titrated to 95% blockade by monitor, children recovered spontaneously within ten minutes after discontinuing the drug. The hemodynamic side effects are limited. Because of its short duration, predictable offset of action, and lack of hemodynamic effects, mivacurium may be a useful drug for short pediatric cases, such as brief, nonoperative procedures requiring a completely still patient.

Rocuronium

Rocuronium has recently been approved for clinical use in the United States. It is a steroidal, nondepolarizing, competitive, neuromuscular blocker that has a more rapid onset of action than vecuronium.[13] The duration of action and recovery from the block are similar to that of vecuronium. Administration of rocuronium is associated with relatively few changes in heart rate or blood pressure. This drug may be useful for rapid sequence intubation when succinylcholine is contraindicated.

Inhalational Anesthetic Agents

Inhalational anesthetics have been the mainstay of general anesthesia techniques for most of the twentieth century and are also occasionally used for sedation in the ICU. These agents are delivered through the respiratory tract and result in relatively rapid and reversible anesthesia. Because the potential exists for serious risk to the patient and the healthcare providers, inhalational anesthetics should be used only by qualified personnel under the supervision of a qualified anesthesiologist.

Two classes of agents are commonly used: nitrous oxide (N_2O) and volatile agents (halothane, enflurane, isoflurane, or desflurane). The precise mechanism of action of the gaseous anesthetics is unclear. All of these agents increase the threshold of cell firing, resulting in decreased neuronal activity. This action is most likely mediated through an effect on the cell membrane.

Inhalational anesthetics are administered via the respiratory tract. The depth of anesthesia is determined by the concentration of the drug in the brain and the CNS. Several factors influence the rate of delivery to the CNS and other tissues. The physicochemical factors include the partial pressure of the agent, which determines the concentration of that gas in a gaseous mixture and the solubility of an anesthetic, which influences the rate of transfer of an agent from the lungs to the blood and from the blood to the tissues. Several physiologic factors influence anesthetic onset of action, such as alveolar ventilation, cardiac output (pulmonary blood flow), and tissue perfusion. The offset action of the inhaled agents occurs when the partial pressure of the agent in the brain falls below the effective dose. The rate and extent of metabolism has little effect on the duration of action.

Inhalational anesthetics can have profound systemic effects. Some of these are listed in Box 1-2. Any patient who is receiving general anesthesia or sedation with an inhalational anesthetic must be cared for by qualified personnel and monitored at the same level as a child undergoing surgery.

BOX 1-2.
Systemic Effects of Inhalational Anesthetics

Decreased airway resistance
Attenuation of hypoxic pulmonary vasoconstriction
Decreased respiratory drive (response to carbon dioxide) and apnea
Decreased systemic blood pressure, myocardial contractility, vascular resistance
Altered cerebral blood flow autoregulation
Decreased renal blood flow, glomerular filtration rate, urine output
Decreased hepatic blood flow
Risk of malignant hyperthermia

SAFETY CONSIDERATIONS

Every sedation attempt carries with it certain risks for the child, such as hypoventilation, apnea, airway obstruction, and cardiovascular compromise. These concerns should not limit the use of sedation but rather highlight the need to assess and prepare the patient appropriately for the procedure.

In 1992 the American Academy of Pediatrics revised its sedation guidelines in an attempt to standardize monitoring practices and encourage high-quality patient care. These guidelines define three levels of sedation: conscious sedation, deep sedation, and general anesthesia.

Conscious sedation is a medically controlled state of depressed consciousness that allows protective reflexes to be maintained, retains the patient's ability to maintain a patent airway independently and continuously, and permits appropriate response by the patient to physical stimulation or verbal command (e.g., "open your eyes").

Deep sedation is a medically controlled state of depressed consciousness or unconsciousness from which the patient is not easily aroused. It may be accompanied by a partial or complete loss of protective reflexes and includes the inability to maintain a patent airway independently and respond purposefully to physical stimulation or verbal command.

General anesthesia is a medically controlled state of unconsciousness accompanied by a loss of protective reflexes, including the inability to maintain a patent airway independently and respond purposefully to physical stimulation or verbal command.

In order to provide adequate sedation or analgesia for a child and at the same time ensure the patient's safety, the practitioner must address several issues: details about the procedure, details of the patient's history and physical examination, and details of the equipment available for airway support and monitoring. Finally, the patient and the family must be properly instructed regarding the scheduled procedure and the plan for sedation and monitoring of the child. The specifics of a particular procedure, such as the level of sedation, patient positioning, and the degree of pain or stimulation, are discussed under the various sections in this book.

Patient Assessment

Before medicating a child for any procedure, it is important to briefly review the patient's medical history and perform a physical examination. The information obtained should include previous and ongoing illnesses, drug allergies, family history of anesthetic problems, such as postoperative fevers, which may suggest a family history of malignant hyperthermia, and the patient's current drug regimen. The last is important since many medications may potentiate the sedative effects of the drugs used.

The possibility of pregnancy in a girl of child-bearing age is often overlooked but must be investigated during the evaluation. The physical examination includes vital signs and a determination of oxygen saturation in room air. The remainder of the examination is focused primarily on the child's airway and the cardiorespiratory system. It is important to determine if the patient may be difficult to intubate in the unlikely event of oversedation or other undesirable side effects. Potential airway problems should be suspected in patients with micrognathia, limited mouth opening, or limited neck mobility. The Mallampati classification of the upper airway is a useful method for gauging the difficulty of intubation in a patient (Fig. 8-1). If the tonsillar pillars and the uvula cannot be visualized (Mallampati grade III or IV), the patient's trachea may be difficult to intubate. Prior records should be reviewed to determine if there have been previous airway problems. The possibility of a difficult airway does not preclude the use of sedation, but it may be appropriate to discuss such patients with a pediatric anesthesiologist. It is important to assess the cardiovascular condition of the child since certain sedative and analgesic drugs may adversely affect the hemodynamic status of patients with large intracardiac shunts, congestive heart failure, pulmonary hypertension, or valvular disease.

The history and physical examination can be summarized as the child's physical status according to the American Society of Anesthesiologists' (ASA) classification (Box 1-3). The classification permits the practitioner to gauge the relative risk of sedating or anesthetizing a patient. In particular, Class 3 and 4 patients may be at significant risk if sedated and may benefit from a consultation with a pediatric anesthesiologist.

Monitoring

The three different levels of sedation are associated with a different degree of risk to the patient and, therefore, require different types of monitoring. At the least, a child undergoing sedation should be monitored with a pulse oximeter and blood pressure cuff. If the patient will be far removed from the observer, such as

BOX 1-3.
Physical Status Classification of the American Society of Anesthesiologists (ASA Classification)

ASA 1: No underlying medical problems:	Normal, healthy patient
ASA 2: Mild systemic illness:	Well controlled asthmatic, Corrected congenital heart disease
ASA 3: Severe systemic illness:	Sickle cell disease, Severe asthmatic, steroid dependent, Uncorrected acyanotic congenital heart disease
ASA 4: Severe systemic illness that is a constant threat to life:	Uncorrected cyanotic congenital heart disease
ASA 5: Patient who is unlikely to survive 24 hours with or without surgery	

in the CT or MR scanner, an end-tidal carbon dioxide (CO_2) capnometer monitor should also be used. Specialized nasal cannulae may be used to permit end-tidal CO_2 sampling from one prong and oxygen delivery to the other. CO_2 monitoring is used to demonstrate an adequate respiratory rate and pattern. End-tidal CO_2 monitoring alerts the caregiver immediately if airway obstruction or apnea occurs. Desaturation measured by pulse oximetry may not occur for 30 to 90 seconds after apnea. Supplemental oxygen should be administered to all patients during sedation. For deep sedation and general anesthesia, in addition to a pulse oximeter, blood pressure cuff, and end-tidal CO_2 monitor, the child should have an electrocardiograph monitor in order to watch for arrhythmias.

It is essential to have resuscitative equipment, appropriate for the child's size and age, and medications readily available before sedating a child for any procedure. Box 1-4 lists the minimum supplies that are needed.

BOX 1-4.
Minimal Equipment and Drugs for Sedation

Personnel
- Practitioner performing procedure
- Trained person to monitor the child and administer drugs
- Must be able to provide basic cardiopulmonary resuscitation
- Must have immediate access to and familiarity with the use of emergency equipment

Suction apparatus including large bore (Yankaur) suction tip
- (At least two functioning suction systems are recommended)

Suction catheters (various size)

Oxygen source and delivery system

Airway equipment
- Mask and bag (proper size) with adjustable "pop off"
- Oral airways (various sizes)
- Endotracheal tubes of various sizes
- Stylet (various sizes)
- Laryngoscope blades and handles of appropriate sizes

Premedication
- Aspiration Prophylaxis
- +/− Antisialogogue

Drugs
- Epinephrine
- Sodium bicarbonate
- Atropine, glycopyrrolate
- Lidocaine, bretylium
- Glucose
- Reversal agents: naloxone, flumazenil
- Anticonvulsants: thiopental, midazolam or diazepam
- Muscle relaxants: succinylcholine, vecuronium or rocuronium

Monitoring equipment
- Electrocardiograph
- Blood pressure monitor with proper size cuff
- Pulse oximeter
- Capnometer (end-tidal CO_2 monitor)
- (for selected conscious sedation and all deep sedation and general anesthesia cases)

Modified from the Guidelines of the Committee on Drugs, American Academy of Pediatrics, *Pediatrics* 89:1110, 1992.

Personnel

In order to provide the appropriate level of care for a child, an adequate number of properly trained personnel must be available. Physicians routinely depend on other physicians, nurses, and auxiliary personnel to assist in patient preparation, transport, and recovery. A specific person who does not have other concurrent responsibilities and who is able to provide basic life support should be assigned to monitor a patient during the procedure and the recovery period. Parents must have detailed instructions at discharge about how to deal with possible side effects and ongoing risks, including the risks of airway compromise or vomiting and aspiration.

Fasting Guidelines

Any child undergoing sedation, particularly deep sedation or general anesthesia, may lose the protective airway reflexes and is at risk for reflux or vomiting and pulmonary aspiration. Therefore, before any elective procedure that requires sedation, the practitioner must ensure that the patient has had an adequate period of fasting. The NPO (nil per os) guidelines that are presently in use are designed to provide a sufficient duration of fasting and minimizing the discomfort for young patients. Previously it was common to withhold clear liquids for up to 6 hours before surgery in children under a year of age and for up to 8 hours in older children. It has been demonstrated more recently that the ingestion of clear liquids may actually promote gastric emptying and raise gastric pH, while decreasing hunger, thirst, and irritability in the patient. The guidelines used for fasting are listed in Table 1-10. These guidelines should be reviewed with the parents to ensure that they understand what to do for the child. On the day of the procedure, the parents should be questioned about when the child last ate or drank anything in order to ensure that the patient has had an adequate fast.

Summary

This chapter has discussed several general considerations that form the basis of a safe practice of sedation and pain management

TABLE 1-10. NPO Guidelines for Children

Age	Milk/Solids	Clear Liquids*
Preterm	4	2
Full term to 6 months	6	3
6 months to 12 months	8	4
12 months to 36 months	8	4
More than 36 months	8	4

*Clear liquids may include breast milk, apple juice, Pedialyte, water, or Sprite.
NPO, Nil per os.

for infants and children. First, in order to understand why infants and children deserve adequate pain management and sedation for procedures, the current understanding of the developmental neurobiology of pain in children was outlined. Second, the pediatric pharmacology of different classes of medications that are commonly used was reviewed. The final section discussed issues of proper preparation that are essential to assure that the child is not placed at undue risk during the treatment of anxiety or pain. The subsequent chapters consider specific clinical conditions and some specific techniques that can be used to provide comfort for the infant or child.

References

1. Anand KJS, Carr DB: The neuroanatomy, neurophysiology and neurochemistry of pain, stress, and analgesia in newborns, infants, and children, *Pediatr Clin North Am* 36:795, 1989.
2. Anand KJS, Hickey PR: Pain and its effects in the human neonate and fetus, *N Engl J Med* 317:1321, 1987.
3. Fitzgerald M: Development of pain mechanisms, *Br Med Bull* 47:667, 1991.
4. Fitzgerald M, Millard C, McIntosh N: Cutaneous hypersensitivity following peripheral tissue damage in newborn infants and its reversal with topical anaesthesia, *Pain* 39:31, 1989.
5. Schecter NL, Berde CB, Yaster M, editors: *Pain in infants, children and adolescents,* Baltimore, 1993, Williams and Wilkins.

6. Stoelting RK: *Pharmacology and physiology in anesthetic practice,* ed. 2, Philadelphia, 1991, JB Lippincott.
7. Watcha MF, Jones MB, Lagueruela R et al: Comparison of ketorolac and morphine as adjuvants during pediatric surgery, *Anesthesiology* 76:368, 1992.
8. Vetter TR, Heiner EJ: Intravenous ketorolac as an adjuvant to pediatric patient-controlled analgesia with morphine, *J Clin Anesth* 6:110, 1994.
9. Yaster M, Deshpande JK, Maxwell LG: The pharmacologic management of pain in children, *Compr Ther* 15:14, 1989.
10. Yamamura T, Haruda K, Okamura A et al: Is the site of action of ketamine anesthesia the N-methyl-D-aspartate receptor? *Anesthesiology* 72:704, 1990.
11. Yaster M, Tobin JR, Fisher QA et al: Local anesthetics in the management of acute pain in children, *J Pediatr* 24:165, 1994.
12. Soliman JE, Braodman LM, Hanallah RS et al: Comparison of the analgesic effects of EMLA (eutectic mixture of local anesthetics) to intradermal lidocaine infiltration prior to venous cannulation in unpremedicated children, *Anesthesiology* 68:804, 1988.
13. Lambalk LM, DeWit AP, Wierda JM et al: Dose-response relationship and time course of action org 9426, *Anaesthesia* 46:907, 1991.

POSTOPERATIVE PAIN MANAGEMENT 2

Joseph D. Tobias

PROSTAGLANDIN SYNTHESIS INHIBITORS
NONSTEROIDAL ANTIINFLAMMATORY DRUGS
Adverse effects of nonsteroidal antiinflammatory drugs
OPIOIDS
Nonintravenous routes of opioid administration
Adverse effects of opioids

The past 10 years have witnessed many changes and advances in the understanding, identification, and treatment of pain in children. The first of many steps was to refute previously held misconceptions that children do not feel or react to pain like adults. These beliefs, compounded by unfounded fears of addiction and side effects, led to the ineffective treatment of pain in children. However, recent clinical studies have demonstrated that children experience severity of postoperative pain similar to adults[1] and that even premature infants demonstrate alterations in heart rate, blood pressure, and oxygen saturation in response to pain.

The issues of controlling postoperative pain extend far beyond purely humanitarian concerns. Recent clinical studies by Anand and colleagues at the Boston Children's Hospital have focused on the adverse effects of the postsurgical stress response, which has been characterized as a metabolic, hormonal, and hemodynamic response to major injury or surgery.[2-4] This neuroendocrine cascade with the release of catecholamines, cortisol, glucagon, and other catabolic hormones results in increased oxygen consumption, increased carbon dioxide production, hyperglycemia, and a generalized catabolic state with a negative nitrogen balance.[5] Additional effects, such as tachycardia, systemic hypertension, and increases in pulmonary artery pressure, may be caused by the liberation of endogenous catecholamines.

Anand and colleagues have demonstrated that the postsurgical stress response occurs even in preterm infants, with the greatest response observed in those with the highest mortality.[2] These investigators were also the first to demonstrate that alterations in intraoperative and postoperative analgesic techniques may influence patient outcome.[3,4] The first of these studies involved preterm infants undergoing ligation of patent ductus arteriosus.[3] The infants received 50% nitrous oxide in oxygen with curare for muscle relaxation and were randomized to receive either 10 μg/kg fentanyl or a placebo. There was a significant decrease in indicators of the stress response in those patients who received fentanyl. Additionally, there was an increased incidence of postoperative complications in the nonfentanyl group, such as increased ventilatory requirements, cardiovascular instability, metabolic acidosis, and intraventricular hemorrhage.

The results of the initial study are further magnified by the more recent trial comparing high-dose sufentanil with halothane-morphine anesthesia in infants undergoing cardiac surgery.[4] Neonates were randomized to receive anesthesia with either high-dose sufentanil followed by continuous sufentanil infusion for 24 hours after surgery or halothane-morphine intraoperatively, followed by intermittent morphine and diazepam for postoperative sedation and analgesia. Again, in infants who received sufentanil, there was a significant decrease in the parameters of the postsurgical stress response and a significant reduction in the incidence of metabolic acidosis, sepsis, disseminated intravascular coagulation, and postoperative mortality (0 of 30 in the sufentanil group versus 4 of 15 in the halothane-morphine group).

In addition to the effects mediated by the postsurgical stress response, pain after thoracic and abdominal surgery can have significant deleterious effects on respiratory function, such as decreased tidal volume, functional residual capacity, and forced expiratory volume.[6,7] These changes, combined with decreased cough effort and the residual effects of anesthetic agents, may result in ventilation-perfusion mismatch with postoperative hypoxemia and respiratory failure. Inadequate analgesia may also delay postoperative ambulation, thereby further compromising postoperative pulmonary function and increasing the risk of postoperative pulmonary complications. With such effects in mind, the need for providing postoperative analgesia becomes readily apparent.

This chapter discusses the options available for the treatment of postoperative pain in children, including the nonopioid analgesic agents (prostaglandin synthesis inhibitors) and opioids. (Regional anesthetic techniques used in the control of pain are discussed in Chapters 3 and 4.) Although this chapter focuses on the control of postoperative pain, many of the techniques used are also valuable in the control of acute pain from other etiologies, including that caused by medical illnesses such as sickle cell disease (see Chapter 5).

PROSTAGLANDIN SYNTHESIS INHIBITORS

When attempting to control postoperative pain, a graded approach using a three-step ladder (Box 2-1) described by the World Health Organization provides a basic guideline.[8] Mild pain, such as that after a soft-tissue procedure (e.g., lymph node biopsy), can usually be controlled with a nonopioid analgesic agent, such as a prostaglandin synthesis inhibitor. Moderate pain, such as that after a bony orthopedic procedure or inguinal herniorrhaphy in an adolescent, can usually be controlled with a combination of a prostaglandin synthesis inhibitor and a weak opioid (e.g., an acetaminophen with codeine preparation). More severe pain, such as that after a thoracotomy or an exploratory laparotomy, requires either a regional anesthetic technique or a parenteral opioid.

Prostaglandin synthesis inhibitors may be classified as paraaminophenol derivatives (acetaminophen), nonsteroidal antiinflammatory drugs (NSAIDs) (ibuprofen), or salicylates (acetylsali-

BOX 2-1.
Strategies for the Treatment of Postoperative Pain

Mild Pain

NSAIDs

Moderate Pain

NSAIDs with opioid (oxycodone or codeine)
Intravenous opioid
- Intravenous opioid by PCA
- Continuous infusion of opioid with p.r.n. rescue doses
- Fixed-interval dosing of opioid

Regional anesthetic technique

Severe Pain

Intravenous opioid by PCA
Regional anesthetic technique

NSAID, Nonsteroidal antiinflammatory drug; *PCA,* patient-controlled analgesia; *p.r.n.,* as needed.

cylic acid, choline magnesium trisalicylate) (Box 2-2). Because of the association of Reye's syndrome with acetylsalicylic acid, this agent is rarely used for postoperative analgesia in children. The major action of these agents is the inhibition of the enzyme cyclooxygenase, thereby blocking the synthesis of prostaglandins that stimulate free nerve endings of the peripheral nervous system. More recent evidence suggests that inhibition of central prostaglandin synthesis may account for part of the analgesic actions of prostaglandin synthesis inhibitors.

Although there are several NSAIDs currently available in the United States, only tolmetin, naproxen, and ibuprofen are approved for pediatric use. NSAIDs are weak organic acids that are rapidly and completely absorbed after oral administration. Metabolism occurs via the cytochrome P-450 system of the liver with renal excretion of 5% to 10% of unmetabolized drug. There is a ceiling effect with all NSAIDs so that increased analgesia is not achieved with increasing doses.

BOX 2-2.
Classification of Nonopioid Analgesics
THE PROSTAGLANDIN SYNTHESIS INHIBITORS

Paraaminophenol Derivatives

Acetaminophen
Phenacetin

Nonsteroidal Antiinflammatory Drugs

Ibuprofen	Indomethacin
Tolmetin	Fenoprofen
Naproxen	Mefenamic acid
Ketorolac	Sulindac

Salicylates

Acetylsalicylic acid
Choline magnesium trisalicylate

The role of prostaglandin synthesis inhibitors in controlling postoperative pain includes their use as the sole agent to control minor pain, their combination with weak opioids for oral administration to control moderate pain, and their addition to parenteral opioids to control severe pain. In the last situation, their use does not replace opioids but instead provides adjunctive analgesia, thereby limiting the dose of opioid and opioid-associated adverse effects.

In the control of minor postoperative pain, decisions regarding prostaglandin synthesis inhibitors concern the agent to be used, the mode of administration, and the route of administration. One of two agents is generally used: acetaminophen or ibuprofen. Both are available in several preparations that include chewable tablets, elixirs, and drops. Acetaminophen is also available in suppositories. These agents can be administered preoperatively, intraoperatively, or postoperatively.

For preoperative administration it is useful to include oral premedication (e.g., midazolam in the operating room) with the acetaminophen or ibuprofen elixir (15 mg/kg). This combination is commonly used for outpatient procedures, such as lymph node biopsies or myringotomies and placement of pressure equalizing (PE) tubes. This not only allows the patient to have some analgesic available when he or she wakes up, but it is also useful to mask the bitter taste of the midazolam premedication.

If preoperative administration is not chosen, the use of a suppository (20 to 30 mg/kg acetaminophen) is recommended after anesthetic induction. Another option is the administration of either ibuprofen or acetaminophen after complaints or displays of pain in the recovery room. This latter option is least desirable since the onset of activity of any of these agents occurs 20 to 30 minutes after oral or rectal administration. The administration of a small dose of intravenous (IV) opioid (0.5 μg/kg fentanyl or 0.02 mg/kg morphine) can be used to provide immediate analgesia along with the oral or rectal prostaglandin synthesis inhibitor. When the patient is ready for discharge home, ongoing analgesia is provided with either acetaminophen or ibuprofen. Although it is most common to administer these agents on a p.r.n. (as needed) basis, fixed-interval dosing may provide more effective analgesia. This requires administering the medication around the clock and not waiting for the child to complain of pain. For this purpose 15 mg/kg of either ibuprofen or acetaminophen is used every 4 to 6 hours for the initial 48 postoperative hours.

When moderate pain needs to be treated on an outpatient basis, the NSAID or acetaminophen can be combined with a weak opioid such as codeine, oxycodone, or hydrocodone. Several preparations are available, and the use of a liquid or tablet is determined by the patient's age and preference. For younger patients, acetaminophen with codeine elixir containing 120 mg acetaminophen and 12 mg codeine per 5 ml is preferred. Dosing is based on the codeine component ranging from 0.5 to 1.0 mg/kg every 4 to 6 hours. Tablet preparations contain 325 mg acetaminophen with 15 mg codeine (Tylenol #2), 30 mg codeine (Tylenol #3), or 60 mg codeine (Tylenol #4). Another effective alternative is oxycodone with acetaminophen preparations. These are available in both liquid and tablet forms. The dosage is generally based on the oxycodone preparation starting at 0.1 to 0.15 mg/kg every 4 to 6 hours. Regardless of the preparation used, it should be noted that with dose escalations the amount of acetaminophen may exceed the recommended dose of 15 mg/kg. When higher doses are needed, switching to preparations that contain either codeine or oxycodone, without the acetaminophen or NSAID, is recommended to avoid toxicity.

NONSTEROIDAL ANTIINFLAMMATORY DRUGS

NSAIDs may also have a role in controlling severe postoperative pain. In this setting NSAIDs are used to decrease the postoperative opioid requirements, thereby decreasing opioid-related adverse effects. Although there has been significant interest in the use of the new, parenteral agent ketorolac for this purpose, older and cheaper preparations, such as ibuprofen and acetaminophen, may also be beneficial.

When oral administration is feasible, the addition of either ibuprofen or acetaminophen (15 mg/kg) every 4 to 6 hours is suggested on a fixed-interval schedule. The optimal combination is the fixed-interval NSAID and an opioid administered by either continuous infusion or a patient-controlled analgesia (PCA) device. When oral administration is not possible, rectal administration should be considered. Maunuksela and colleagues evaluated the efficacy of rectal ibuprofen (40 mg/kg/day) in children after inpatient surgery.[9] The children who received ibuprofen had lower pain scores and decreased opioid requirements in the recovery room, during the day of operation, and during the 72 hours after the procedure. Additionally, the incidence of opioid-related adverse effects was lower in the group that received ibuprofen. Similar results have been reported in both children and adults using rectal ibuprofen. Although indomethacin is available in suppository form in the United States, ibuprofen is not.

The use of NSAIDs in acute postoperative pain has been limited by the reluctance to use rectal administration and the inability in many cases for oral dosing. However there are currently two parenteral agents available: indomethacin and ketorolac tromethamine, of which only the latter is available for parenteral use in the United States.[10] The Food and Drug Administration (FDA) has recently given approval for IV administration of ketorolac in adults.

Maunuksela and colleagues found that the continuous IV administration of indomethacin improved analgesia and diminished opioid requirements in children after surgery.[11] Watcha and colleagues have demonstrated the efficacy of ketorolac for postoperative analgesia in children.[12] Although initial studies suggest that ketorolac may be as effective as opioids in treating postoperative pain, its real role seems to be similar to that of other NSAIDs—an adjunct to opioid analgesia. Vetter and Heiner evaluated the use of ketorolac to supplement PCA in children.[13] Ketorolac (0.8 mg/kg to a maximum of 60 mg) was administered IV just before the completion of the surgical procedure. Patients who received ketorolac had decreased morphine requirements, lower pain scores, and a decreased incidence of adverse effects during the study period, which included the first 12 postoperative hours.

Other recent studies suggest that improved analgesia could be provided by use of a continuous infusion of ketorolac rather than intermittent bolus dosing.[14,15] Once again, ketorolac effectively decreased the total opioid requirements; however, no advantage was noted when comparing intermittent administration with continuous administration. An additional report documents the use of ketorolac by continuous subcutaneous infusion in a patient population (terminal cancer patients) in whom IV access was not feasible.[16]

Ketorolac may also be effective against inflammatory and musculoskeletal pain in patients with a pleuritic type of pain or vasoocclusive crisis caused by sickle cell disease. For either indication, the use of fixed-interval dosing of ketorolac (0.5 mg/kg to a maximum of 30 mg every 6 hrs) is recommended. In these settings, ketorolac is not meant to replace opioids but to decrease total opioid requirements. Since ketorolac is relatively expensive, future studies are needed to determine its advantages over more inexpensive agents and routes of delivery (oral or rectal). The optimal mode of delivery (intermittent versus continuous infusion) should also be further evaluated.

Adverse Effects of Nonsteroidal Antiinflammatory Drugs

Adverse effects of NSAIDs relate to the inhibition of prostaglandins distant from the site of inflammation (Box 2-3) and may include decreased platelet function, peptic ulcer formation with gastrointestinal bleeding, decreased glomerular filtration rate, and bronchospasm. Acetaminophen or magnesium choline trisalicylate should be used in patients with qualitative or quantitative platelet disorders since neither agent alters platelet function. Alterations in the glomerular filtration rate are uncommon except in patients with preexisting renal dysfunction, with the concomitant administration of other nephrotoxic agents, in the presence of hypovolemia, or with prolonged administration. Clinical experience suggests that the risk of nephrotoxicity may be greater with certain NSAIDs, such as ketorolac. Therefore the use of this agent should be limited to 72 hours or less. The issues surrounding the effects of NSAIDs on coagulation and platelet function remain somewhat controversial as to whether they are clinically signifi-

BOX 2-3.
Adverse Effects of NSAIDs

Headache, dizziness, or drowsiness
Nausea or vomiting
Peptic ulcer formation
Gastrointestinal bleeding
Decreased glomerular filtration rate
Renal dysfunction
Platelet dysfunction
Bronchospasm
Interaction with coumarin preparations (this effect varies from one NSAID to another)

NSAID, Nonsteroidal antiinflammatory drugs.

cant. It is preferable to avoid the use of ketorolac for procedures involving the airway, such as tonsilloadenoidectomy.

OPIOIDS

Opioids can be grouped into three classes: naturally occurring, semisynthetic, and synthetic (Box 2-4). Naturally occurring opioids are derived from the poppy plant, *papaver somni'ferum,* and include papaverine, thebaine, and morphine. Only morphine is used clinically. Chemical manipulation of the base compound gives rise to the semisynthetic opioids, such as codeine, hydromorphone, oxycodone, and oxymorphone. Synthetic compounds resemble morphine chemically but are artificially manufactured. This latter group has seen accelerated growth over the past 10 years and includes many of the commonly used opioids, such as levorphanol, meperidine, methadone, pentazocine. The latest additions to the synthetic opioid group are fentanyl, alfentanil, sufentanil, and remifentanil. Remifentanil is still undergoing initial clinical trials and is not available for routine clinical use. Al-

BOX 2-4.
Classification of Opioids

Naturally Occurring Agents

Papaverine
Thebaine
Morphine

Semisynthetic Agents

Codeine	Oxycodone
Hydromorphone	Oxymorphone

Synthetic Agents

Fentanyl	Levorphanol
Sufentanil	Meperidine
Alfentanil	Methadone
Remifentanil	Pentazocine

though the chemical structure and mode of production can serve to separate the various opioids, the more clinically relevant differences are their potency, duration of action, and the presence or absence of active metabolites (Table 2-1).

Opioids act through interaction with specific opioid receptors in the peripheral nervous system and the central nervous system (CNS) (see Chapter 1). Analgesia is mediated through either mu or kappa receptors. Opioids may act as either pure agonists (binding and activating both mu and kappa receptors) or agonist/antagonists (binding and activating kappa receptors while binding to, but not activating, mu receptors). Some of the commercially available agonist/antagonists are listed in Box 2-5.

In most situations, agonist/antagonists offer little advantage over pure agonists for the treatment of postoperative pain. Agonist/antagonists should never be used in patients who have been chronically receiving opioids, because withdrawal symptoms may ensue. Specific uses of the agonist/antagonists are discussed later in this chapter (nasal butorphanol) and in Chapter 3 (intravenous

TABLE 2-1. Potency and Half-Life of Opioids

Agent	Potency	Half-life (Hours)	Active Metabolites
Agonists			
Morphine	1	2-3	Yes
Meperidine	0.1	2-3	Yes
Hydromorphone	5	2-4	No
Oxymorphone	10	2-4	No
Methadone	1	12-24	No
Fentanyl	100	0.3-0.5	No
Sufentanil	1000	0.2-0.4	No
Alfentanil	20	0.1-0.2	No
Agonists/antagonists			
Butorphanol	5	2-4	No
Nalbuphine	1	5	No
Pentazocine	0.3-0.4	2-3	No

BOX 2-5.
Opioids of the Agonist/Antagonist Class

Butorphanol
Buprenorphine
Nalbuphine
Pentazocine
Dezocine

butorphanol to supplement analgesia in patients receiving epidural/spinal opioids). In the latter situation, clinical evidence suggests that the respiratory depression that may occur with the combination of IV and neuraxial opioids may be minimized if an agonist/antagonist, such as butorphanol, is used rather than a pure agonist, such as morphine.

When opioids are chosen for postoperative analgesia, three choices must be made: the opioid to be used, the mode of administration, and the route of administration. There is relatively little information concerning the optimal opioid for postoperative analgesia, and several acceptable alternatives are available that should provide equipotent analgesia, provided that equipotent doses are administered. In the patient with compromised cardiovascular status or at risk for pulmonary hypertension, such as an infant with a large preoperative systemic to pulmonary shunt, the synthetic opioid with cardiovascular stability, beneficial effects on pulmonary vascular resistance, and ability to blunt the sympathetic stress response may be advantageous. Anand and colleagues suggest that these agents, by blunting the postsurgical stress response, may improve postoperative outcome.

Since synthetic opioids have short plasma half-lives (less than 30 minutes), they are generally administered by a continuous infusion to maintain a plasma concentration adequate to provide analgesia. There seems to be no inherent advantage regarding any of the three commonly used synthetic agents (alfentanil, fentanyl, and sufentanil). However, fentanyl is the least expensive of the three.

Although synthetic opioids can be expected to maintain stable hemodynamics in patients with compromised cardiovascular function, other alternatives, such as morphine, are acceptable and cheaper in patients with normal cardiovascular function. Morphine causes some venodilatation and may decrease blood pressure in hypovolemic patients. However, for the majority of patients, morphine is effective as the first line opioid. The dosing regimen depends on the chosen mode of administration (Box 2-6).

Alternatives to morphine include hydromorphone (Dilaudid), meperidine (Demerol), and methadone (Dolobid). Hydromorphone may be advantageous when adverse effects related to histamine release, such as pruritus, occur with morphine.[17] In such cases, an equipotent dose of hydromorphone should be administered. Hydromorphone is 5 to 7 times as potent as morphine (Table 2-1); therefore, one fifth to one seventh of the morphine dose should be used.

Meperidine is associated with a relatively high incidence of adverse CNS effects, such as dysphoria, agitation, and seizures.[18] In older children and adults, the dysphoric response may manifest

BOX 2-6.
Dosing Guidelines for Morphine Administration*

Initial dose in the recovery room
  0.01 to 0.02 mg/kg every 5 minutes, titrate to effective analgesia
P.r.n./fixed-interval dosing
  0.05 mg/kg every 3 hrs
Continuous infusion
  0.01 to 0.03 mg/kg/hr
Patient-controlled analgesia
  Bolus: 0.02 mg/kg every 10 minutes
  Infusion: 0.005 mg/kg/hr

*The doses listed are guidelines for starting doses in patients who have not previously been receiving opioids. These doses should be adjusted as necessary to achieve the desired level of analgesia while limiting adverse effects. When opioids are used in infants under 6 months of age or patients with severe systemic illnesses (see Box 2-7), the starting dose should be 50% of the above listed doses and monitoring of cardiorespiratory function is suggested.
P.r.n., as needed.

as complaints of "not feeling well" and restlessness, whereas agitation and uncontrollable crying may be the only manifestations in the younger child or infant. CNS toxicity (including seizures) results from the accumulation of normeperidine, which occurs after hepatic N-methylation of the parent compound.[19] Normeperidine has a long half-life (15 to 20 hours) and is dependent on renal excretion. High or toxic levels occur more commonly in the setting of renal insufficiency, with the coadministration of drugs such as phenobarbital that stimulate hepatic microsomal enzymes, and with large doses (greater than 2 g/day in an adult). Toxicity may be a significant problem in the patient who is chronically receiving opioids and requires dose escalations to provide effective analgesia. Since meperidine offers no particular advantage over other opioids, morphine is preferred as the initial opioid for postoperative analgesia.

Methadone, with a plasma half-life of 12 to 24 hours, may provide a prolonged steady state serum concentration after a single bolus administration. Its pharmacokinetic profile is such that prolonged analgesia is provided without the need for a continuous infusion or PCA technique. Gourlay and colleagues administered a single, 20 mg, intraoperative dose of methadone to adults after major surgical procedures.[20] Half of the patients required only acetaminophen for analgesia, and those patients who required supplemental opioid analgesic agents were an average of 17 hours into the postoperative course. Berde and colleagues found that a single dose of 0.2 mg/kg of methadone administered after the induction of anesthesia in children between 3 and 7 years of age resulted in lower pain scores and decreased the need for supplemental opioid analgesic agents over the first 36 postoperative hours.[21] Although there is still limited experience with methadone in children, its longer duration of action offers certain advantages over the intermittent administration of agents with shorter half-lives. It may be useful in situations where PCA devices or continuous infusions are not available. In this setting, the intraoperative administration of 0.1 mg/kg is recommended. Analgesia is then supplemented with p.r.n. bolus doses of a shorter acting agent, such as morphine. Although the prolonged serum half-life of methadone provides longer analgesia, the time frame during which adverse effects may occur is also greater. Therefore, cardiorespiratory monitoring of patients at risk must be continued for up to 24 hours after a dose.

The second choice concerning opioid administration regards the mode of administration. Options include p.r.n. dosing, fixed-interval administration, continuous infusion, or the use of a PCA device. To provide optimal analgesia, opioids should be administered to maintain a steady state serum concentration. Without this concentration an effect cannot occur, and analgesia will be inadequate. The p.r.n. mode is the least likely to provide adequate sedation and analgesia for the patient. With p.r.n. dosing, a significant delay can occur from the time that it is recognized that the child is in pain until the medication is drawn up, administered, and takes effect.[22] Therefore other modes of administration must be used to ensure adequate analgesia. Either a continuous infusion or a PCA device is preferred.

Lynn and colleagues evaluated the respiratory effects of continuous morphine infusion in children after cardiac surgery[23] and found that morphine infusions of 10 to 30 μg/kg/hr resulted in serum concentrations of 10 to 22 ng/ml, provided adequate analgesia, and did not impair weaning from mechanical ventilation. This study demonstrates that adequate analgesia with opioids, even when administered by continuous infusion, does not preclude or hamper weaning from mechanical ventilation.

An alternative to continuous infusion or intermittent IV administration is PCA. This mode of opioid delivery allows the patient to administer a preset amount of opioid at preselected intervals. These devices may be used in children as young as 5 to 6 years of age.[24-26] To start, an opioid is titrated in small, IV bolus doses (0.01 mg/kg morphine every 5 mins). Once the desired level of analgesia is obtained, the PCA device is started. Although any opioid can be used with PCA, morphine is generally used first (0.01 to 0.02 mg/kg every 10 mins as needed). It is usually best to institute PCA in the recovery room so that the serum concentration of opioid does not diminish if there is a delay in starting PCA on the inpatient floor.

PCA may also include a low basal infusion rate in addition to the patient administered bolus doses. This represents one of the most controversial issues concerning PCA. It is suggested that the use of a basal infusion rate is contradictory to the "safety factor" of PCA: if a patient is too sleepy to push the button, no opioid is infused. With the basal infusion rate, the opioid is infused regardless of patient demands. Adult studies suggest no improvement in analgesia with a basal infusion and an increased incidence of adverse effects, such as sedation and respiratory depression.[27,28] Different results have been reported in pediatric patients depending on the dose used for the basal infusion rate. Doyle and colleagues compared PCA (0.02 mg/kg morphine every 5 minutes as needed) with and without a basal infusion rate of 0.02 mg/kg/hr.[29] There was no difference in the pain scores between the two groups, although there were more adverse effects, including nausea, sedation, and hypoxemia, in the patients who received the basal infusion rate. In a follow-up study the same investigators compared three different regimens of PCA.[30] The PCA included 0.02 mg/kg every 5 minutes as needed with no basal infusion rate (group 1), a basal infusion of 0.01 mg/kg/hr (group 2), and a basal infusion rate of 0.004 mg/kg/hr (group 3). Pain scores were equivalent in all three groups. There was an increased time spent asleep during the first two postoperative nights in groups 2 and 3 with no difference in time asleep during the day. There was an increased incidence of nausea and vomiting in the group that received the basal infusion rate of 0.01 mg/kg/hr (group 2). The authors concluded that a low basal infusion of 0.004 mg/kg/hr improved the sleep pattern when compared with no basal infusion rate.

When used in its classic sense, PCA requires an awake, cooperative patient who is able to comprehend its purpose and is able to push the button when additional analgesia is required. Its use may be limited in many of the patients because of age or underlying illness. In these patients, the PCA device may be activated by the bedside nurse, thereby eliminating the delay in opioid administration that occurs as the nurse signs out the medication and draws it up. However, when used in this fashion, one again loses the inherent safety factor of PCA.

Nonintravenous Routes of Opioid Administration

Although the majority of moderate to severe postoperative pain is treated with IV opioids, certain situations may arise that limit or preclude IV administration. In these situations, nonintravenous routes of administration may become necessary to provide ongoing analgesia. These nonintravenous routes include subcutaneous, oral, transdermal, and transmucosal (sublingual, buccal, intranasal, and rectal) administration. The intramuscular route should be avoided since variability in uptake and absorption leads to erratic serum levels and ineffective analgesia. Several investigators have demonstrated superior analgesia with IV administration when compared with intramuscular administration.[31,32] Additionally, children will deny pain to avoid a shot.

The simplest and cheapest nonintravenous route is oral administration. Although this route is frequently chosen for outpatients, its use remains limited in hospitalized patients. The oral use of weak opioids, including codeine and oxycodone, has previously been discussed. Other opioids, including morphine, hydromorphone, and methadone, can be administered orally to control more severe pain. Regardless of the opioid agent chosen, problems that arise with oral administration include a delay in onset of action, the need for larger doses because of decreased bioavailability, and underlying medical or surgical problems that preclude the use of the gastrointestinal tract.

One of the major problems with oral administration of morphine is the controversy concerning its oral bioavailability with estimates ranging from 15% to 50%.[33] More importantly it has been demonstrated that oral bioavailability varies significantly from patient to patient and is dependent on whether administration occurs in the fasting or fed state. These problems can lead to either inadequate analgesia or the occurrence of adverse effects.

With morphine, the IV/oral ratio is 1:3 (oral bioavailability of 33%). Several oral preparations are available, including 10, 15, and 30 mg tablets as well as an elixir. There are also sustained release tablets, but these preparations have no role in the treatment of acute pain and are generally used for the patient with chronic pain. Although the onset of action of the immediate release preparations occurs within 20 to 30 minutes, the sustained release tablets have a significant delay in peak effect of up to 4 to 6 hours and may take 2 to 3 days to reach a steady state serum concentration.

Other options for oral administration include methadone and hydromorphone. Although methadone is equipotent with morphine, its oral bioavailability is greater (70% to 80%) with a longer duration of action (12 to 24 hrs). The parenteral/oral ratio of hydromorphone is similar to that of morphine (1:3). As with morphine, hydromorphone is available in both tablets (2, 4, and 8 mg) and an elixir. One advantage of the hydromorphone elixir is that it is alcohol free and tends to have a more palatable taste than the morphine elixir.

Despite the availability of such preparations, experience with the oral use of any of these opioids to control postoperative pain remains limited. Litman and Shapiro have described their use of oral PCA (hydromorphone or morphine) to treat acute pain of various etiologies in four children.[34] Future studies are needed to define the role and efficacy of oral administration for the treatment of acute pain. Despite limited applications in acute pain, oral administration continues to play a prominent role in the control of cancer pain.[35]

One novel approach to opioid delivery is the recent development of transdermal fentanyl. Despite early success in adults,[36] its use in children remains anecdotal.[37] The transdermal delivery system allows the continuous administration of the potent opioid fentanyl at four different doses (25, 50, 75, and 100 μg/hr). Steady state serum concentrations are reached 8 hours after patch application and maintained for 72 hours.[38] Because of the limitation to only four sizes, titration of doses for children of various sizes may not be practical. Additionally, since the smallest size is 25 μg/hr, its use in smaller patients who are naive to opioids may not be possible. Limited use has been found for the fentanyl patch in controlling postoperative pain, and its use is suggested only for difficult situations when other routes of delivery, such as oral or IV administration, are not feasible.[37] A recent episode of respiratory depression with the use of the fentanyl patch in a child for routine postoperative analgesia stresses its potential complications. These problems have led the Janssen Pharmaceutical Company to advise against its use in children under 12 years of age. It has been used in younger children but only in special circumstances when the options for route of opioid administration are limited.

Subcutaneous administration has generally been reserved for the terminal cancer patient. Limited experience outside the cancer population suggests its efficacy for controlling acute pain. Bruera used subcutaneous infusions of opioids to control pain in an adult intensive care unit (ICU) population.[39] Opioids were administered by either intermittent subcutaneous dosing or by continuous infusion to 13 patients for a total of 60 days. The infusions were delivered through a 25-gauge butterfly needle inserted subcutaneously in the subclavicular area or the anterior abdominal wall. The site was changed if erythema, swelling, or leakage was observed or at seven-day intervals. No infectious complications were noted, and the insertion site was changed only three times because of local problems, such as erythema. They expressed some concern over possible delays in onset of activity or decreased absorption in patients with decreased peripheral perfusion, although they noted no such problems in their patients.

Doyle and colleagues investigated the efficacy of PCA by the subcutaneous route in children after appendectomy.[40] The patients were randomized to receive either IV or subcutaneous administration. The PCA regimen included morphine with bolus doses of 0.02 mg/kg every 5 minutes, as needed, with a basal infusion rate of 0.005 mg/kg/hr. The subcutaneous PCA was delivered through a 22-gauge, IV cannula that was placed into the subcutaneous tissue over the deltoid muscle. There was no difference in the pain scores at rest or with activity between the two groups. However, there was a significantly increased number of hypoxemic events with IV administration when compared with subcutaneous administration.

The authors have had anecdotal experience with switching from IV to subcutaneous fentanyl for sedation during mechanical ventilation in a patient in the pediatric ICU. IV administration was not possible since the fentanyl was not compatible with the antibiotics that the patient was receiving. Adequate sedation by continuous, subcutaneous infusion and bolus dosing of fentanyl was possible during the time that IV administration was not feasible.

For subcutaneous administration, a butterfly needle or a standard IV catheter is inserted into the subcutaneous tissue of the thigh, abdominal wall, subclavicular area, or deltoid. Dosing regimens, including basal infusion rates and boluses, are the same as for IV administration. The fluid volume should generally be kept to a maximum of 1 to 3 ml/hr. The site should be changed at seven-day intervals or sooner if erythema or local tissue reaction is noted. Several different opioids may be administered subcutaneously, including morphine, hydromorphone, and fentanyl. Methadone on the other hand causes significant tissue reaction with erythema and is not recommended for subcutaneous administration.

In addition to transdermal and subcutaneous administration, there has been recent interest in the administration of various opioids across mucous membranes (nasal, sublingual, buccal, or rectal). Systemic effects can be achieved with the transmucosal administration of various nonopioid medications, including synthetic vasopressin, midazolam, calcitonin, and insulin. This route has recently been evaluated with opioids, including fentanyl and butorphanol.[41-43] Striebel and colleagues evaluated the efficacy of intranasal fentanyl in controlling pain resulting from lumbar laminectomy. Patients were randomized to receive either IV or intranasal fentanyl when they first complained of severe pain. The fentanyl was delivered intranasally via a premetered spray bottle that delivered 0.09 ml per spray of a 50 μg/ml fentanyl solution. Therefore each spray contained 4.5 μg of fentanyl. The dose of fentanyl was the same in both groups (27 μg) and was repeated every 5 minutes. Analgesia was assessed using a visual analogue score ranging from 0 to 100. The onset of analgesia was comparable between the groups. The dose of fentanyl was greater (although not statistically significant) with the intranasal administration as opposed to the IV administration (110 versus 73 μg). Intranasal fentanyl decreased the pain scores from a mean of 60 down to 10 to 20. The pain scores were lower at the 10, 20, and 30 minute intervals in the IV group when compared with the intranasal group but were similar between the two groups throughout the remainder of the study (90 minutes after the dose). The authors concluded that intranasal fentanyl has a rapid onset and provides effective postoperative analgesia.

The other opioid agent that has been used by the intranasal route is the agonist/antagonist butorphanol (Stadol). Butorphanol is an opioid of the agonist/antagonist class that is five times as potent as morphine. It provides analgesia through its agonistic activity at the kappa receptor while competitively blocking the mu receptor. Butorphanol is commercially available in a metered dose spray that delivers 1 mg of butorphanol per spray.

Abboud and colleagues evaluated the efficacy of intranasal versus IV butorphanol following gynecologic surgery.[42] When intranasal administration was compared with IV administration, the onset of action was slower (15 versus 5 mins); however, the duration of analgesia was longer (4.5 versus 3 hrs). Somnolence was the only significant adverse effect encountered during the study.

There has been similar success with intranasal butorphanol in a prospective, open-label trial.[43] Intranasal butorphanol was used to control postoperative pain after pediatric surgery in eight adolescents in an underdeveloped country. In that setting the use of parenteral opioids is limited because of the high patient/nurse ratio, the unavailability of parenteral medications, and the inability to maintain IV access. Given these restraints, intranasal butorphanol is far superior to the usual technique that involved exclusively oral opioids and NSAIDs. Adverse effects were limited, although some of the patients did complain of a burning sensation or irritation in the back of the throat. Although nasal butorphanol does provide adequate analgesia, it has certain limitations in the pediatric population. Since each milliliter contains 1 mg of butorphanol, it cannot be used in patients who weigh less than 30 to 40 kg. Since a wide range of weights are encountered in pediatric practice, changing the concentration of the solution is necessary to allow appropriate adjustment of the dose.

Success has also been reported with the administration of opioids across more distal parts of the respiratory system.[44-46] Farncombe and Chater reported the use of nebulized morphine to treat dyspnea in four patients with either end-stage lung disease or congestive heart failure. In these patients the standard IV morphine preparation was diluted in 2 ml of sterile water. The initial dose was 2.5 mg morphine, which was increased to 10 mg as needed. All four patients received subjective relief of their dyspnea. The authors speculate that the morphine was either acting centrally after absorption across the respiratory mucosa or binding to opioid receptors that have been identified in lung tissue. Regardless of the mechanism of action, the authors emphasize that the major advantage of this technique is avoiding the need for IV access and thereby, perhaps, eliminating the need for hospitalization for terminal patients who prefer to stay at home. Although nebulized morphine may be effective, certain problems can occur with administration, such as the loss of a significant amount of the drug with exhalation, adherence of the drug to the nebulizer and tubing, and swallowing of the drug that lands on the oropharynx.

Other transmucosal routes that may allow the rapid, nonparenteral absorption of opioids are buccal administration and sublingual administration.[47] Although the surface of these spaces is relatively limited, the rich vascular and lymphatic drainage allows for the rapid absorption of medications. Additionally, these routes, as with the other transmucosal routes previously described, avoid first-pass hepatic metabolism. The primary disadvantage of this route is the need to keep the medication in contact with either the buccal mucosa or the sublingual area. Since there are no special preparations for buccal and sublingual administration, standard orally administered tablets are used. Dissolution of the tablet takes 15 to 20 minutes. During administration the patient is asked not to talk, chew, eat, or drink. Additionally, many of the opioids have a bitter taste. These factors make the task of delivery of the medication difficult in children. Because of the problems of delivery, there remains relatively little enthusiasm and hence little scientific information concerning the buccal and sublingual administration of opioids.

The newest addition to the transmucosal opioid line is the Fentanyl Oralet. This preparation incorporates the synthetic opioid into a raspberry-flavored oral lozenge. There are currently three preparations available (200, 300, and 400 μg). Dosing recommendations include 5 to 10 μg/kg with a maximum of 400 μg. Onset time varies from 10 to 20 minutes after administration. It has been used most commonly as a premedicant for children before anesthetic induction; however, it may also have a role in the treatment of postoperative or procedure-related pain. Although the preparation is ingested like a standard lollipop, its systemic effects result from the absorption of fentanyl across the buccal mucosa. The portion of the preparation that is swallowed has limited bioavailability (15% to 25%). Experience with the Oralet and its possible adverse effects remains limited. Since there have been reports of respiratory depression, careful monitoring of the patient's cardiorespiratory function is recommended regardless of the route of delivery of the opioid.

Adverse Effects of Opioids

Several different adverse effects may occur with opioids and thereby interfere with the delivery of effective analgesia (Table 2-2). Although the life threatening effects of opioids, such as respiratory depression, cause the greatest worry, it is more commonly the nonlife-threatening problems that prevent their use. The respiratory depressant activity is directly related to potency and occurs with all opioids. Equianalgesic doses of opioids produce equal amounts of respiratory depression. Factors that may predispose patients to respiratory depression include extremes of age, severe underlying systemic diseases, a preexisting altered mental status,

TABLE 2-2. Adverse Effects of Opioids and Suggested Therapies*

Adverse Effect	Treatment Options
Respiratory depression	Stop opioid Airway management if severe Naloxone 2 to 4 μg/kg up to 0.2 mg
Sedation	Stimulant medication such as methylphenidate
Dysphoria	Change opioid
Constipation or ileus	Stool softeners Cathartic agents Motility agent (methoclopramide or cisapride)
Nausea or vomiting	Phenothiazine (0.25 mg/kg promethazine up to 25 mg) Butyrophenone (0.01 mg/kg droperidol up to 0.625 mg) Ondansetron (0.1 mg/kg up to 4 mg)
Pruritus	Diphenhydramine (0.5 mg/kg up to 25 mg)
Seizures	Stop opioid Symptomatic treatment Airway intervention if needed Benzodiazepines to control seizures
Tolerance or physical dependence	See Chapters 6 and 7

*Regardless of the adverse effects, the incidence can be limited by adjusting the dose of opioid to the least amount necessary to provide optimal analgesia. Certain adverse effects like nausea, vomiting, and pruritus may be controlled in severe cases by changing to a different opioid.

and the addition of other medications that potentiate the central respiratory depressant effects of opioids (Box 2-7).

Respiratory depression may also occur in the setting of renal failure in patients receiving morphine. Although the parent compound (morphine) undergoes primarily hepatic metabolism, one of the metabolites (morphine-6-glucuronide) possesses half of the respiratory depressant activity of the parent compound and is dependent on renal excretion. In the setting of altered renal function, opioids such as fentanyl or hydromorphone, which are not depen-

BOX 2-7.
Patients at Risk for Opioid-Related Adverse Effects*

Extreme age (infants less than 6 months of age)
Patients with severe underlying systemic illness
- Cardiorespiratory dysfunction
- Hepatic insufficiency
- Renal insufficiency
- Altered mental status
- Airway obstruction
- Central or obstructive apnea

Concomitant use of other medications
- Barbiturates
- Phenothiazines
- Benzodiazepines

*The presence of these problems does not preclude opioid administration. When opioids are used in these patients, 50% of the usual dose is recommended in addition to continuous monitoring of cardiorespiratory function.

dent on renal function, may offer a safer alternative. In any of the above situations, cardiorespiratory monitoring is recommended. In the "at risk" group, the dose should be 50% of the usual starting dose and titrated up as needed.

Naloxone is recommended for the treatment of severe respiratory depression related to opioids. Naloxone is available in several different dilutions and therefore particular attention must be paid to the individual ampule. Standard pediatric ampules include either 0.4 or 1.0 mg/ml. Respiratory depression should be treated with incremental doses of 2 to 4 μg/kg (maximum dose of 0.2 mg) repeated every 3 to 5 minutes as needed. Small, incremental doses are suggested since it may be possible to reverse respiratory depression without reversing analgesia. Once respiratory depression is reversed, continued monitoring of the patient is important since the half-life of naloxone is only 20 to 30 minutes compared to 2 to 3 hours for the majority of opioids.

Inadequate analgesia may occur, especially in younger children and infants, because of healthcare providers' unfounded fears of addiction. The incidence of addiction in patients receiving opioid analgesic agents for postoperative pain control has been shown to be exceedingly rare.[48] Physical dependence can be seen after the prolonged administration of opioids and sedative agents. (Options to deal with physical dependency are discussed in Chapters 6 and 7.) These problems should not limit the use of opioids but rather act as a reminder of the need to slowly taper their use after prolonged administration (greater than 7 to 10 days).

Additional adverse effects of opioids include sedation, constipation, pruritus, nausea, and vomiting. Careful attention to the patient's bowel habits and the use of stool softeners concurrently with opioid therapy may help to avoid constipation. Although tolerance to some of the other adverse effects of opioids such as sedation may develop, it does not occur with the opioids' effects on gastrointestinal motility. Cathartic agents (cascara) or osmotic agents (milk of magnesia) may be needed for refractory cases or when constipation has already developed. When opioids are used for sedation in the ICU, the addition of metoclopramide or cisapride (0.1 mg/kg every 6 hrs) may also be used to prevent the opioids from exacerbating the altered gastrointestinal motility, which may occur as a result of acute illnesses. The addition of these agents may allow for earlier and continued enteral feeding in such patients.

Tolerance to opioid sedation generally occurs over a period of two to three days. Although sedation is a beneficial side effect when the opioids are used to control agitation during mechanical ventilation, it may be undesirable if it interferes with the activities of daily life in chronic pain patients. One option for the prevention of opioid-induced sedation is the addition of stimulant medications such as methylphenidate, pemoline, or dextroamphetamine. Stimulant medications are contraindicated in patients with hypertension, cardiac arrhythmias, coronary artery disease, and psychiatric disorders.

Nausea and vomiting are probably the most bothersome of the nonlife-threatening adverse effects of opioids. Three different mechanisms may be involved: a direct stimulation of the central, chemoreceptor trigger zone of the medulla, decreased gastrointestinal motility and increased pyloric tone, and sensitization of the vestibular apparatus. Regardless of the mechanisms involved, treatment is primarily symptomatic and may include phenothiazines, butyrophenones, metoclopromide, and ondansetron. Although there is more experience with the phenothiazines (promethazine 0.25 to 0.5 mg/kg up to 25 mg) and the butyrophenones (droperidol 0.01 to 0.02 mg/kg up to 0.625 mg), adverse effects may occur with these agents, such as dystonic reactions, lowering of the seizure threshold, and potentiation of opioid-induced respiratory depression. When phenothiazines are used to treat nausea in patients receiving PCA, because of the issues of potentiation of opioid-induced respiratory depression, stopping the PCA pump for 30 minutes before and after the dose is recommended.

Other options include either metoclopramide (0.1 mg/kg to 10 mg) or one of the new serotonin antagonists (ondansetron or granisetron). Ondansetron is administered in a dose of 0.1 mg/kg IV (maximum of 4 mg) every 6 hours as needed. Unlike the phenothiazines, ondansetron and granisetron do not cause sedation or potentiate the respiratory depressant effects of opioids.

When nausea or vomiting persists despite symptomatic treatment, changing opioids may be helpful. Although there does not seem to be any particular opioid with a higher incidence of nausea and vomiting, some patients may vomit with one opioid and not another.

Pruritus may occur as an isolated symptom or in association with urticaria. The mechanisms of opioid-induced pruritus are multifactorial and include a direct central effect as well as histamine release. One strategy to control pruritus is the administration of an antihistamine, such as diphenhydramine (0.5 mg/kg to 25 mg), or changing to another opioid. The sedative properties of diphenhydramine may also potentiate opioid-induced sedation. When pruritus is not controlled with antihistamines, changing to another opioid may be helpful. For IV use, these include hydromorphone, oxymorphone, and the synthetic agent, fentanyl. Oxycodone preparations are recommended for oral administration.

When switching opioids equipotent doses should be used. The initial approach for severe pruritus is symptomatic treatment with diphenhydramine. If this fails, switching to hydromorphone is frequently successful. Patients with severe skin diseases, such as cutaneous involvement of graft-versus-host disease, may be particularly likely to develop opioid-induced pruritus.[49] In this group of patients it may be necessary to use fentanyl to provide analgesia and prevent pruritus.

Summary

Recent evidence has documented the deleterious physiologic effects of pain and the beneficial results of effective postoperative analgesia. As outlined in this chapter, a three-step approach is recommended depending on the severity of pain. This approach utilizes a combination of NSAIDs, oral opioids, and IV opioids. In addition to selecting a particular opioid to use, the practitioner must also consider the route of administration and the mode of administration. All three choices may significantly impact the efficacy of analgesia. Although IV opioids are the primary treatment for moderate and severe pain in the hospital setting, future formulations and developments may allow for the increased use of nonparenteral routes.

References

1. Mather L, Mackie J: The incidence of postoperative pain in children, *Pain* 15:271, 1983.
2. Anand KJS, Hansen DD, Hickey PR: Hormonal-metabolic stress responses in neonates undergoing cardiac surgery, *Anesthesiology* 73:661, 1990.
3. Anand KJS, Sippell WG, Aynsley-Green A: Randomized trial of fentanyl anesthesia in preterm babies undergoing surgery: effects on the stress response, *Lancet* 2:243, 1987.
4. Anand KJS, Hickey PR: Halothane-morphine compared with high-dose sufentanil for anesthesia and postoperative analgesia in neonatal cardiac surgery, *N Engl J Med* 326:1, 1992.

5. Weissman C: The metabolic response to stress: an overview and update, *Anesthesiology* 73:308, 1990.
6. Marshall BE, Wyche MQ: Hypoxia during and after anesthesia, *Anesthesiology* 37:178, 1972.
7. Craig DB: Postoperative recovery of pulmonary function, *Anesth Analg* 60:46, 1981.
8. Schug SA, Zech D, Dorr U: Cancer pain management according to WHO analgesic guidelines, *J Pain Symptom Manage* 5:27, 1990.
9. Maunuksela EL, Ryhanen P, Janhunen L: Efficacy of rectal ibuprofen in controlling postoperative pain in children, *Can J Anaesth* 39:226, 1992.
10. O'Hara DA, Fragen RJ, Kinzer M et al: Ketorolac tromethamine as compared with morphine sulfate for treatment of postoperative pain, *Clin Pharmacol Ther* 41:556, 1987.
11. Maunuksela EL, Olkkola KT, Korpela R: Does prophylactic intravenous infusion of indomethacin improve the management of postoperative pain in children? *Can J Anaesth* 35:123, 1988.
12. Watcha MF, Jones MB, Lagueruela R et al: Comparison of ketorolac and morphine as adjuvants during pediatric surgery, *Anesthesiology* 76:368, 1992.
13. Vetter TR, Heiner EJ: Intravenous ketorolac as an adjuvant to pediatric patient-controlled analgesia with morphine, *J Clin Anesth* 6:110, 1994.
14. Ready LB, Brown CR, Stahlgren LH et al: Evaluation of intravenous ketorolac administered by bolus or infusion for treatment of postoperative pain, *Anesthesiology* 80:1277, 1994.
15. Klein DS, Edwards LW. Continuous intravenous ketorolac infusion for the treatment of cancer pain, *American Journal of Pain Management* 3:179, 1993.
16. De Conno F, Zecca E, Martini C et al: Tolerability of ketorolac administered via continuous subcutaneous infusion for cancer pain: a preliminary report, *J Pain Symptom Manage* 9:119, 1994.

17. Rosow CE, Moss J, Philbin DM et al: Histamine release during morphine and fentanyl anesthesia, *Anesthesiology* 56:93, 1982.
18. Shochet RB, Murray GB: Neuropsychiatric toxicity of meperidine, *Intensive Care Med* 3:246, 1988.
19. Goetting MG, Thirman MJ: Neurotoxicity of meperidine, *Ann Emerg Med* 14:1007, 1985.
20. Gourlay GK, Wilson PR, Lamberty J: A double-blinded comparison of morphine and methadone in postoperative pain control, *Anesthesiology* 64:322, 1986.
21. Berde CB, Beyer JE, Bournaki MC et al: Comparison of morphine and methadone for prevention of postoperative pain in children, *J Pediatr* 119:136, 1991.
22. Nayman J: Measurement and control of postoperative pain, *Ann R Coll Surg Engl* 61:419, 1979.
23. Lynn AM, Opheim KE, Tyler DC: Morphine infusion after pediatric cardiac surgery, *Crit Care Med* 12:863, 1984.
24. Berde CB, Lehn BM, Yee JD et al: Patient-controlled analgesia in children and adolescents: a randomized, prospective comparison with intramuscular administration of morphine for postoperative analgesia, *J Pediatr* 118:460, 1991.
25. Lawrie SC, Forbes DW, Akhtar TM et al: Patient-controlled analgesia in children, *Anaesthesia* 46:1074, 1990.
26. Gaukroger PB, Omkins DP, Van Der Walt JH: Patient-controlled analgesia in children, *Anaesth Intensive Care* 17:264, 1989.
27. Parker RK, Holtmann B, White PF: Patient-controlled analgesia: does a concurrent opioid infusion improve pain management after surgery? *JAMA* 266:1947, 1991.
28. Parker RK, Holtmann B, White PF: Effects of a nighttime opioid infusion with PCA therapy on patient comfort and analgesic requirements after abdominal hysterectomy, *Anesthesiology* 76:362, 1992.
29. Doyle E, Robinson D, Morton NS: Comparison of patient-controlled analgesia with and without a background infusion after lower abdominal surgery in children, *Br J Anaesth* 71:670, 1993.

30. Doyle E, Harper I, Morton NS: Patient-controlled analgesia with low dose background infusions after lower abdominal surgery in children, *Br J Anaesth* 71:818, 1993.
31. Stapleton JV, Austin KL, Mather LE: A pharmacokinetic approach to postoperative pain: continuous infusion of pethidine, *Anaesth Intensive Care* 7:25, 1979.
32. Rutter PC, Murphy F, Dudley HAF: Morphine: controlled trial of different methods of administration, *Br Med J* 280:12, 1980.
33. Gourlay GK, Plummer JL, Cherry DA et al: The reproducibility of bioavailability of oral morphine from solution under fed and fasted conditions, *J Pain Symptom Manage* 6:431, 1991.
34. Litman RS, Shapiro BS: Oral patient-controlled analgesia in adolescents, *J Pain Symptom Manage* 7:78, 1992.
35. Miser AW, Miser JS: The use of oral methadone to control moderate and severe pain in children and young adults with malignancy, *Clin Pain* 1:243, 1986.
36. Holley FR, van Steenis C: Postoperative analgesia with fentanyl: pharmacokinetics and pharmacodynamics at constant intravenous and transdermal delivery, *Br J Anaesth* 63:56, 1989.
37. Tobias JD: Transdermal fentanyl: applications and indications in the pediatric patient, *Pain Management* 2:30, 1992.
38. Duthie DJR, Rowbotham DJ, Wyld R et al: Plasma fentanyl concentrations during transdermal delivery of fentanyl in surgical patients, *Br J Anaesth* 60:614, 1988.
39. Bruera E, Gibney N, Stollery D et al: Use of the subcutaneous route of administration of morphine in the Intensive Care Unit, *J Pain Symptom Manage* 6:263, 1991.
40. Doyle E, Morton NS, McNicol LR: Comparison of patient-controlled analgesia in children by i.v. and s.c. routes of administration, *Br J Anaesth* 72:533, 1994.
41. Striebel HW, Koenigs D, Kramer J: Postoperative pain management by intranasal demand-adapted fentanyl, *Anesthesiology* 77:281, 1992.

42. Abboud TK, Zhu J, Gangolly J et al: Transnasal butorphanol: a new method for pain relief in post-cesarean section pain, *Acta Anaesthesiol Scand* 35:14, 1991.
43. Tobias JD, Rasmussen GE: Transnasal butorphanol for post-operative analgesia following pediatric surgery in a third world country, *Pediatr Anaesth* (in press).
44. Farncombe M, Chater S: Case studies outlining use of nebulized morphine for patients with end-stage chronic lung and cardiac disease, *J Pain Symptom Manage* 8:221, 1993.
45. Chrubasik J, Wust H, Friedrich et al: Absorption and bioavailability of nebulized morphine, *Br J Anaesth* 61:228, 1988.
46. Irazuzta J, Ahmed U, Gancayco A et al: Intratracheal administration of fentanyl in rabbits: pharmacokinetics and local effects, *Crit Care Med* 22:A220, 1994 (abstract).
47. Edge WG, Cooper GM, Morgan M: Analgesic effects of sublingual buprenorphine, *Anaesthesia* 34:463, 1979.
48. Porter J, Jick J: Addiction rare in patients treated with narcotics, *N Engl J Med* 302:123, 1980.
49. Tobias JD, Baker DK: Patient-controlled analgesia with fentanyl in children, *Clin Pediatr* 31:177, 1992.

3

EPIDURAL AND SPINAL ANESTHESIA AND ANALGESIA

Gail E. Rasmussen

LOCAL ANESTHESIA
Local anesthetic toxicity
OPIOIDS FOR REGIONAL ANESTHESIA
EPIDURAL ANESTHESIA
Caudal anesthesia
Adverse effects of epidural anesthesia
SPINAL ANESTHESIA

The popularity and applications of epidural and spinal anesthetic techniques in the pediatric population continue to increase. The indications include preemptive analgesia to decrease the surgical stress response and perioperative pain management. These regional anesthetic techniques may be used in conjunction with general anesthesia or as the primary anesthetic technique. As with any technique, there are inherent risks and contraindications that must be taken into consideration (Box 3-1). It should also be noted that these techniques should be performed only by anesthesiologists. With these caveats in mind, spinal and epidural anesthesia are a valuable adjunct in the prevention and treatment of pain in children. This chapter discusses the most frequently used local anesthetics and opioids for pediatric epidural and spinal blockade, as well as the techniques and applications of spinal and epidural anesthesia in children.

BOX 3-1.
Absolute/Relative Contraindications to Regional Anesthesia

- Systemic infection
  - Septicemia
  - Meningitis
- Bleeding diathesis
  - Coagulopathy
  - Thrombocytopenia
  - Qualitative coagulation defect
- Allergy to local anesthetics
- Patient, parent, or guardian refusal
- Hypovolemia
- Progressive and degenerative central nervous system diseases
- Other considerations in pediatric patients
  - Malformation of the vertebral column (meningomyelocele, spina bifida)
  - Hydrocephalus or raised intracranial pressure
  - Severe seizure disorder
  - Poorly controlled seizures
  - Spinal instrumentation (Harrington rods)

LOCAL ANESTHESIA

Local anesthetics can be separated into two groups based on their chemical structure: esters and amides (Box 3-2). The mechanism of action of local anesthetics is similar between adults and children. Local anesthetics bind to sodium channels of the neurons, preventing depolarization, thereby blocking nerve impulse conduction. The subsequent uptake and metabolism of the local anesthetic determine the duration of action and peak blood levels (Box 3-3). The primary modes of metabolism are plasma cholinesterases for the ester group and hepatic metabolism for the amides. Local anesthetic metabolism is affected by age, especially in the premature infant and neonate where the hepatic, microsomal enzyme system is not fully mature. Decreased protein binding, which may occur in infants less than 6 months of age, results in an increased free fraction of a local anesthetic. The free moiety of

BOX 3-2.
Classification of Local Anesthetics

- Amides
  - Bupivacaine
  - Etidocaine
  - Lidocaine
  - Mepivacaine
  - Prilocaine
  - Ropivacaine
- Esters
  - Chloroprocaine
  - Cocaine
  - Procaine
  - Tetracaine

BOX 3-3.
Determinants of Local Anesthetic Toxicity

Total dose of drug
Peak plasma concentration
Time to peak level
Free fraction of drug (influenced by alterations in protein binding)
Vascularity of injection site
Pharmacokinetic and pharmacodynamic profile of local anesthetic

the local anesthetic is responsible for its clinical effect as well as its toxicity.

Local anesthetic toxicity correlates with the serum concentration of the local anesthetic, whether from a direct intravascular injection or absorption from the injection site. The time it takes for the drug to be absorbed is also a consideration since a rapid rise of the serum concentration is more likely to result in toxicity. The primary factor that affects local anesthetic absorption and subsequent serum levels is the vascularity of the site of injection. Use of a vasoconstrictor, such as epinephrine or phenylephrine, with a local anesthetic solution can retard the absorption rate and lower the peak serum concentration by 10% to 20%.[1]

With the use of any local anesthetic, regardless of the concentration of the solution, the practitioner must calculate the milligram dose on a per kilogram basis to avoid toxic blood levels. This is especially important in neonates and infants. For example, if a 0.25% concentration of bupivacaine is used for a caudal anesthetic on a 3 kg baby, the maximum dose that should be used is 3 mg/kg (3 mg/kg × 3 kg = 9 mg). A 0.25% solution has 2.5 mg/ml, thus a maximum of 3.6 ml of the solution should be used. Recommended maximum doses for local anesthetics are outlined in Table 3-1.

In addition to the properties of local anesthetics, the type of block and site of injection also affect serum concentration.[2] The highest concentration and fastest absorption of local anesthetics occur after interpleural analgesia and intercostal nerve blocks (Table 3-2).

TABLE 3-1. Maximum Recommended Doses of Local Anesthetics

	Without Epinephrine	With Epinephrine
Lidocaine	5 mg/kg	7 mg/kg
Bupivacaine	2.5-3 mg/kg	3-3.5 mg/kg
Tetracaine	1.5-2 mg/kg	1.5-2 mg/kg
Chloroprocaine	8 mg/kg	8-10 mg/kg
Mepivacaine	5 mg/kg	7 mg/kg

TABLE 3-2. Rate of Local Anesthetic Absorption According to Site of Injection

Fastest absorption	Interpleural
	Intercostal
	Paracervical
	Caudal epidural
	Lumbar/thoracic epidural
	Axillary
	Brachial plexus
	Subarachnoid
	Sciatic-femoral
	Distal peripheral block
Slowest absorption	Subcutaneous infiltration

Local Anesthetic Toxicity

Even with extreme caution and careful calculation of doses, local anesthetic toxicity can occur. The anesthesiologist must be prepared to deal with such problems (Box 3-4). Although local anesthetic toxicity can result from vascular absorption of local anesthetics during continuous infusion techniques, the majority of complications occur with the administration of the initial or subsequent bolus doses. Local anesthetic toxicity may result from inadvertent intravascular or intraosseous administration. Before injection of the local anesthetic solution, careful aspiration for blood is suggested. Even with negative aspiration, inadvertent intravascular injection may still occur. Therefore a test dose is administered (0.5 μg/kg of epinephrine or 0.1 ml/kg of local anesthetic solution with 1:200,000 epinephrine). Even if no increase in heart rate or blood pressure is noted, the remainder of the dose should

BOX 3-4.
Management of Local Anesthetic Toxicity

- Stop administration of local anesthetic
- Airway management with delivery of 100% oxygen
  - Bag-valve-mask ventilation
  - Endotracheal intubation
- Maintenance of cardiac output
  - Cardiopulmonary resuscitation
  - Support intravascular volume
  - Inotropic support
- Anticonvulsant therapy (one of the following)
  - Diazepam 0.1 mg/kg (maximum 10 mg)
  - Midazolam 0.05 to 0.1 mg/kg (maximum 5 mg)
  - Lorazepam 0.05 mg/kg (maximum 4 mg)
  - Sodium pentothal (2 to 4 mg/kg)
- Defibrillation
  - 2 J/kg up to 6 J/kg
- Antiarrhythmic therapy for ventricular fibrillation and tachycardia
  - Bretylium 5 mg/kg (maximum 300 mg)
  - Magnesium 50 to 100 mg/kg (maximum 2 g)
  - Phenytoin 10 to 20 mg/kg (maximum 1 g)

be fractionated and administered slowly over 2 to 3 minutes. Repeated aspiration is recommended before each injection. Although there has been some question as to whether the test dose will produce tachycardia in patients anesthetized with halothane who have not received atropine, ST-T wave and axis changes on the electrocardiogram may occur in the absence of tachycardia as signs of intravascular injection of epinephrine. The use of a test dose costs nothing and may offer some protection for the patient. Because of the risk of toxicity, it is recommended that all blocks be performed with age- and size-appropriate emergency airway and resuscitation equipment. This precaution is necessary whether the blocks are performed in the operating room, procedure room, or at another location. (The signs and symptoms of local anesthetic toxicity are discussed in detail in Chapter 1.)

Bupivacaine is one of the most frequently used local anesthetics because of its long duration of action and its relative selectivity for sensory neurons, as opposed to motor neurons. However, it is also the most cardiotoxic. Bupivacaine binds avidly to the sodium channels in the myocardium, and in toxic doses it can precipitate cardiovascular collapse as a result of myocardial depression and ventricular arrhythmias.[3,4] Resuscitation from bupivacaine toxicity should be continued for up to 60 minutes to allow the bupivacaine time to disassociate from the sodium channels. Agents that may be effective in the treatment of ventricular tachycardia and fibrillation related to bupivacaine include bretylium (5 mg/kg up to 3 g), phenytoin (10 to 20 mg/kg up to 1 g), and magnesium (50 to 100 mg/kg up to 2 g). Also of great importance in immediate resuscitation is prevention or correction of hypoxia, hypercarbia, and acidosis by adequate airway management and cardiopulmonary resuscitation. Hypoxia, hypercarbia, and acidosis have all been shown to potentiate bupivacaine toxicity.

A final adverse effect of local anesthetics that must be considered is the rare allergic or anaphylactic reaction. A true allergy to the local anesthetic is more common with the ester group, whose chemical structure is similar to that of paraamino benzoic acid (PABA), which is known to be allergenic. A true allergy to the amide class is much less common and usually represents a response to the preservative, methylparaben. The latter compound also shares a similar chemical structure with PABA. Regardless of the agent involved, the allergic reaction may range in severity from urticaria and pruritus to bronchospasm and respiratory arrest. The treatment is primarily to stop the inciting agent (i.e., to stop injection of the local anesthetic). Supportive care may also be required (Box 3-5).

OPIOIDS FOR REGIONAL ANESTHESIA

Opioids have been used parenterally to treat postoperative pain. In the last decade they have been used with increased frequency in

BOX 3-5.
Management of Anaphylaxis

- Recognition
  - Flushing
  - Urticaria
  - Bronchospasm
  - Tachycardia
  - Hypotension
- Initial therapy
  - Identification and stoppage of antigenic exposure
  - Maintenance of airway (endotracheal intubation if compromised) with 100% O_2
  - Intravascular volume expansion
  - Titration of epinephrine 0.5 μg/kg intraveneously as needed to prevent cardiovascular collapse
- Second line therapy
  - Catecholamine infusions
    - Epinephrine (0.05 to 1 μg/kg/min)
    - Isoproterenol (0.05 to 1 μg/kg/min)
    - Norepinephrine (0.05 to 1 μg/kg/min)
  - Antihistamines (diphenhydramine 0.05 to 2 mg/kg)
  - H_2 Blockers (ranitidine 1 to 1.5 mg/kg)
  - Corticosteroids (solumedrol 10 mg/kg)
  - Bronchodilators (albuterol metered dose inhaler)

regional blockade, either solely or in conjunction with local anesthetics. Opioids bind to receptors in the dorsal horn of the spinal cord and modulate the synapse between first and second order neurons. Unlike local anesthetics, opioids affect sensory neurons without affecting motor or sympathetic functions. When used with local anesthetics there is a synergistic effect with an increase in the duration of the regional anesthetic and an improvement in the quality of analgesia while allowing the use of more dilute solutions of local anesthetics. Thus, opioids may lessen the potential for local anesthetic toxicity and side effects, such as motor blockade. This is particularly beneficial for postoperative pain control where dilute solutions of local anesthetics and opioids are being used as continuous infusions. Neuraxial opioids are also beneficial in high risk pediatric patients, such as infants who were born prematurely or those with a compromised respiratory status, where the doses of parenteral opioids to achieve adequate pain control may be too high to be both safe and effective.

The two most frequently used neuraxial opioids are morphine and fentanyl. These two agents have different properties that allow for versatility in the management of postoperative analgesia. Preservative-free morphine is frequently used in a single dose by epidural or intrathecal administration and can provide up to 24 hours of postoperative pain control. Because of its hydrophilic nature, morphine tends to stay in the cerebrospinal fluid (CSF) and travel cephalad. As a result, caudal or lumbar administration may be used to provide analgesia for thoracic or even craniofacial procedures.[5] For intrathecal administration, it is generally recommended to use 5 to 10 μg/kg of preservative-free morphine. The medication is best administered at the start of the procedure since onset of action may take 20 to 60 minutes, depending on the level of surgery.

On the other hand, fentanyl is more lipophilic with a more rapid onset of action (5 to 15 minutes) and a shorter duration of action (4 to 6 hours) when used as a single dose. Since it has a quicker onset of action than morphine, these two agents may be given simultaneously for pain control in an epidural injection at the end of a surgical case. Fentanyl provides a rapid onset of analgesia, whereas epidural morphine provides a longer duration. Because of its shorter duration of action, fentanyl is used more commonly in continuous infusions with dilute local anesthetic solutions for postoperative analgesia (e.g., 2 μg/ml fentanyl in 0.1% bupivacaine). Box 3-6 outlines the various opioids that are used in epidural and spinal anesthesia and analgesia and suggested doses for children. A summary of adult dosing is listed in Table 3-3.

Although neuraxial opioids can provide more effective analgesia than parenteral opioids, certain adverse effects may occur, such as delayed respiratory depression. This is particularly true

BOX 3-6.
Neuraxial Opioids

Epidural

Morphine (Preservative-free)
Single dose
(abdominal incision: 30-50 μg/kg)
(thoracic incision: 50-70 μg/kg)
Infusion: 0.1% bupivacaine + morphine 0.1-0.2 mg/kg/24 hr

Butorphanol
Single dose: 20-40 μg/kg. May be combined with morphine to limit adverse effects such as pruritus, nausea, and vomiting.

Fentanyl
Single dose: 0.5-1 μg/kg
Infusion
0.1% bupivacaine + fentanyl (2-5 μg/ml) at 0.3 ml/kg/hr (thoracic) to a maximum of 12 ml/hr or 0.4 ml/kg/hr (abdominal) to a maximum of 15 ml/hr

Sufentanil
Single dose: 0.75 μg/kg
Infusion: little information available

Intrathecal

Morphine 5-20 μg/kg
Fentanyl 0.2-0.5 μg/kg

TABLE 3-3. Opioids for Adult Epidural and Intrathecal Analgesia

	Epidural	Intrathecal
Morphine	1-10 mg	0.1-1 mg
Meperidine	20-200 mg	10-30 mg
Methadone	1-10 mg	
Hydromorphone	1-2 mg	
Diamorphine	4-6 mg	1-2 mg
Fentanyl	5-25 μg	5-50 μg
Sufentanil	25-150 μg	10-25 μg
Butorphanol	1-2 mg	

for morphine since significant concentrations persist in the CSF for up to 24 hours after administration, which may lead to central respiratory depression. Because of its lipophilic nature, the risks for delayed respiratory depression are limited with fentanyl. These effects are reversible with parenteral naloxone.

Pruritus also tends to be more common with spinal morphine. Although the patient may be pain free, he or she may have significant distress from the pruritus and may require treatment with diphenhydramine or a low-dose naloxone infusion. The latter can be used to treat the side effect without diminishing the analgesic effect of the opioid (Table 3-4). Another method that has recently been described to prevent the adverse effects associated with epidural morphine is the addition of the agonist/antagonist butorphanol.[6] The combination of epidural morphine (30 to 50 μg/kg) with butorphanol (20 to 30 μg/kg) has been shown to provide effective, long-lasting analgesia while limiting problems such as nausea, vomiting, pruritus, and respiratory depression.[6] This technique is effective when using a single-shot, caudal, epidural block after a major surgical procedure. The local anesthetic is combined (1 to 1.2 ml/kg of 0.25% bupivacaine with morphine and butorphanol). The standard intravenous (IV) solution of butorphanol is free of preservatives and can be used for epidural analgesia.

All patients who have received neuraxial opioids require respiratory monitoring in the postoperative period. In the past, chil-

TABLE 3-4. Side Effects of Neuraxial Opioids and Treatment

Side effect	Treatment
Pruritus (0%-20%)	Diphenhydramine 1-2 mg/kg Naloxone infusion 0.5-1 μg/kg/hr
Nausea and vomiting (25%-50%)	Metoclopramide 0.1-0.3 mg/kg q 8h Ondansetron 0.15 mg/kg Droperidol 10-30 μg intravenously Naloxone infusion 0.5-1 μg/kg/hr
Respiratory depression and somnolence*	Stop infusion Maintain ventilation 100% O_2 Naloxone bolus 0.5-1 μg/kg Naloxone infusion 3-5 μg/kg/hr
Urinary retention (30%-40%)	Naloxone infusion 3-5 μg/kg/hr Bethanecol 0.05 mg/kg SQ q 8h Straight catheterization or indwelling Foley catheter

*When continuous infusions of local anesthetics and opioids are used, the infusion rate or the opioid concentration in the infusion may need to be decreased.

dren who had received opioids were sent to the pediatric intensive/intermediate care unit (PICU). With proper training and inservicing of the nursing staff in the inpatient wards, these children should not require ICU admission. Monitoring should include pulse oximetry when the child is asleep with an evaluation of respiratory rate every 2 hours and sedation scores every 6 hours. With these parameters, changes in respiratory status and increased sedation can be detected early, and appropriate treatment can be instituted. This may mean simply decreasing the infusion rate, decreasing the amount of opioid in the infusion, or using a low-dose naloxone infusion. Monitoring should be continued for 24 hours after neuraxial morphine and 8 hours after fentanyl.

Although parenteral opioids may be needed to supplement the analgesia of spinal or epidural opioids, their use may increase the incidence of respiratory depression. When it becomes necessary to use parenteral opioids in patients who have received neuraxial opioids, a mixed agonist-antagonist, such as butorphanol (0.01 to

0.02 mg/kg up to 1 mg), may have less effect on respiratory function than pure agonists, such as morphine.

EPIDURAL ANESTHESIA

The epidural space lies between the dura mater and the ligamentum flavum and extends from the base of the skull to the sacrococcygeal membrane (Fig. 3-1). The epidural space may be approached anywhere along the spinal axis for regional blockade. The level at which the epidural block is performed depends on the type of surgery and the medications that are used. As discussed previously, morphine can be administered caudally and provide thoracic analgesia, whereas fentanyl should be placed nearer to the level of incision. Likewise, local anesthetics should be placed near the dermatomes that are to be anesthetized. Although a midthoracic block can be achieved with the caudal administration of local anesthetics, the dosing requirements to maintain the block for a protracted period of time result in high serum concentrations and toxicity. The placement of the catheter near the level of surgery allows for the use of a combination of a local anesthetic and fentanyl, which provides superior analgesia to the use of opioids alone. The administration of fentanyl near the level of surgery also decreases the dose needed, thereby limiting systemic levels and adverse effects.

Several decisions must be made in planning for epidural anesthesia in children. These include the use of a single shot or placement of a catheter, the choice of medications (opioids, local anesthetics, or a combination of the two), and the level of puncture (caudal, lumbar, or thoracic). Although it is preferable to place the catheter directly at the level of the surgery, it may be placed at the thoracic or lumbar level by advancing the catheter up the epidural space from a caudal approach.[7] The latter technique is less than optimal since the catheter may kink or coil during advancement. The techniques used depend on the experience and training of the anesthesiologist performing the block.

Several different local anesthetics and concentrations may be used for epidural anesthesia. Higher concentrations are used intra-

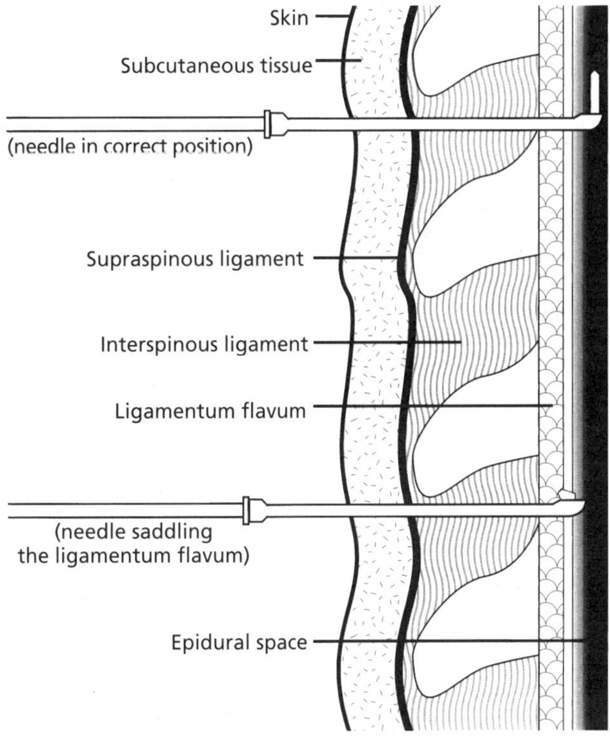

FIG 3-1.
Anatomy of the epidural space with proper needle placement *(above)* and the bevel of the epidural needle saddling the ligamentum flavum *(below).*

operatively to achieve surgical anesthesia, whereas more dilute solutions are used in postoperative infusions to provide analgesia and avoid motor blockade. After epidural administration, local anesthetics act on the spinal cord, spinal nerves, and the dorsal root ganglia to provide anesthesia and analgesia. Although dilute concentrations (0.125% or 0.1% bupivacaine) may provide selective sensory blockade, motor and sympathetic functions may also be affected. Although sympathetic blockade may cause hypotension in adults, its effects in children are generally well tolerated even without preoperative fluid administration. Epidural opioids provide selective analgesia without affecting sympathetic or motor function.

Epidural blocks are performed under sterile conditions after betadine or iodine preparation. In children the majority of blocks are placed after the induction of general anesthesia, and therefore the lateral decubitus position is generally used. Occasionally the sitting position may be possible in older, cooperative children. There are several commercially available kits with 18- or 20-gauge Tuohy or Weiss epidural needles. The traditional adult kits with a 17-gauge, 3.5-inch needle can be used even in 2 to 3 kg infants. Although several companies manufacture suitable catheters, the Arrow Theracath is preferred since it is radiopaque and its position can be easily confirmed by routine x-ray examination without the need to inject contrast material (Fig. 3-2).

The technique of catheter placement in children is somewhat different from that in adults. The distance from the skin to the epidural space is shorter in children; therefore a small skin nick is made at the site before placing the epidural needle. In this way, the pressure required to get the epidural needle through the skin does not cause the needle to advance too far and puncture the dura. The loss-of-resistance technique is most often used with either air or normal saline to identify passage of the needle into the epidural space. Recent evidence suggests that the saline loss-of-resistance technique may be preferred because of the risks of air embolism and patchy blockade if air is injected into the epidural space. It can be used with either continuous or intermittent pressure on the plunger. The latter technique is preferred. The depth of the epidural space in children is less than in adults, and entry into the epidural space is often more subtle in pediatric patients. Several different formulas based on age or body weight have been suggested to calculate the skin-to-epidural distance. Uemura and Yamashita have suggested that the skin-to-epidural distance can be

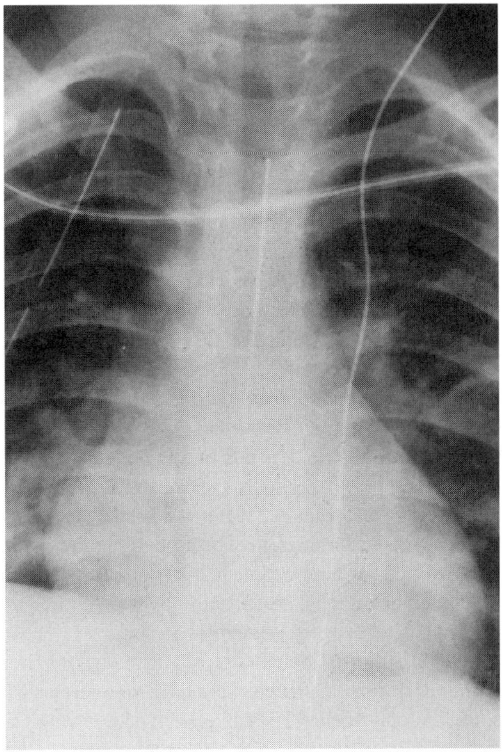

FIG 3-2.
X-ray film demonstrating the radiopaque appearance of the Arrow Theracath.

calculated by this formula: (weight + 10) $\times$ 0.8 = distance (mm) from the skin to the epidural space.[8] As a rule, such formulas have not been very helpful or accurate.

In children a characteristic "pop" may not be noted as the needle enters the epidural space. In infants the needle is frequently placed through the skin and ligaments directly into the epidural space during the initial insertion. Therefore when the syringe is attached, there is no resistance. At this point the injection of 1 to 2 ml of fluid is useful since it will frequently drip out of the needle, confirming that the needle is in the epidural space. Careful aspiration for blood or CSF and testing of the catheter must be performed before medications are administered. A 1 ml test dose is given through the needle after aspiration, the catheter is placed in the desired position, and aspiration is repeated. The catheter is then hung below the level of the heart to look for the return of CSF or blood through the catheter. The test dose (0.1 ml/kg of 0.25% bupivacaine with epinephrine 1:200,000 or 0.5 μg/kg epinephrine) is repeated through the catheter before the bolus dose is given. Even with a negative response to the test dose, the bolus dose should be administered in increments.

The initial bolus dose depends on the patient's size and the level of catheter placement. When the catheter is placed as an adjunct to general anesthesia, 0.25% or 0.5% bupivacaine is used. Although either concentration may be used to supplement general anesthesia, even 0.5% bupivacaine may not provide surgical anesthesia. Supplemental, inhalational anesthetic agents are generally needed. Suggested starting guidelines for bupivacaine (0.25%) dosing include an initial bolus dose of 0.3 ml/kg (maximum 12 ml) for thoracic epidural placement and 0.5 ml/kg (maximum 15 ml) for lumbar placement.[9] The catheter is secured out of the surgical field with benzoin and a bioocclusive dressing.

Lumbar and thoracic epidural catheters can be maintained and used for postoperative analgesia. The authors' current practice and dosing guidelines are outlined in Table 3-5. A continuous infusion of fentanyl and bupivacaine is preferred. The infusion is delivered by a PCA (patient-controlled analgesia) device and allows the patient to administer epidural bolus doses as needed. The bolus doses may be particularly valuable when used before coughing and breathing exercises or ambulation. If such devices are not available, standard IV pumps may be used to deliver the continuous infusion. These should be labeled carefully, and the

TABLE 3-5. Epidural Doses and Infusions of Bupivacaine

Single bolus with bupivacaine (0.25% with epinephrine)	
Caudal	
Midthoracic block	1.3 ml/kg
Low thoracic block	1.0 ml/kg
Lumbar/sacral	0.5-0.75 ml/kg (max 25 ml)
Lumbar	0.5-0.75 ml/kg (max 20 ml)
Thoracic	0.3-0.5 ml/kg (max 12 ml)
*Infusions with bupivacaine 0.1% with 2-5 μg/ml of fentanyl**	
Caudal†	
Neonates	0.2-0.25 ml/kg/hr
<30 kg:	0.4 ml/kg/hr
>40 kg:	15 ml/hr
Lumbar†	
Neonates	0.2-0.25 ml/kg/hr
<30 kg	0.3-0.4 ml/kg/hr
>40 kg	15 ml/hr
Bolus dose	1/3 of hourly rate every 1 hr p.r.n.
Thoracic‡	
<30 kg	0.3 ml/kg/hr
>40 kg	12 ml/hr
Bolus dose	1/3 of hourly rate every 1 hr p.r.n.

*Regardless of the site of administration, the dose of bupivacaine should not exceed 0.4 to 0.5 mg/kg/hr in patients older than 3 months of age and 0.2 to 0.25 mg/kg/hr in patients younger than 3 months of age. If opioids are added to the solution for neonates, the starting dose should be one third to one half that used in older patients.

†For lumbar/caudal administration, the starting fentanyl concentration is 2.5 μg/ml with an infusion rate of 0.4 ml/kg/hr resulting in a fentanyl dose of 1 μg/kg/hr. In patients greater than 40 kg the infusion is maintained at 15 ml/hr while the fentanyl concentration in the solutions is increased as needed to deliver 1.0 μg/kg/hr.

‡For thoracic infusions the starting fentanyl concentration is 2 μg/ml with an infusion rate of 0.3 ml/kg/hr resulting in a fentanyl dose of 0.6 μg/kg/hr. In patients greater than 40 kg the infusion is maintained at 12 ml/hr while the fentanyl concentration in the solution is increased as needed to deliver 0.6 μg/kg/hr.

infusion ports should be taped over so that inadvertent injections do not occur. Supplemental analgesia, if required, may be accomplished with IV opioids. Again, this may increase the likelihood of respiratory depression. Another option is to teach the nursing staff to administer epidural fentanyl.[10] Since regulations vary from state to state, this practice should first be reviewed by the state board of nursing.

The epidural catheters are usually left in place for 3 days, but in certain circumstances they may remain in place for up to 7 days. The catheter site should be inspected daily, and the dressing should be changed after 48 hours and after each subsequent 48-hour period.

Caudal Anesthesia

Perhaps the most popular regional technique now employed in pediatric patients is the caudal epidural block. A caudal epidural block is relatively easy to perform once the proper landmarks have been identified. It can be used in combination with general anesthesia, placed at the completion of the surgical procedure for post-operative analgesia, or used instead of general anesthesia for lower abdominal and extremity procedures. When placed at the onset of the surgical procedure, it can decrease the requirements for inhalational anesthetic agents, allowing quicker emergence and extubation. Caudal epidural blocks have been used for intraabdominal procedures, herniorrhaphies (both inguinal and umbilical), urologic procedures, and orthopedic procedures. The versatility and ease of performance have made this the most popular regional technique in children.

To perform a caudal epidural block, the patient is placed in either the prone position or the lateral decubitus position. If the patient is to be placed prone for the surgical procedure (e.g., bone marrow harvesting or club foot repair), the caudal block should be placed with the patient in this position, thereby avoiding the need to position the patient twice. The landmarks to identify are the coccyx and the sacral hiatus marked by the two sacral cornua (Figs. 3-3 and 3-4). Using the aseptic technique, the cornua are identified. Midway between the two cornu and 1 to 2 mm caudad, a 22-gauge, short-beveled needle is directed rostrally to contact bone at a 45- to 60-degree angle and then redirected, parallel with the skin, and advanced through the sacrococcygeal membrane with the characteristic "pop" (Figs. 3-5, 3-6, and 3-7). After care-

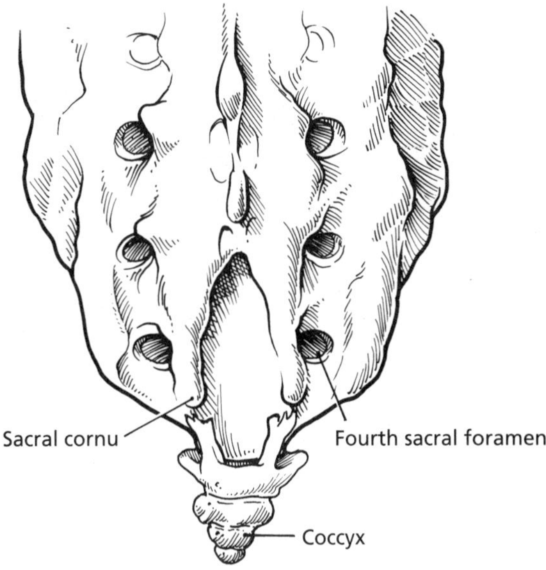

FIG 3-3.
Anatomy of the sacrum and coccyx with identification of the sacral cornu.

ful aspiration to test for blood or CSF, a test dose of local anesthetic with epinephrine is given. Sixty seconds is allowed to elapse to assess for either intravascular or intraosseous injection. The rest of the calculated dose is titrated in over 3 minutes while the vital signs are continuously monitored.

A caudal epidural block may be achieved using any available local anesthetics. The concentration and volume are determined by the dermatome level and density of blockade that is required. The volume of local anesthetic determines the height of the block and should be determined by the level of surgical incision (Table 3-5). Volumes of 1.2 to 1.3 ml/kg provide analgesia and

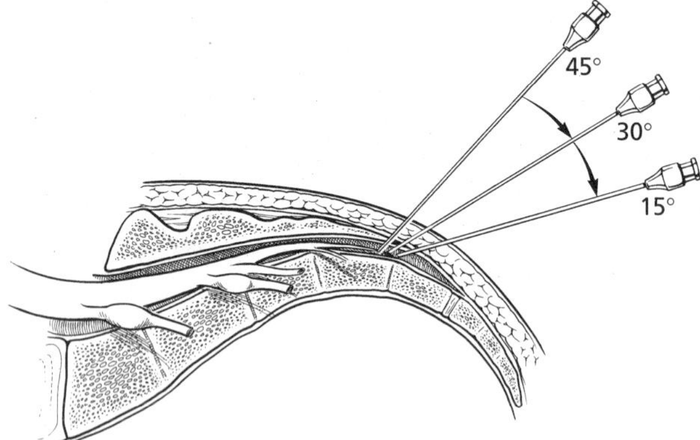

FIG 3-4.
Coronal view of the sacrum showing proper needle placement for performance of a caudal epidural block. The needle is advanced at a 45 degree angle to the skin until the bone is contacted. The angle is then decreased to 15 to 30 degrees, and the needle is advanced through the sacrococcygeal ligament into the epidural space.

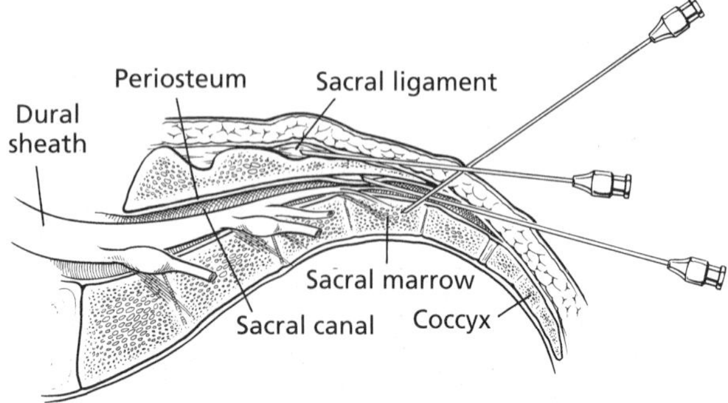

FIG 3-5.
Coronal view of the sacral anatomy demonstrating potential improper needle locations during a caudal epidural block.

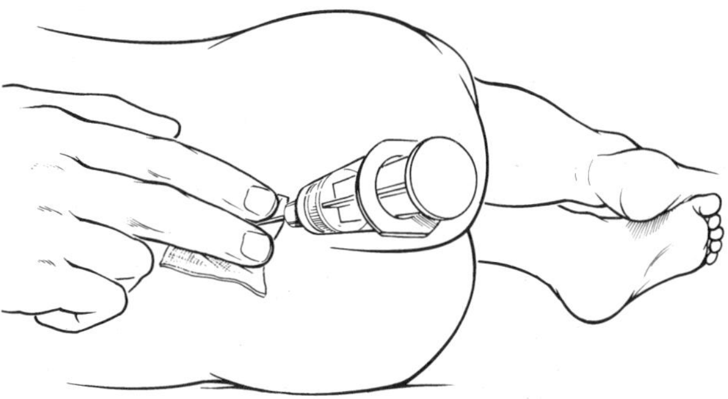

FIG 3-6.
No-touch technique for a caudal epidural block using an alcohol swab to palpate landmarks.

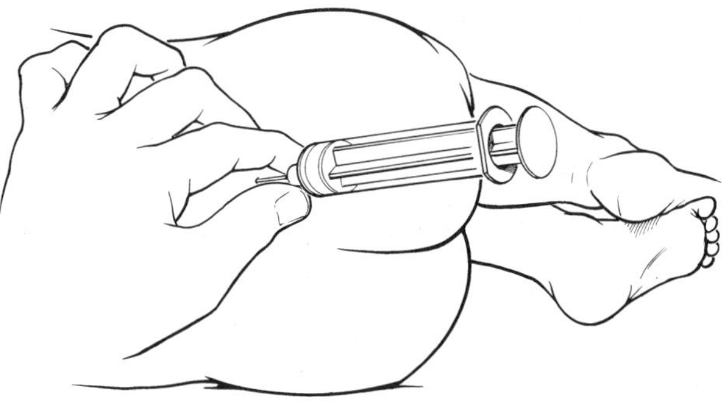

FIG 3-7.
Technique to secure the needle and syringe after entry into the caudal epidural space.

anesthesia to the $T_{4\text{-}6}$ dermatome and may be needed to provide analgesia after pyloromyotomy. Doses of 1 ml/kg provide postoperative analgesia for inguinal incisions, and 0.5 to 0.75 ml/kg are sufficient for lower extremity and urogenital procedures.

Although the majority of experience is with 0.25% bupivacaine, it has been suggested that equivalent analgesia can be achieved with 0.125% after routine herniorrhaphy. There remains limited experience with more dilute solutions for other surgical procedures. The current preference is to use 0.25% bupivacaine. The volume should be limited to a maximum of 1.3 ml/kg up to 20 ml to avoid toxic serum concentrations of bupivacaine.

Continuous catheter techniques are preferred to provide analgesia after major surgical procedures, such as laparotomy and thoracotomy. If these are not feasible because of logistical problems, the addition of preservative-free morphine to the local anesthetic used for caudal block may provide prolonged analgesia after major surgical procedures. The mixture of morphine (30 to 70 μg/kg) with butorphanol (20 to 30 μg/kg) is preferred to limit the side effects associated with morphine.

The caudal epidural block is generally performed as a "single-shot" technique for inguinal herniorrhaphies and outpatient urologic procedures. It can also be used as a continuous epidural technique either by placing a standard IV catheter into the caudal space or by using one of the commercially prepared kits for continuous caudal anesthesia.[11] These kits contain catheters (22- or 24-gauge) and needles (20-gauge) that are small enough to use in neonates. Although these techniques are used intraoperatively, leaving these catheters in for postoperative analgesia is not recommended. The primary problem with the use of continuous caudal catheters for postoperative analgesia is the difficulty in keeping the catheter site free from fecal contamination despite the use of tape and clean bioocclusive dressings.

Although the caudal block is most often used with general anesthesia, certain situations may arise in which a caudal block is used alone (see Chapter 8). Since there may be an increased risk of postoperative respiratory complications in this group of patients, there is a continued interest in the use of regional anesthesia (epidural or spinal) as a means of avoiding general anesthesia. Many of these procedures can be performed with either a single-shot caudal anesthetic or a spinal anesthetic (Box 3-7 and Table 3-6). Various dos-

BOX 3-7.
Spinal Versus Caudal Anesthesia

Spinal Anesthesia

Advantages
- Lower dose of local anesthetic (1 mg/kg vs. 3-4 mg/kg bupivacaine)
- Definitive endpoint (aspiration of cerebrospinal fluid)
- Rapid onset
- Dense sensory and motor block

Disadvantages
- Limited duration of action (60 minutes)
- Technical difficulties placing block
- Potential for high block with change in patient position

Caudal Anesthesia

Advantages
- High rate of success
- Longer duration (90 minutes)
- Limited change in level of block with change in patient position

Disadvantages
- High doses of local anesthetic needed
- Slow onset
- Incomplete motor block with 0.25% bupivacaine

TABLE 3-6. Local Anesthetics for Spinal Anesthesia*

Local Anesthetic	Dose	
Lidocaine (5%)	2-3 mg/kg	
Bupivacaine (0.75%)	0-5 kg:	0.5-1.0 mg/kg
	6-15 kg:	0.5-0.7 mg/kg
	15-30 kg:	0.4-0.5 mg/kg
	>30 kg:	0.4 mg/kg (max 15 mg)
Tetracaine (1.0%)	0.4-0.7 mg/kg	

*All local anesthetics are administered with an epinephrine wash in an equal volume of 10% dextrose in water.

ing regimens have been suggested for caudal anesthesia for patients with volumes ranging from 1 to 1.5 ml/kg and concentrations of bupivacaine from 0.2% to 0.375%.[12] The higher volumes are required to provide a T_2 block, and the higher concentrations are needed to provide surgical anesthesia. The combination of high volumes and high concentrations can result in toxicity. The authors use 1.3 ml/kg of 0.25% bupivacaine.

Although 0.25% bupivacaine provides sensory block, it may provide only partial motor block. Another problem with the technique is that the duration of surgical anesthesia is limited to 90 minutes. Since many surgical procedures last longer, repeated dosing is needed, which may result in toxic serum levels if bupivacaine is used. To avoid such problems, Henderson and colleagues at the Boston Children's Hospital suggest the use of chloroprocaine for continuous caudal anesthesia. After placement of a catheter in the caudal epidural space, an initial bolus dose of 1.5 to 2.0 ml/kg of 3% chloroprocaine was followed by a continuous infusion of 1.5 to 2.0 ml/kg/hr. Serum levels of chloroprocaine were well below the toxic level after 2 to 3 hours of surgical anesthesia. Additional advantages of 3% chloroprocaine include a rapid onset of action and dense motor blockade. This technique is used for procedures lasting as long as 3 hours on infants as small as 1.44 kg.[13]

Although caudal epidural kits with catheters are commercially available, standard IV catheters are preferred (22- or 24-gauge) for this technique. Catheter placement is accomplished with the infant in the lateral decubitus position after sterile betadine preparation and local infiltration with 0.2 to 0.3 ml of 1% lidocaine or 3% chloroprocaine. Another option is the application of EMLA (eutetic mixture of local anesthetics) cream over the site 1 to 2 hours before the procedure. The catheter is advanced through the sacrococcygeal membrane and a t-piece flushed with 3% chloroprocaine is attached to the catheter. The catheter and t-piece are secured in place with a transparent bioocclusive dressing. The initial dose includes up to 2 ml/kg of 3% chloroprocaine (administered in fractionated doses of 0.5 ml/kg at 3 minute intervals) followed by a continuous infusion of 3% chloroprocaine. The infusion rate is set in ml/kg/hr to equal the initial bolus dose (ml/kg). Subsequent bolus doses of 0.3 ml/kg are administered if the infant appears to be in pain or the sensory level regresses to T_6.

The continuous caudal technique may also be combined with general anesthesia. The advantage of this technique is that it limits the need for inhalational anesthetic agents and avoids the use of opioids that may necessitate postoperative mechanical ventilation. The authors have had experience with this technique in several neonates ranging in age from 1 to 28 days and in weight from 2.2 to 4.9 kg.[14] After anesthetic induction and endotracheal intubation, the caudal catheter was placed using the previously described technique. The initial dose of 3% chloroprocaine included either 1.0 or 1.5 ml/kg administered in increments of 0.5 ml/kg in 3 minute increments. After the initial bolus dose, an infusion was started at a rate equivalent to the initial bolus dose (1.0 or 1.5 ml/kg/hr). Maintenance anesthesia consisted of either 0.2% isoflurane (expired concentration) in 40% oxygen and air or 70% nitrous oxide in oxygen. If the level of surgical anesthesia was judged inadequate, as demonstrated by an increase in heart rate or blood pressure in response to surgical stimulation, an additional bolus dose of 3% chloroprocaine (0.5 ml/kg) was administered, and the infusion was increased by 0.5 ml/kg/hr. The two patients who initially received a bolus dose of 1.0 ml/kg, followed by an infusion of 1.0 ml/kg/hr, required an additional bolus dose, followed by an increase in the infusion to 1.5 ml/kg/hr. No infant required more than 0.2% isoflurane or 70% nitrous oxide in oxygen. Within 10 minutes of the completion of the surgical procedure, 16 of the 18 infants were extubated in the operating room.

Chloroprocaine may also be an acceptable alternative outside of the neonatal population. When surgical anesthesia is required from the epidural block 3% chloroprocaine has been used. This may be the case when epidural anesthesia is used instead of general anesthesia. In such cases, the doses of bupivacaine may be limited because of the risk of toxicity. Larger doses of chloroprocaine (volume and concentration) can be used because of its rapid metabolism by serum cholinesterases. Outside of the neonatal and infant age range, 0.5 ml/kg via a lumbar epidural catheter should be followed by a continuous infusion of 0.5 ml/kg/hr. If needed, the bolus may be repeated, and the infusion may be increased to 1.0 ml/kg/hr.

Previously, some practitioners were hesitant to use chloroprocaine because of reported cases of neurotoxicity and arachnoiditis. These were thought to be the result of the low pH and the preservative sodium metabisulfite that were present in the original formulation. The currently available preparation contains ethylenediaminetetraacetic acid (EDTA) as the preservative and, although not recommended for intrathecal use, it has not been reported to cause neurotoxicity. The advantages and disadvantages of chloroprocaine are listed in Box 3-8.

Adverse Effects of Epidural Anesthesia

Despite a long safety record, adverse effects may occur with epidural anesthesia.[15] They can be grouped into two main categories: those related to catheter placement and those related to medication administration (Box 3-9). Placement problems include bleeding, dural puncture, infection, and abscess formation. Since the epidural space is vascular with numerous epidural veins, the needle or catheter can disrupt a blood vessel leading to epidural hematoma formation. The hematoma can cause a compromise of spinal cord perfusion and ultimately lead to paralysis. Because of the risks of bleeding, these techniques are contraindicated in patients with an ongoing coagulopathy (platelet count less than 100,000/mm^3 or prothrombin time (PT) or partial thromboplastin time (PTT) greater than 1.5 control) or qualitative bleeding dysfunction (e.g., hemophilia or von Willebrand's disease). Ongoing evaluation of neurologic function and patient status is performed to quickly identify patients with progressive neurologic dysfunction or back pain, which are the early signs of epidural hematoma formation.

The adverse sequelae of drug administration are related to either the local anesthetics or the neuraxial opioids. (The toxicity of local anesthetics has been previously discussed.) The most prob-

BOX 3-8.
Advantages and Disadvantages of Chloroprocaine

Advantages

Rapid onset
Dense sensory and motor block
Provides surgical anesthesia
Rapid metabolism limits risk of toxicity
Rapid metabolism even in neonates
Less cardiac toxicity than bupivacaine

Disadvantages

Rapid onset of tachyphylaxis
Back pain related to EDTA*
May limit efficacy of epidural opioids (morphine)

*The back pain after chloroprocaine use is thought to be the result of tetany in the paraspinus muscles related to calcium binding by the preservative EDTA.
EDTA, ethylenediaminetetraacetic acid.

lematic complications related to local anesthetics are inadvertent intrathecal injection and intravascular injection. An intrathecal injection can cause a total spinal blockade with the patient requiring airway management and cardiovascular support until the effects of the local anesthetic have dissipated. An intravascular injection can cause cardiovascular and CNS toxicity requiring airway and cardiovascular support. Adverse effects related to neuraxial opioids include respiratory depression (early and delayed), pruritus, nausea, vomiting, and urinary retention.

Fortunately, complications are uncommon and the benefits of superior, postoperative analgesia for children undergoing major surgical procedures are numerous. To maintain the highest level of safety, the practitioner should be meticulous in the performance of the regional technique and in choosing which drugs are administered. Careful observation for subtle changes in cardiorespiratory parameters may herald problems early on so that appropriate measures may be taken before potential complications fully manifest.

BOX 3-9.
Adverse Effects of Epidural Anesthesia

Catheter placement
- Local infection or epidural abscess
- Epidural hematoma
- Dural puncture

Local anesthetic effects
- Motor blockade
- Sympathetic blockade
- Horner's syndrome
- Urinary retention
- Intrathecal injection (total spinal)
- Systemic toxicity (CNS or cardiovascular toxicity)*

Opioid effects
- Respiratory depression (early and late)
- Pruritus
- Nausea or vomiting
- Urinary retention
- Possible reactivation of herpes simplex infection

Failed block or inadequate analgesia

*Systemic toxicity can result from inadvertent intravascular or intraosseous injection or vascular uptake of local anesthetic from the epidural space. This may be seen with bolus dosing or use of excessive doses by continuous infusion.
CNS, Central nervous system.

SPINAL ANESTHESIA

Spinal anesthetic techniques are useful for infants and children undergoing a surgical procedure where general anesthesia with endotracheal intubation is best avoided (i.e., neonates with severe bronchopulmonary dysplasia or children with severe cystic fibrosis). Specialized equipment, such as 1.5-inch, 24- and 22-gauge spinal needles are now available for neonates and infants.

Spinal anesthesia is performed under the aseptic technique with the child either sitting or in the lateral decubitus position. The former position is better tolerated by the infant and also provides a greater chance of success. Application of a small amount of EMLA cream over the lumbar spine 1 hour before the procedure may make needle insertion less painful in the infant or child who has received no sedative or systemic analgesic. Placement of IV access before performing the block is recommended. Although cardiorespiratory effects are uncommon after spinal block in infants, total spinal blockade can occur and may be particularly dangerous in a patient without IV access.

Once the block has been performed, the patient must be carefully placed on the operating room table. Tape is then placed across the legs to prevent them from being lifted up, which may result in total spinal block. This has occurred when the legs were inadvertently lifted to place the electrocautery pad. Placing the blood pressure cuff on the lower extremity is also recommended since the periodic pressure on the upper extremity with cuff inflation may be bothersome to the conscious infant.

A number of different local anesthetics and doses have been suggested for spinal anesthesia (Table 3-6). The type of local anesthetic is determined by the desired duration of anesthesia. Surgical anesthesia lasts 30 to 60 minutes with lidocaine and 60 to 90 minutes with tetracaine or bupivacaine.[16] Except for the briefest of procedures (less than 30 minutes), either tetracaine or bupivacaine is used. For infants and neonates, 1% tetracaine or 0.75% bupivacaine in a dose of 0.7 to 1 mg/kg with an epinephrine wash provides effective spinal anesthesia. The epinephrine wash is prepared by drawing epinephrine (1 mg/ml) into a tuberculin syringe and then squirting it out. A small amount of epinephrine is left in the syringe. The local anesthetic is then drawn up and diluted with an equal volume of 10% dextrose in water ($D_{10}W$). No parenteral sedation is administered to these infants since the addition of such medications may increase the risks of postoperative respiratory complications.

Even with a successful block, the anesthesiologist is still left with an awake neonate who must be entertained for 1 to 2 hours. Many infants sleep during the procedure or calm down when offered a pacifier dipped in $D_{10}W$ or Pedialyte.

In addition to local anesthetics, opioids may be administered into the intrathecal space for postoperative analgesia (Box 3-6,

Table 3-3). Although not recommended for routine procedures such as herniorrhaphy, it is a more widely used technique for thoracic, cardiac, craniofacial, and major intraabdominal procedures. For most cases, intrathecal morphine (5 to 10 μg/kg) is administered and provides 18 to 24 hours of postoperative analgesia. These patients require close postoperative monitoring of respiratory function because of the risk of delayed respiratory depression. Respiratory depression may be treated with a low-dose naloxone infusion, which generally does not interfere with the analgesic effects of the opioid.

Spinal anesthesia may also be used in combination with general anesthesia. This technique may be useful in neonates undergoing major intraabdominal procedures such as gastroschisis repair. The combination of spinal anesthesia with general anesthesia may be used to limit the intraoperative requirements for inhalational agents, to avoid the use of parenteral opioids, to provide preemptive analgesia, or to blunt surgical stress response. Spinal anesthesia, using the above outlined doses, is performed after the induction of general anesthesia and endotracheal intubation. As with the combination of general anesthesia and caudal anesthesia, the requirements for inhalational agents are usually minimal (0.2% isoflurane). Preservative-free morphine may be added to the local anesthetic to provide postoperative analgesia.

Other authors suggest that spinal anesthesia may be used as the sole technique for gastroschisis repair, thereby avoiding the need for general anesthesia.[17] However, there are significant potential risks to not having a secured airway in neonates undergoing intraabdominal procedures.

Summary

The interest and applications of spinal and epidural anesthesia continue to increase in children. These techniques may be used to provide postoperative analgesia, as an alternative to general anesthesia, or as an adjunct to general anesthesia. With proper preparation of the physician and nursing staff, these techniques may be used safely and effectively to improve the quality of analgesia provided for patients.

For major surgical procedures, an epidural catheter can be placed near the level of surgery and a combination of bupivacaine and fentanyl can be delivered with a PCA device for postoperative analgesia. When this is not possible, a combination of caudal epidural morphine and butorphanol may provide prolonged analgesia without the need for a catheter technique. Another option is the intraoperative administration of intrathecal morphine. The latter may be used even for head, neck, or craniofacial surgery.

REFERENCES

1. Dalens B: Regional anesthesia in children, *Anesth Analg* 68:654, 1989.
2. Broadman LM: Pediatric regional anesthesia, *Clin Anesth Updates* 3:1, 1992.
3. McCloskey JJ, Haun SE, Deshpande JK: Bupivacaine toxicity secondary to continuous caudal epidural infusion in children, *Anesth Analg* 75:287, 1992.
4. Agarwal R, Gutlove DP, Lockhart CH: Seizures occurring in pediatric patients receiving continuous infusion of bupivacaine, *Anesth Analg* 75:284, 1992.
5. Tobias JD, Deshpande JK, Wetzel R et al: Postoperative analgesia: use of intrathecal morphine in children, *Clin Pediatr* 29:44, 1990.
6. Lawhon CD, Brown RE: Epidural morphine with butorphanol in pediatric patients, *J Clin Anesth* 6:91, 1994.
7. Yaster M, Maxwell LG: Pediatric regional anesthesia, *Anesthesiology* 70:324, 1989.
8. Uemura A, Yamashita M: A formula for determining the distance from the skin to the lumbar epidural space in infants and children, *Paediatric Anaesthesia* 2:305, 1992.
9. Tobias JD, Lowe S, O'Dell N et al: Thoracic epidural anaesthesia in infants and children, *Can J Anaesth* 40:879, 1993.

10. Tobias JD, Oakes L, Austin BA: Pediatric analgesia with epidural fentanyl citrate administered by nursing staff, *South Med J* 85:384, 1992.
11. Tobias JD, Lowe S, O'Dell N et al: Continuous regional anesthesia in infants, *Can J Anaesth* 40:1065, 1993.
12. Gunter JB, Watcha MF, Forestner JE et al: Caudal epidural anesthesia in conscious premature and high risk infants, *J Ped Surg* 26:9, 1991.
13. Tobias JD, Hersey S: Continuous caudal anaesthesia during inguinal herniorrhaphy in an awake, 1440 g infant, *Paediatric Anaesthesia* 4:187, 1994.
14. Tobias JD, Rasmussen GE, Holcomb GW III et al: Continuous caudal anesthesia with chloroprocaine as an adjunct to general anesthesia in neonates, *Can J Anaesth* (submitted).
15. Wood CE, Goresky GV, Klassen KA et al: Complication of continuous epidural infusions for postoperative analgesia in children, *Can J Anaesth* 41:613, 1994.
16. Rice LJ, DeMars PD, Whalen TV et al: Duration of spinal anesthesia in infants less than one year of age, *Reg Anesth* 19:325, 1994.
17. Vane DW, Abajian JC, Hong AR: Spinal anesthesia for primary repair of gastroschisis: a new and safe technique for selected patients, *J Ped Surg* 29:1234, 1994.

4

REGIONAL NERVE BLOCKS AND INTERPLEURAL ANALGESIA

Joseph D. Tobias

INTERPLEURAL ANALGESIA
- Technique
- Adverse effects

INTERCOSTAL BLOCKADE
- Technique
- Adverse effects

LOWER EXTREMITY BLOCKADE
- Lumbar and sacral plexus
- Femoral nerve block
- Lateral femoral cutaneous nerve
- Obturator nerve/lumbar plexus blockade
- Sciatic nerve block

UPPER EXTREMITY BLOCKADE
- Brachial plexus
- Interscalene block
- Axillary block

BIER BLOCK

PERIPHERAL NERVE BLOCK
- Ilioinguinal and iliohypogastric blocks
- Digital blocks
- Ankle block
- Wrist block

The anatomic distribution of the peripheral nervous system lends itself to neural blockade at various points from the periphery until entry into the spinal cord. These techniques may be used to provide postoperative analgesia, intraoperative anesthesia instead of general anesthesia, or analgesia during various procedures outside of the operating room, such as fracture reduction in the emergency room. Additionally, these techniques may be used as therapeutic modalities in the treatment of vascular compromise of various etiologies.[1] In these instances, the associated sympathetic blockade that is achieved with regional anesthesia may improve regional blood flow (Table 4-1). The applicability of such techniques for correcting vascular compromise is discussed later in this chapter.

Although regional anesthesia may provide effective analgesia in children, careful consideration must be given to the volume and concentration of the local anesthetic used (Table 4-2). Furthermore, the technique significantly impacts on the resultant serum concentration since some areas are more vascular, allowing for more rapid uptake of the local anesthetic (Table 4-3). Blood levels

TABLE 4-1. Therapeutic Uses of Regional Blockade

Ref No.	Type of Regional Blockade	Etiology of Ischemia
16	Interpleural anesthesia	Thromboembolic/Raynaud's disease
28	Caudal epidural anesthesia	Meningococcemia
29	Lumbar epidural anesthesia	Meningococcemia
30	Stellate ganglion block	Vascular malformation/status post embolization
31	Axillary block	Surgical repair of radial club hands
32	Caudal epidural/axillary block	Kawasaki's disease
33	Stellate ganglion block	Pneumococcal sepsis
34	Lumbar sympathetic block	Vascular cannulae

TABLE 4-2. Dosing Guidelines for Local Anesthetic Agents

Local Anesthetic	Dose*
Amide Group	
Lidocaine	5-7 mg/kg
Mepivacaine	4-7 mg/kg
Bupivacaine	2.5-3.5 mg/kg
Ester Group	
Chloroprocaine	8-10 mg/kg
Procaine	7-8.5 mg/kg
Tetracaine	1.5 mg/kg
Cocaine (topical)	2 mg/kg

*The first number represents the dose when epinephrine is not added to the solution, whereas the second number represents the dose with the addition of epinephrine (1:200,000 or 5 μg/ml).

TABLE 4-3. Local Anesthetic Absorption from Regional Blockade

Systemic Absorption	Type of Blockade
Most	Interpleural
	Intercostal
	Caudal epidural
	Lumbar, thoracic epidural
	Brachial plexus
	Sciatic/femoral
	Distal peripheral nerve
Least	Subcutaneous

are greatest with interpleural and intercostal blockade and least with subcutaneous or peripheral nerve blockade. Excessive dosing regimens can result in local anesthetic toxicity and its resultant cardiovascular or central nervous system (CNS) toxicity. With such cautions in mind and careful monitoring of patients, these techniques have wide applicability in the pediatric population. This chapter discusses interpleural analgesia, several types of peripheral nerve blockade (intercostal, brachial plexus, femoral, digital, ankle, and wrist), and the Bier block.

INTERPLEURAL ANALGESIA

Technique

Interpleural analgesia (IPA) involves the placement of a catheter, either percutaneously after upper abdominal procedures or under direct vision during thoracic procedures, in the paravertebral space between the visceral and parietal pleurae[2] (Figs. 4-1

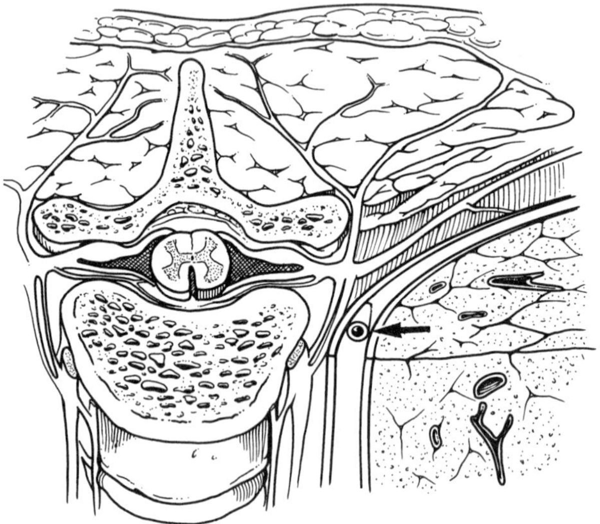

FIG 4-1.

Transverse section through the intervertebral body with *arrow* showing optimal placement of an interpleural catheter in the paravertebral space. Analgesia is obtained by the diffusion of a local anesthetic through the parietal pleura to the intercostal nerve, spinal root, and sympathetic chain.

and 4-2). Analgesia is obtained by the administration of local anesthetics (bolus or continuous infusion) leading to multiple, ipsilateral, intercostal nerve blocks as the local anesthetic diffuses from the pleural space through the parietal pleura.[3] Local anesthetic effects on afferents in the greater and lesser splanchnic, phrenic, and vagus nerves may also provide additional visceral analgesia after upper abdominal procedures.

Although there is considerable experience with this technique in adults, its use in children has been limited.[4,5] Reports in the pediatric population are restricted to patients undergoing thoracotomy. There are no reports of percutaneous placement of an IPA catheter for upper abdominal procedures. Most importantly, in both adults and children, there remains a debate over the analgesic efficacy of this technique after thoracotomy. Although IPA may be effective, it

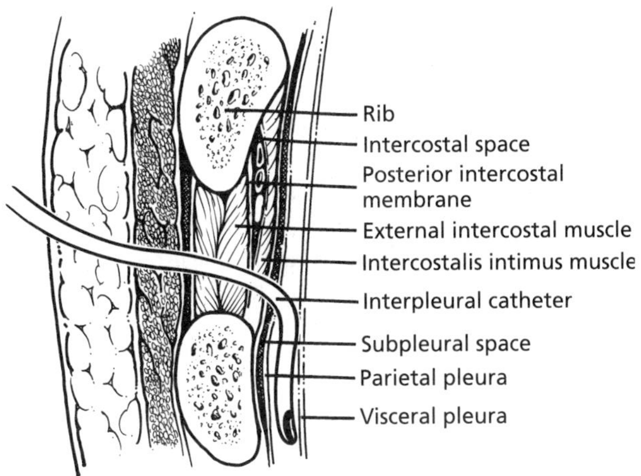

FIG 4-2.

Cross section of an intercostal space showing placement of an interpleural catheter over the top border of a rib, into the interpleural space, with the tip lying between the parietal and visceral pleurae.

is less effective than thoracic epidural analgesia after thoracotomy.[6] Interpleural analgesia decreases the requirements for intravenous (IV) opioids after thoracotomy when compared with patients who receive no regional anesthetic; however, when compared with epidural analgesia, interpleural analgesia is less effective.[6] The true efficacy of IPA has also been questioned by adult studies, suggesting that although it may be effective after upper abdominal procedures, such as cholecystectomy, it has limited utility after thoracotomy. One problem with many of the studies evaluating IPA is that the technique of catheter placement has varied.

A standard epidural catheter is usually used, although some manufacturers do make a specialized catheter for IPA. The Arrow Theracath epidural catheter offers the advantage of being radiopaque; therefore, its position can be verified by chest x-ray examination. For intraoperative placement, the catheter is inserted by the surgeon 1 or 2 interspaces below the surgical incision, 4 to 8 centimeters from the posterior midline. Placing the catheter in the posterior aspect of the thoracic cavity with the tip 2 to 4 centimeters above and posterior to the incision may provide optimal analgesia. A loose suture placed around the catheter tip may help keep it in place. When possible, anterior placement of the chest tube delays drainage of the local anesthetic out of the thoracic cavity. Clamping the chest tube for an hour after a bolus dose may produce better analgesia. Another factor affecting analgesia is patient positioning. Bolus dosing is best accomplished with the patient supine or the operative side up, thereby allowing the local anesthetic to pool in the paravertebral space.

Considerations for the use of IPA include the choice of a local anesthetic, its concentration, and the mode of administration (continuous versus bolus dosing). Although many adult studies have administered initial doses of up to 40 ml of 0.5% bupivacaine, the use of such concentrated solutions is not recommended in children. Stromskag and colleagues demonstrated no difference in analgesic efficacy when comparing 0.5%, 0.375%, and 0.25% bupivacaine.[7] Starting with an initial bolus dose of 1 ml/kg of 0.25% bupivacaine with epinephrine (maximum dose of 30 ml) is recommended. This can be followed by a continuous infusion of 0.125 ml/kg/hr of 0.25% bupivacaine (0.31 mg/kg/hr bupivacaine). Although some authors advocate bolus doses if the analgesia is inadequate, IV opioids should be used as needed to supplement analgesia, thereby limiting the risk of local anesthetic toxicity (Table 4-4).

Adverse Effects

Complications during placement of the interpleural catheter include pneumothorax, bleeding, and infection. Bleeding is readily controlled when these catheters are placed under direct vision, and to date no significant episodes of hemorrhage or infection related to IPA have been reported. In fact, this technique is useful in patients with platelet dysfunction or bleeding dyscrasias in whom epidural anesthesia is contraindicated.[8] Pneumothorax is primarily a concern when the catheter is placed for analgesia after an upper abdominal procedure. The minimal amount of air that is entrained is rarely of clinical consequence.

The major toxicity related to IPA results from the systemic absorption of a local anesthetic by the rich pleural vasculature. Toxic manifestations of local anesthetics include both CNS effects (seizures) and cardiovascular manifestations (hypotension and arrhythmias). Toxic levels have been reported in both adults and children during IPA[4] with plasma bupivacaine levels greater than 2 μg/ml in 11 of 14 children and greater than 4.0 μg/ml in 5 of 14 children. Bupivacaine infusion rates in these patients varied from 1.25 to 2.5 mg/kg/hr. No clinical evidence of cardiovascular or CNS toxicity was noted in either of these two studies. Although these high infusion rates were tolerated in this small group of patients, current recommendations advise against bupivacaine infusion rates greater than 0.4 to 0.5 mg/kg/hr.[9] These recommendations should be closely followed since seizures have been reported during IPA in both adults and children.[10] There have also been an inordinate number of complications, such as seizures, in patients receiving IPA when compared with other regional anesthetic techniques.[9] The risk of local anesthetic toxicity may be increased by

TABLE 4-4. Suggested Starting Guidelines for Dosing of Regional Blocks

Block	Bolus Dose	Continuous Infusion	Comments
Interpleural	1 ml/kg of 0.25% bupivacaine (maximum 30 ml)	0.125 ml/kg/hr of 0.25% bupivacaine	Supplement analgesia with intravenous opioids to limit risk of local anesthetic toxicity.
Intercostal	0.1 to 0.15 ml/kg/interspace of 0.25% bupivacaine (maximum of 3 ml/interspace)		Inject at the involved interspace in addition to 2 interspaces above and 2 below.
Femoral	0.5 to 0.7 ml/kg of 0.25% bupivacaine (maximum 25 ml)	0.15 ml/kg/hr of 0.2% bupivacaine 0.3 ml/kg/hr of 0.125% bupivacaine	For denser motor block, consider using 0.5 ml/kg of 3% chloroprocaine + 0.5 ml/kg of 0.5% bupivacaine (maximum volume of 20 ml of each).
Lateral femoral cutaneous	0.1 to 0.2 ml/kg of 0.25% bupivacaine (maximum 5 ml)		
Fascia iliaca block 3-in-1 block	1 ml/kg of 0.25% bupivacaine (maximum 40 ml)		
Psoas compartment	0.5 ml/kg of 0.5% bupivacaine 0.7 ml/kg of 0.375% (maximum 30 ml)		May also result in sacral plexus block anesthesia of entire leg.

Sciatic nerve	0.5 ml/kg of 0.25% bupivacaine		
Interscalene axillary	0.75 ml/kg of 0.25% bupivacaine (maximum 30 ml)	Same as for continuous femoral	For denser motor block, consider a combination of 3% chloroprocaine and 0.5% bupivacaine as for femoral block.
Bier block	Upper extremity: 0.6 ml/kg Lower extremity: 1 ml/kg (0.25% or 0.5% lidocaine or prilocaine)		Addition of fentanyl (1 μg/kg) to the solution may improve the quality of the block. The addition of pancuronium (0.01 mg/kg) may increase motor block.
Ilioinguinal iliohypogastric	0.5 to 1.0 ml/year of age of 0.25% bupivacaine (maximum 5 to 7 ml)		
Ankle or wrist	0.1 to 0.15 ml/kg of 0.25% bupivacaine for each nerve (maximum 5 ml for ankle and 3 ml for wrist)		No vasoconstrictor (epinephrine) is added to the solution for these blocks.
Digital	0.2 to 0.3 ml/year of age for each side of the digit (maximum 3 ml)		No vasoconstrictor (epinephrine) is added to the solution for these blocks.

inflammatory processes of the pleura, which increase its vascularity and absorptive capabilities. Because of the concerns of local anesthetic toxicity and the superior analgesia with thoracic epidural anesthesia, the latter technique is preferred after major thoracic procedures in children.

The disadvantages of IPA are listed in Box 4-1. Analgesia is unilateral; therefore, other techniques are needed for procedures that involve or cross the midline. IPA provides analgesia, but not anesthesia. Therefore, it cannot be used instead of general anesthesia but only as a postoperative analgesic technique. As discussed previously, several factors may interfere with analgesia. Despite these problems, IPA may be useful in situations that contraindicate epidural anesthesia.

In addition to its use for postoperative analgesia, IPA has been suggested as a means of dealing with pain of other etiologies (Box 4-2). In the adult population it has been used to treat pain related to pancreatitis,[11] cancer,[12] and postherpetic neuralgia.[13] One report details the effective, protracted (2 months) use of this technique to treat chronic, cancer-related pain.[14] The sympathetic blockade related to IPA has been used as a therapeutic modality to treat upper extremity, reflex-sympathetic dystrophy,[15] or ischemia.[16]

BOX 4-1.
Disadvantages of Interpleural Analgesia

Provides only unilateral analgesia, not effective for midline procedures
Provides analgesia and not anesthesia
Is of questionable efficacy after thoracotomy
Needs large doses of local anesthetics
The analgesia is affected by:
- Patient position
- Catheter position
- Drainage of local anesthetic by chest tube
- Binding of local anesthetic to blood and protein in pleural space
- Pleural disease and fibrotic changes

BOX 4-2.
Additional Uses of Interpleural Analgesia

Postherpetic neuralgia[13]
Cancer-related pain[12,14]
Chronic pancreatitis[11]
Upper extremity reflex sympathetic dystrophy[15]
Upper extremity ischemia[16]

INTERCOSTAL BLOCKADE

Another alternative for providing analgesia after thoracic and upper abdominal analgesia is intercostal nerve blockade. Intercostal blocks may be used to provide postoperative analgesia after thoracotomy and upper abdominal procedures, such as cholecystectomy, or to decrease the discomfort and respiratory compromise associated with rib fractures of various etiologies. When compared with parenteral opioids, intercostal blocks have been shown to more effectively alleviate postoperative pain, to decrease postoperative opioid requirements, and to improve pulmonary function and arterial blood gases.[17,18] Although intercostal blocks provide effective dermal analgesia for thoracic and upper abdominal dermatomes, they do not provide effective analgesia for intraperitoneal procedures, since nociception from this area is also transmitted via the celiac plexus. Intercostal blocks may be performed either percutaneously or intraoperatively under direct vision and offer a means of providing postoperative analgesia when central blockade (spinal or epidural anesthesia) is contraindicated.

Technique

The intercostal nerves arise from the first 11 thoracic spinal nerves. Before entering the intercostal space, gray and white rami communicantes branch off and enter the adjoining sympathetic ganglia forming the thoracic sympathetic chain. Another branch, the posterior cutaneous branch, travels posteriorly and innervates the paraspinus muscles. Since intercostal blocks are performed more anteriorly, this latter branch, which may be involved in nociception after thoracotomy, is not blocked. However, it is effectively blocked by epidural and interpleural analgesia. The anterior ramus of the second thoracic nerve has branches that contribute to the brachial plexus (posterior branch), innervation of the arm (intercostobrachial nerve), and the second intercostal nerve. The anterior ramus of the twelfth thoracic spinal nerve travels below the last rib and is not thought of as an intercostal nerve, but is referred to as the subcostal nerve.

The intercostal nerves run in a groove below the corresponding rib (i.e., the sixth intercostal nerve runs underneath the sixth rib). The nerves are contained posteriorly between the posterior intercostal membrane and the pleura until they reach the angle of the ribs. At this point they are held between the internal intercostal (oblique) muscle and the posterior intercostal membrane/innermost intercostal muscle. The intercostal space under each rib contains, from outside to inside, the intercostal vein, artery, and nerve. The anterior border is formed, from outside to inside, by the external intercostal (oblique) muscle and the internal intercostal muscle, and the posterior border is formed by the posterior intercostal membrane and the innermost intercostal muscle (Fig. 4-3).

The intercostal space can be approached anywhere along the lower border of the rib. The lateral decubitus or the sitting position is preferred in children (Figs. 4-4 and 4-5). The lateral decubitus position is used when the blocks are performed after thoracotomy, whereas the sitting position may be easier for the awake or awake-sedated patient. In the lateral decubitus position, the arm is elevated onto a pillow (Fig. 4-4) so that the midaxillary and posterior axillary lines are uncovered. Regardless of the patient's position, the technique remains similar. Although several approaches are possible, the posterior axillary line approach is the easiest technique to learn. After sterile preparation of the area, local anesthesia is applied if the patient is awake. A 22- or 25-gauge needle (for patients less than 3 years of age) is inserted and advanced to contact the lower border of the rib. Once contact is made, the needle is withdrawn and advanced slightly inferiorly and cephalad until the external and internal oblique muscles are penetrated. At this

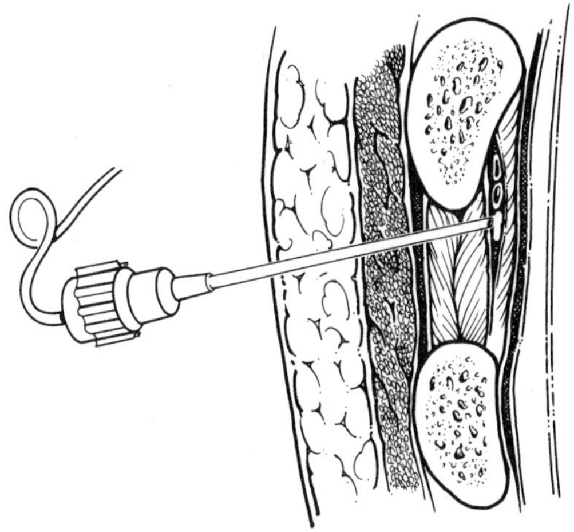

FIG 4-3.
Cross section of an intercostal space showing needle placement for an intercostal block. The needle is walked off the inferior edge of the rib into the intercostal space.

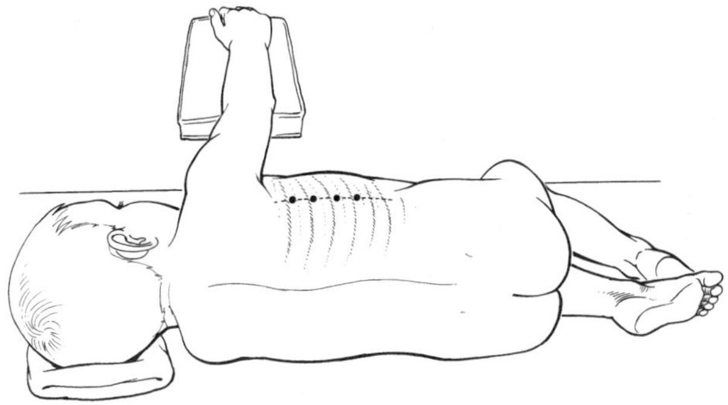

FIG 4-4.
Patient positioning in the lateral decubitus position for placement of intercostal blocks with needle entry at the posterior axillary line.

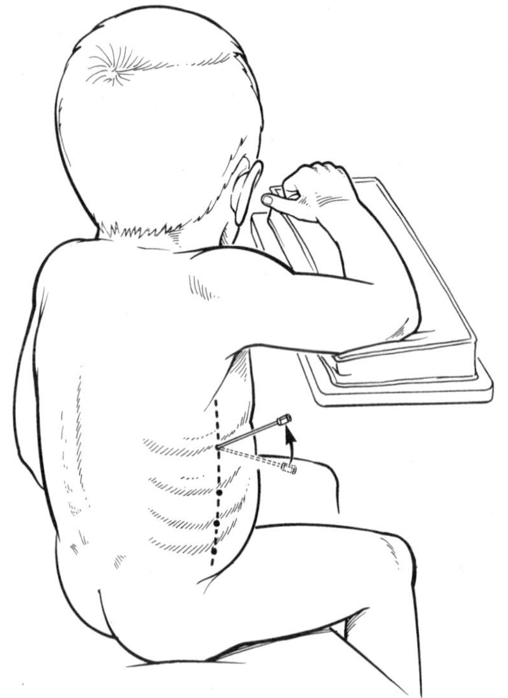

FIG 4-5.
Patient positioning for placement of intercostal blocks in a sitting position with needle entry at the posterior axillary line. The needle is inserted perpendicular to the skin and walked off the inferior border of the rib.

point a loss of resistance is felt. The depth at which the loss of resistance is felt is dependent on the age and weight of the patient.

After needle placement and negative aspiration for blood, the local anesthetic agent is injected. The intercostal space is vascular and, as a result, plasma concentrations of the local anesthetic are higher after intercostal block than other peripheral nerve blocks (Table 4-2). The amount of bupivacaine should be limited to 2 to 2.5 mg/kg. Although other local anesthetic agents may be used, bupivacaine offers the advantage of a duration of action of up to 12 hours.[19] Doses of 0.1 to 0.15 ml/kg/interspace up to a maximum of 3 ml provides effective analgesia (Table 4-4). To achieve the best response, injections are recommended at the involved interspace, two interspaces above, and two below.

Adverse Effects

As with any regional anesthetic technique, adverse effects may occur with intercostal blocks. Aside from the previously mentioned problems with local anesthetic toxicity, other adverse effects include pneumothorax, puncture of intercostal vessels, and spread of the block to the epidural or spinal space. Pneumothorax may occur when the needle traverses the posterior aspect of the intercostal space and punctures the dura. Careful monitoring of the patient during and after the block is required to identify and treat this complication. Although most adult series report an incidence of pneumothorax of less than 0.1%, a postprocedure chest x-ray examination is recommended in children. The same mechanism can result in a puncture of the peritoneum or viscera when the lower interspaces are approached.

Excessive spread of the local anesthetic from the intercostal space to the epidural, subdural, or spinal space may occur. This is more likely when the blocks are performed closer to the midline (posterior) approach and may represent injection into a dural sleeve that covers the spinal root as it exits the vertebral column. Excessive spreading of the block may lead to respiratory failure or hemodynamic instability related to sympathetic blockade.

The major disadvantage of intercostal blocks is that even with long acting agents, such as bupivacaine, the duration of action is only 8 to 12 hours. Repeated blocks are needed to provide ongoing analgesia. Aside from being relatively labor intensive, this necessitates multiple needle sticks to achieve the 4 to 5 dermatomes of analgesia.

An alternative approach to decrease provider time and obviate the need for repeated needle sticks involves the placement of an intercostal catheter into the intercostal space during surgical closure of the wound.[20] A standard epidural catheter is usually placed into the intercostal space during surgical closure and brought out through the wound. The disadvantage of this technique is that it provides analgesia only for the single interspace.

LOWER EXTREMITY BLOCKADE

Lumbar and Sacral Plexus

The lower extremity is supplied by two plexuses. Anterior innervation is supplied by the lumbar plexus, and the posterior aspect is supplied by the sacral plexus. The lumbar plexus is formed by the union of the ventral branches of the first four lumbar spinal nerves with a small input from the T_{12} root. The plexus lies in a fascial plane, or the "psoas compartment," and is bordered posteriorly by the quadratus lumborum muscle and anteriorly by the psoas major muscle. The lumbar plexus gives rise to the femoral, lateral femoral cutaneous, and obturator nerves.

Different approaches (3-in-1 or fascia iliaca block) allow the blockade of the lumbar plexus and its three major branches or the individual nerves as they arise from the plexus. One of the more common techniques involves blockade of the femoral nerve as it passes under the inguinal ligament (Fig. 4-6). The femoral nerve provides sensory innervation to the anterior aspect of the thigh and the periosteum of the femur. The periosteum is the source of nociceptive input after femur fracture. This technique can be used to provide analgesia in the pediatric trauma patient and, if placed in the emergency department, offers analgesia during patient transport, imaging procedures, and orthopedic fixation. Direct blockade of either the obturator or lateral femoral cutaneous branches is rarely indicated. Because of the deep location of the obturator nerve, blockade is best obtained with an approach that blocks the entire lumbar plexus.

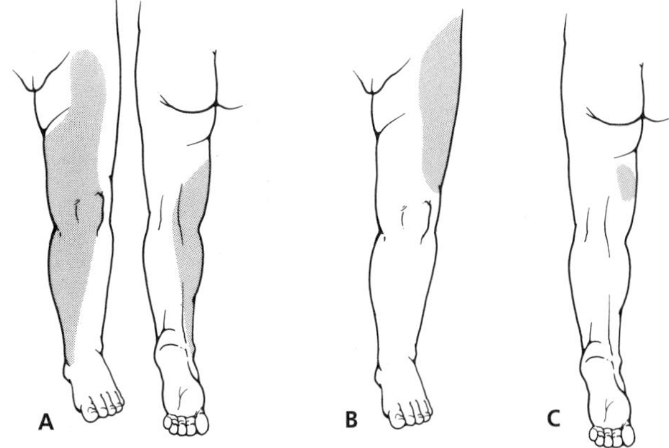

FIG 4-6.
Cutaneous sensory innervation of the femoral nerve **(A),** the lateral femoral cutaneous nerve **(B),** and the obturator nerve **(C).**

Femoral Nerve Block

The femoral nerve is blocked as it passes lateral to the femoral artery at the inguinal ligament (Fig. 4-7). A standard, 22-gauge, short-beveled needle or an insulated block needle may be used. The femoral nerve is blocked just lateral to the femoral artery, 1 cm below the inguinal ligament. After sterile preparation of the area, local anesthesia is applied to the skin and soft tissue if the patient is awake. The needle is advanced at a 30 to 45 degree angle to the skin, parallel to the pulsation of the femoral artery. A double loss of resistance, or "pop," is felt as the needle traverses the fascia lata, which lies under the subcutaneous tissue of the skin, and then the fascia iliaca, which covers the femoral nerve. With this and other peripheral nerve blocks, an alternative approach involves the use of a nerve stimulator set at 0.1 to 1 mA. For this technique, an insulated block needle is needed. The ground (+)

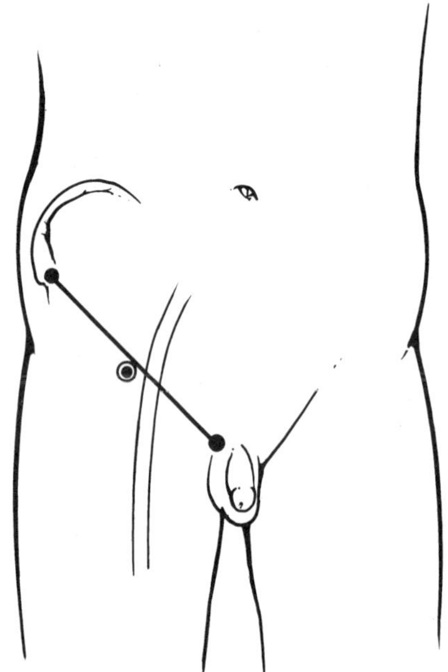

FIG 4-7.
Location of the femoral nerve immediately lateral to the femoral artery. For femoral nerve block, a needle is inserted at a 45 to 60 degree angle to the skin, 1 to 2 centimeters below the inguinal crease. The femoral artery pulsation is located midway between the anterosuperior iliac crest and the pubic tubercle.

electrode is placed on the patient, whereas the negative electrode is attached to the needle with an alligator clip. Muscle movement is sought in the rectus femoris muscle.

Once the femoral nerve is identified, the local anesthetic is injected. Several options have been suggested as to which and how much anesthetic should be used. Grossbard and Love recommend the use of 0.2 ml/kg of 0.5% bupivacaine to a maximum of 10 ml.[21] Lower concentrations of bupivacaine (0.25%) provide effective analgesia and the administration of 0.5 to 0.7 ml/kg up to 25 ml of 0.25% bupivacaine with epinephrine 1:200,000 is recommended. When more profound motor blockade is desired, such as during pin application for traction, the combination of 3% chloroprocaine (0.5 ml/kg) plus 0.5% bupivacaine with epinephrine 1:200,000 (0.5 ml/kg) to a maximum of 40 ml provides effective analgesia and motor blockade. The major disadvantage of this technique is that, like other regional anesthetic techniques, the block can be expected to last a maximum of 8 hours and repeated injections are needed to provide ongoing analgesia.

Two recent studies document the efficacy of continuous infusion via a catheter placed next to the femoral nerve.[22,23] A standard central line, polyethylene catheter (3 French, 5 or 8 centimeter, Cook Critical Care, Bloomington, Indiana) is preferred.[22] The needle is advanced in the manner described above. When the femoral sheath is identified, the local anesthetic solution is injected followed by placement of the guidewire into the sheath. The catheter is inserted using the Seldinger technique. Analgesia may be provided by intermittent doses of local anesthetic (0.5 to 0.75 ml/kg of 0.25% bupivacaine) or a continuous infusion of 0.15 ml/kg/hr of 0.2% bupivacaine (0.3 mg/kg/hr)(Table 4-4). Another technique, described by Johnson, entails the use of the same double-loss-of-resistance technique using a standard Tuohy needle and an 18-gauge epidural catheter.[23] In the latter study, which included 23 patients ranging from 15 months to 14 years of age, analgesia was provided by an infusion of 0.3 ml/kg/hr of 0.125% bupivacaine. Bupivacaine levels were measured in three patients and ranged from 0.67 to 0.93 mg/L. The catheters were left in place for 2 to 5 days. Local infection developed in one patient who was treated with oral antibiotics. No other complications were noted.

Lateral Femoral Cutaneous Nerve

The lateral femoral cutaneous nerve is a purely sensory nerve that supplies the lateral aspect of the thigh (Fig. 4-6). Blockade of the nerve may be used to provide analgesia for various procedures, including harvesting of skin grafts or after percutaneous hip pinning. The nerve emerges in a fascial canal, medial to the anterosuperior iliac spine. A 22-gauge needle is inserted perpendicular to the skin and medial to the spine. A double loss of resistance is felt as the needle passes through the aponeurosis of the external oblique and the fascial canal containing the nerve. After the second loss of resistance, the local anesthetic (3 to 5 ml of 0.25% or 0.5% bupivacaine with epinephrine) is injected.

Obturator Nerve/Lumbar Plexus Blockade

Blockade of the obturator nerve is most frequently required during procedures on the knee joint. When compared to blockade of either the femoral or lateral femoral cutaneous nerves, blockade of the obturator nerve tends to be more difficult because of its deeper course. Therefore an approach that blocks the entire lumbar plexus is recommended. Three techniques are available: the 3-in-1, fascia iliaca, and psoas compartment blocks.

The 3-in-1 block is a modification of the technique used for femoral nerve blockade and is performed by holding distal pressure during injection of the local anesthetic. With this maneuver, the local anesthetic spreads up the femoral sheath and blocks not only the femoral nerve, but also the obturator and lateral femoral cutaneous nerves. A slightly larger volume of local anesthetic is used (1 ml/kg of 0.25% bupivacaine with epinephrine 1:200,000 to a maximum of 40 ml) than for the femoral nerve block.

The fascia iliaca block is another modification of injection below the inguinal ligament that results in spread of the local anesthetic up the sheath to block all three nerves. The patient is positioned supine, as for a femoral nerve block. The landmarks include the pubic tubercle and the anterosuperior iliac spine. The site of needle injection is along the line connecting these two landmarks at a point between the lateral third and the medial two thirds of the line (Fig. 4-8). The needle is inserted at this point perpendicular to the skin. A double loss of resistance is felt as the needle first pierces the fascia lata and then the fascia iliaca. An aspiration

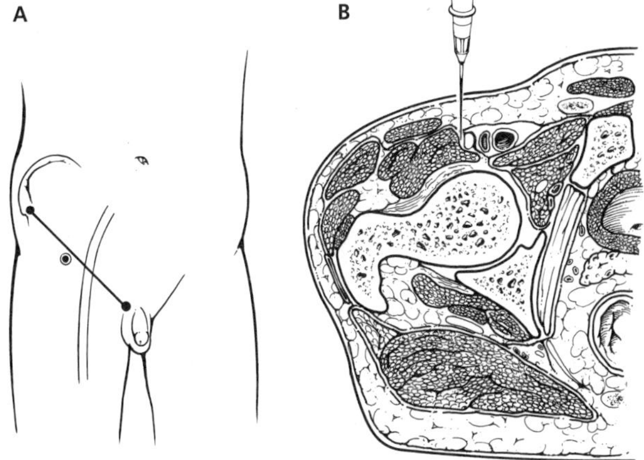

FIG 4-8.
Location of needle insertion **(A)** for fascia iliac block. The site of needle entry is identified as a point between the lateral third and medial two thirds of a line connecting the anterosuperior iliac crest and the pubic tubercle. The technique involves a double "pop" as the needle passes through the fascia lata and the fascia iliaca. The fascia lata passes over the femoral nerve, artery, and vein, and the fascia iliaca passes over the femoral nerve and under the femoral artery and vein **(B).**

test is performed to verify that the needle is not in a blood vessel and the local anesthetic (1 ml/kg of 0.25% bupivacaine with epinephrine 1:200,000) is administered. Placement of a tourniquet around the upper aspect of the thigh may improve the density of block by favoring spread of the local anesthetic up the fascial plane (Fig. 4-8). With either the 3-in-1 or fascia iliaca block, the same sensory blockade can be expected (Fig. 4-9), and it includes distribution to the femoral, lateral femoral cutaneous, and obturator nerves.

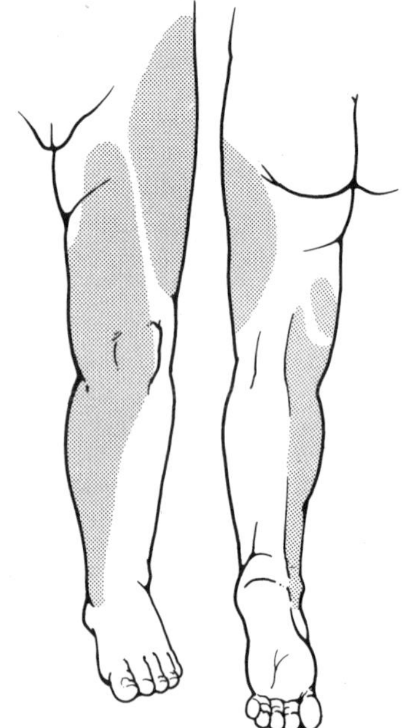

FIG 4-9.
Sensory distribution anesthetized by a 3-in-1 block. The sensory pattern includes the distribution of three nerves (femoral, lateral femoral cutaneous, and obturator).

The third approach to the lumbar plexus is the psoas compartment block. It is the most direct method and involves blockade of the lumbar plexus as it lies in a fascial plane within the psoas muscle, bordered posteriorly by the quadratus lumborum muscle and anteriorly by the psoas major muscle. For this block, the patient is positioned on his or her side with the side to be blocked facing up. The knees and thighs are flexed (Fig. 4-10). The point of needle in-

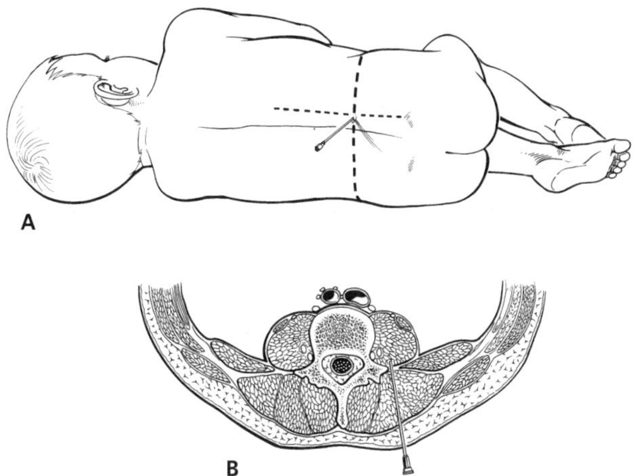

FIG 4-10.
Site of needle entry for a psoas compartment block of the lumbar plexus **(A).** The point of needle insertion is determined by the intersection of two lines. The first is a line drawn through the posterosuperior iliac spine parallel to the spinous processes. The second is a line drawn between the two iliac crests. The needle is inserted perpendicular to the skin, through the quadratus lumborum muscle, into the psoas compartment **(B).**

sertion is determined by the intersection of two lines. The first is a line drawn through the posterosuperior iliac spine, parallel to the spinous processes. The second is a line connecting the two iliac crests. The needle is inserted perpendicular to the skin, through the quadratus lumborum muscle, and into the psoas compartment (Fig. 4-10). If the needle hits the transverse process of the vertebrae, it should be withdrawn and reinserted in a more caudad direction. Penetration into the correct plane can be determined by either loss of resistance, eliciting paresthesias, or twitches in the foot, ankle, or thigh with a nerve stimulator. Recommended doses of local anesthetic include 0.5 ml/kg of 0.5% bupivacaine or 0.7 ml/kg of 0.375% bupivacaine. Unlike the other two approaches to the lumbar plexus, this block may also include the sacral plexus, resulting in anesthesia of the entire leg. Unfortunately, this approach is the most difficult and the least likely to result in successful blockade, especially in smaller children.

Sciatic Nerve Block

Blockade of the lumbar plexus with either a 3-in-1 or a fascia iliaca block may be combined with a sciatic nerve block for surgery of the knee or lower extremity. The sciatic nerve is a branch of the sacral plexus ($L_{4,5}$ and $S_{1,2,3}$). It supplies motor innervation to the extensors of the hip and flexors of the knee. Its sensory distribution includes the back of the thigh and leg to the dorsum of the foot. Although both an anterior and posterior approach have been described in children, the posterior approach is most often used. The patient is positioned in the Sims' position with the side to be blocked facing up. The landmarks for the block include the posterosuperior iliac spine, the greater trochanter, and the sacral cornu (Fig. 4-11). A line is drawn connecting the greater trochanter and the posterosuperior iliac spine. From its midpoint, a perpendicular line is dropped, which intersects a line drawn from the greater trochanter to the ipsilateral sacral cornu (Fig. 4-11). The intersection of these points is the site of needle entry. A 22- or 25-gauge, 3.5 inch spinal needle is inserted perpendicular to the skin and advanced until a paresthesia is obtained. More commonly, since the majority of pediatric patients are anesthetized during the procedure, a nerve stimulator is used and a twitch is elicited in the foot. The depth of the nerve depends on the weight and size of the patient. When the nerve is identified, 0.5 ml/kg to a maximum of 20 ml of 0.25% bupivacaine with epinephrine 1:200,000 is injected. As with any of these blocks, aspiration for blood before injection, the use of a test dose, and fractionating the total dose are recommended to prevent inadvertent intravascular injection.

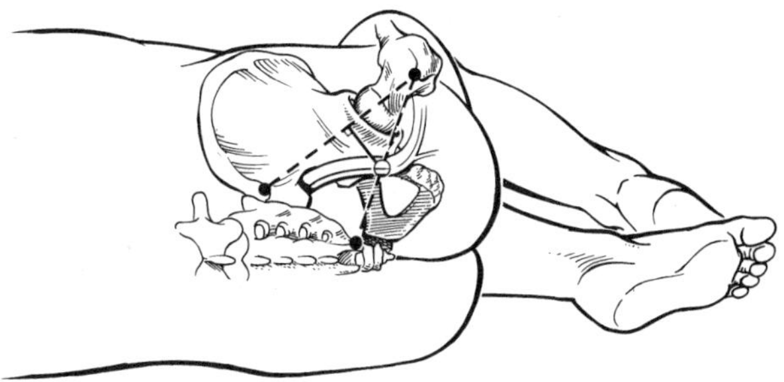

FIG 4-11.
Site of needle entry for posterior approach to the sciatic nerve. A line is drawn connecting the greater trochanter and the posterosuperior iliac spine. From its midpoint, a perpendicular line is dropped that intersects a line drawn from the greater trochanter to the ipsilateral sacral cornu. The intersection of these points is the site of needle entry.

UPPER EXTREMITY BLOCKADE

Brachial Plexus

The brachial plexus is derived from the ventral branches of spinal roots C_{5-8} and T_1, providing the motor supply to the upper extremity. It also provides sensory innervation to that entire area except for a small part of the shoulder that is innervated by descending branches of the cervical plexus and the posterolateral aspect of the upper arm, which is supplied by a branch of the second intercostal nerve (intercostobrachial nerve). As the spinal roots leave the vertebral body, they are contained between the anterior and middle scalene muscles and unite to form three trunks (superior, middle, and inferior). The trunks of the brachial plexus are blocked when the interscalene approach is used. The trunks split into anterior and posterior divisions, which then unite to form cords (lateral, posterior, and medial) that surround the axillary artery. It is at this level that an axillary approach to the brachial plexus is used. The cords further divide to form the various nerves of the brachial plexus.

Several approaches to the brachial plexus have been described, such as axillary, interscalene, supraclavicular, and infraclavicular blockade. The latter two approaches are not routinely used because of the increased risk of adverse effects, such as pneumothorax. As with the other regional blocks, this block may be used alone to provide surgical anesthesia, as an adjunct to general anesthesia, or for postoperative analgesia. The approach depends on the age of the patient and the level of surgery. Although axillary blockade may be effective for procedures of the elbow and hand, procedures involving the shoulder usually require an interscalene approach. The interscalene approach does not require special positioning of the arm, thereby making it useful in situations when arm movement is limited.

Interscalene Block

An interscalene block may be placed with the patient awake, sedated, or after the induction of general anesthesia. For the last purpose, a nerve stimulator is used to identify correct placement, whereas elicitation of paresthesias is frequently used for the awake or sedated patient. With the use of a nerve stimulator, movement should be elicited distally (i.e., in the hand or forearm) before injection of the medication. The landmarks for the block include the anterior and middle scalene muscles and Chassaignac's tubercle (the transverse process of the sixth cervical vertebra). Since deep palpation to identify this latter structure may be painful in the awake patient, its location can also be determined by the intersection of a line drawn from the cricoid cartilage to the posterior border of the sternocleidomastoid muscle (Fig. 4-12). This point should lie between the anterior and middle scalene muscles. After correct needle placement, 0.75 ml/kg of 0.25% bupivacaine with epinephrine 1:200,000 is injected to a maximum of 30 ml. In larger patients, 0.375% or 0.5% bupivacaine may be used, provided that the total dose does not exceed 2.5 mg/kg. Another al-

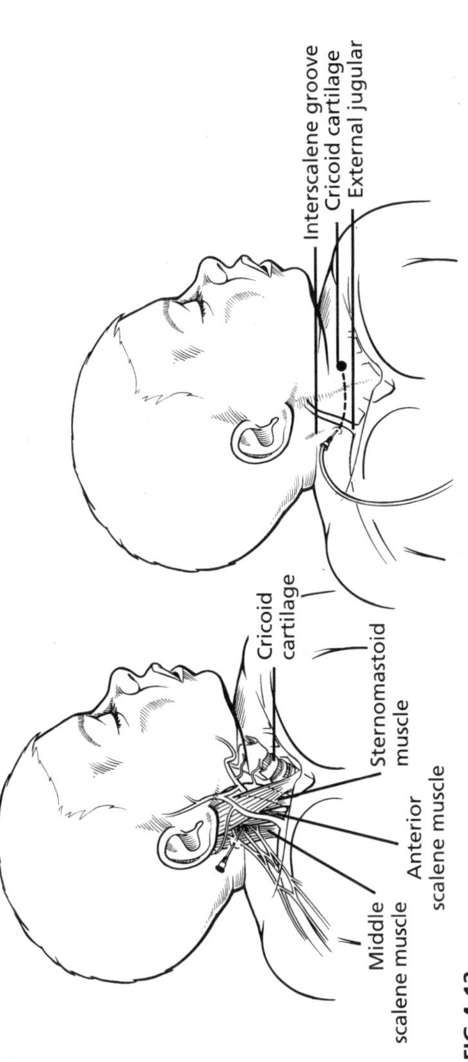

FIG 4-12.
Site of needle entry for an interscalene block. Since deep palpation to identify Chassaignac's tubercle is painful in the awake patient, its location can also be determined by the intersection of a line drawn from the cricoid cartilage to the posterior border of the sternocleidomastoid muscle. This point should lie between the anterior and middle scalene muscles.

ternative is the addition of 0.5 ml/kg of 3% chloroprocaine to 0.5 ml/kg of 0.5% bupivacaine up to a maximum of 40 ml total. Chloroprocaine is added when a rapid onset of block is desired, such as when the block is being used instead of general anesthesia. The addition of 3% chloroprocaine also results in a motor block, thereby eliminating the immediate evaluation of postoperative motor function.

Complications related to the interscalene approach in children include inadvertent epidural, spinal, and intravascular injections. Careful aspiration before an injection should identify the majority of these problems; however, ready access to resuscitation equipment is mandatory. Cardiovascular or CNS toxicity may result from an inadvertent intravascular injection. Spinal or epidural injections may result in a high motor block causing a respiratory arrest and hypotension from sympathetic blockade. Even with correct needle placement, phrenic nerve blockade occurs in up to 40% of interscalene blocks. Although inconsequential in healthy, adult patients, in the pediatric patient, especially the infant, significant respiratory compromise may develop because the infant is more dependent on the diaphragm for ventilatory function. Spread of the local anesthetic to the area near the recurrent laryngeal nerve may result in temporary hoarseness or vocal cord paralysis with aspiration. Pneumothorax, although less common than with the supraclavicular approach, may also occur, especially in young children where the dome of the pleura lies higher in the neck.

Inadequate or incomplete block may be a problem even with correct needle placement. Since the trunks are located in a superior-to-inferior fashion in the interscalene groove, the inferior trunk, which gives rise to sensory innervation of the lateral aspect of the arm to the little finger (C_8 and T_1 dermatomes), may not be effectively blocked. This block is less effective than the axillary approach for these areas.

Axillary Block

The most commonly used brachial plexus block in children is the axillary approach. For this procedure, the patient's arm is abducted 90° from the body and, if possible, the elbow is flexed and the hand is placed behind the head (Fig. 4-13). This block may be performed using one of three different approaches: the transarterial, single injection, or two-injection technique.

The transarterial approach includes fixation of the artery against the humerus. The needle is inserted at a 45 degree angle to the skin toward the arterial pulsation until the artery is identified by the presence of arterial blood in the syringe. The needle is advanced through the artery until blood is no longer aspirated and half of the local anesthetic is injected. The needle is withdrawn until blood flow again ceases and the other half of the anesthetic solution is injected. The advantage of this technique is that the posterior cord, which may be missed with other axillary approaches since it lies behind the artery, is effectively blocked. The major disadvantage is the risk of vascular trauma. Although no

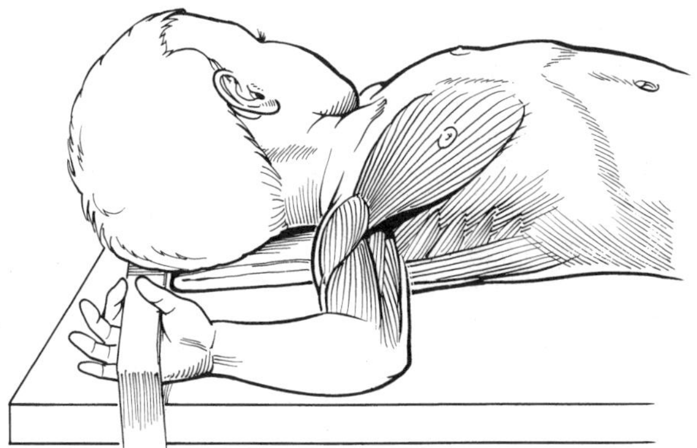

FIG 4-13.

Patient positioning for the axillary approach to the brachial plexus. The patient's arm is abducted to 90°, the elbow is flexed, and the hand is placed above or behind the head. Needle entry is at a 45° angle to the skin and should be as high in the axilla as possible.

controlled studies have demonstrated an increased risk with this technique, it is best to avoid direct arterial puncture.

The other approaches are the one- and two-injection techniques. After palpation of the artery, the needle is advanced at a 45 degree angle to the skin, just above the arterial pulsation. Entry into the neurovascular bundle is identified by a "pop," or a loss of resistance. When the pop is felt, correct placement can be confirmed with a nerve stimulator or elicitation of a paresthesia. The entire volume of local anesthetic solution is injected at this point for the single-injection technique. For the two-injection technique, half of the solution is injected above the artery, and the procedure is repeated with the needle directed below the arterial pulsation for the second injection. It is preferred to leave the first needle in place and to use a second needle for the inferior injection. At that time, a small amount of the local anesthetic solution may drip out of the first needle, further confirming correct location of both needles. During injection, pressure is held distal to the injection site and facilitates the spread of the local anesthetic up the neurovascular sheath.

The single-dose or "one-shot" technique is able to provide only a limited duration of analgesia. In some circumstances, such as a more prolonged surgical procedure or to provide ongoing analgesia into the postoperative period, a catheter can be placed into the neurovascular bundle using the axillary approach to allow for either intermittent bolus dosing or a continuous infusion. The technique and dosing regimen are the same as those described for a continuous femoral nerve block.

The axillary approach is more effective than the interscalene approach in providing analgesia along the ulnar side; however, the posterior cord may be more difficult to anesthetize, leading to inadequate anesthesia of the radial side. The musculocutaneous nerve, which provides sensory innervation to the lateral aspect of the forearm, may be missed with the axillary approach since it branches higher up from the plexus.

If a tourniquet is used for this procedure, a ring of local anesthetic is injected high around the arm to avoid tourniquet pain. The ring infiltration blocks the intercostobrachial branch of T_2 which innervates this area.

BIER BLOCK

The Bier block is a regional anesthetic technique that involves the IV administration of a local anesthetic distal to an inflated tourniquet. This technique is used only for intraoperative analgesia, most frequently as an alternative to general anesthesia. After tourniquet deflation, the block dissipates rapidly with no potential for providing postoperative analgesia. Although it has been widely applied in adult anesthesia practice, its use in pediatric anesthesia is somewhat limited.

Advantages of the Bier block include ease of placement, rapid onset of block, and the use of a tourniquet, which provides a bloodless field. Disadvantages include a limited duration of action (60 minutes) because of the onset of tourniquet pain and the risk of local anesthetic toxicity.

This procedure should be used outside of the operating room only by trained personnel with the availability of appropriate airway equipment and resuscitation medication. In older patients and adults, the block may be used without accompanying IV sedation in patients that may have an increased risk for general anesthesia, such as those with a full stomach. In younger patients, IV sedation is frequently required. However, it should be remembered that conscious sedation may quickly become deep sedation with loss of airway reflexes. Any regional anesthetic technique that requires deep sedation in a patient with a full stomach may entail even greater risks than those of a general anesthetic.

After placement of IV access in the limb not to be operated on, a double tourniquet is applied to the involved extremity (Fig. 4-14). IV access is obtained in the involved limb, preferably in a distal site. The limb is elevated above the heart for 3 minutes and, if possible, an elastic bandage is wrapped around the extremity starting distally and proceeding proximally. The proximal tourniquet is

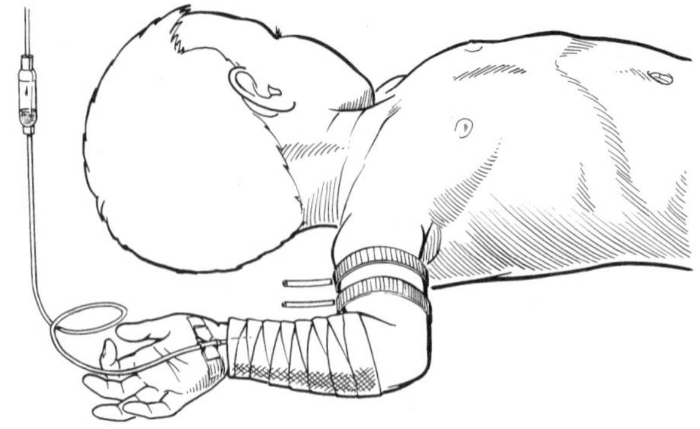

FIG 4-14.
Technique for a Bier block with a double tourniquet, an elastic bandage to exsanguinate the extremity, and intravenous access in a distal portion of the extremity.

then inflated. Various recommendations exist for inflation pressure for the tourniquet with values as high as 300 mm Hg for adults. Carrel and Eyring recommend inflation pressures of 180 to 240 mm Hg for upper extremity procedures and 350 to 500 mm Hg for the lower extremity,[24] but Fitzgerald reported successful blockade without complications with lower pressures (50 mm Hg above systolic blood pressure).[25] Inflation of the proximal cuff to 50 to 80 mm Hg above systolic blood pressure is adequate.

After proximal cuff inflation, the local anesthetic solution is injected. The solution should be injected slowly without excessive pressure, since this may push the anesthetic out of the involved limb and into the systemic circulation. Although the concentration of the anesthetic is important, an adequate volume is necessary to prevent patchy blockade.

With a Bier block, there is a rapid onset of blockade within 5 minutes of the injection of the local anesthetic. The patient usually complains of tourniquet pain after 5 to 10 minutes. At that time, the distal tourniquet is inflated. Once it is assured that the distal tourniquet is inflated, the proximal tourniquet is deflated. The area under the distal tourniquet should be adequately anesthetized by the block and the patient should not experience pain.

At the completion of the procedure, the cuff is deflated for 15 seconds and then reinflated. This procedure is repeated two or three times. This prevents the sudden release of a large quantity of local anesthetic into the systemic circulation. Motor and sensory function return in 5 minutes. Regardless of the length of the procedure, the cuff should not be deflated until at least 20 minutes from the time the block was placed.

Because of the risk of toxicity, volumes and concentrations of the local anesthetic solution are limited in the pediatric population. Current practice includes 0.5% lidocaine (without epinephrine) in a volume of 0.6 ml/kg (3 mg/kg) for the upper extremity and 1 ml/kg (5 mg/kg) for the lower extremity. Prilocaine, a local anesthetic, may be preferable for IV regional anesthesia. With its larger volume of distribution, it is the least toxic of the amide anesthetics. However, prilocaine may induce methemoglobin. Although this effect is clinically insignificant in most patients, prilocaine is contraindicated in patients receiving other drugs that induce methemoglobin, in the rare patient with hereditary methemoglobinemia, and in neonates, since their ability to reduce methemoglobin back to the ferrous state is limited. Bupivacaine is absolutely contraindicated for IV regional anesthesia because of its cardiovascular toxicity. Likewise, mepivacaine is not recommended since local acidosis and hyperkalemia may develop in the anesthetized limb. Chloroprocaine, although it has the advantage of rapid metabolism and minimal blood levels, is not desirable in this setting because it may lead to thrombophlebitis.

Several investigators suggest an improvement in the quality of anesthesia by the addition of either opioids (morphine or fentanyl) or small doses of neuromuscular blocking agents to the local anesthetic solution. Although the majority of analgesia provided by opioids relates to their binding to receptors in the spinal cord or CNS, opioid receptors have also been demonstrated in the peripheral nervous system. These findings support the addition of fentanyl (1 μg/kg) to the local anesthetic solution. With lower concentrations of local anesthetic (0.25% or 0.5% lidocaine), motor block may be incomplete and the patient may move during the procedure. The addition of pancuronium (0.01 mg/kg) to the local anesthetic solution may improve the degree of motor block regionally without producing systemic signs.

Amiot and colleagues have described the use of ketamine for Bier block.[26] An injection of 40 ml of a 0.5% solution was used for upper extremity surgery. The onset of blockade was rapid (less than 5 minutes) and provided adequate analgesia in 18 of 20 patients. The two failures were in patients with extensive wounds in whom adequate exsanguination of the extremity could not be performed. However, with release of the tourniquet, all patients developed a loss of consciousness (average duration of 10 minutes) as a result of the systemic effects of ketamine. This problem severely limits the applicability of ketamine for Bier block.

Although the techniques described are safe and effective, certain contraindications exist to the performance of the Bier block. These include an underlying seizure disorder, cardiac arrhythmias, and ongoing sepsis. Other contraindications are related more to the use of the tourniquet than the local anesthetic and include sickle-cell disease, vascular insufficiency of the involved extremity, and procedures that will last longer than 90 minutes.

PERIPHERAL NERVE BLOCKS

Distal blockade of major sensory nerves can be used alone to provide analgesia and anesthesia or to supplement another technique. For example, a radial nerve block may supplement an axillary block when anesthesia in the radial distribution is insufficient. Several different peripheral blocks may be performed, including ilioinguinal, iliohypogastric, digital, ankle, and wrist blocks. Another commonly performed block, the penile block, is discussed in Chapter 8.

Ilioinguinal and Iliohypogastric Blocks

Ilioinguinal and iliohypogastric blocks may be used to provide anesthesia and analgesia for operations of the inguinal region, including herniorrhaphy, orchiopexy, and hydrocoelectomy. Although these blocks decrease anesthetic requirements when placed before surgical incision, they do not block visceral pain produced during peritoneal traction and manipulation of the spermatic cord. The ilioinguinal (L_1) and iliohypogastric (T_{12} and L_1) nerves are branches of the lumbar plexus and supply sensory innervation to the scrotum and inner aspect of the thigh. The two nerves run along the posterior aspect of the external oblique muscle, anterior to the transversus abdominis. They are blocked by inserting a 22- or 23-gauge needle perpendicular to the skin, 1 cm lateral and 1 cm inferior to the anterosuperior iliac crest. A "pop" is felt as the needle pierces the external oblique muscle, and the local anesthetic is injected in a fanwise manner at right angles to the nerve (medial to lateral). The amount and concentration of local anesthetic varies with the age of the patient (0.5 to 1.0 ml/year of age of 0.25% or 0.5% bupivacaine with epinephrine 1:200,000). The advantage of the ilioinguinal and iliohypogastric blocks is that it does not affect motor or sensory function of the lower extremities. When compared with caudal block for analgesia after routine herniorrhaphy, it has been suggested that ilioinguinal and iliohypogastric blocks provide equal analgesia.[27] However, for bilateral procedures two injections are required. Therefore the caudal block is preferred for younger patients (less than 8 years of age) and ilioinguinal and hypogastric blocks are performed percutaneously by the anesthesiologist before the start of the procedure or under direct vision by the surgeon during operative repair for patients more than 8 years of age.

Digital Block

Digital blocks of either the fingers or toes may be used for brief procedures, such as removal of ingrown nails, suturing lacerations, debridement of injuries, or removal of foreign bodies. This technique has also been suggested as a means of improving pulse oximetry waveform readings intraoperatively in patients who are poorly perfused or cold. They may be used alone in older patients or after sedation in younger patients. Since the arteries supplying the fingers and toes are end-arteries, vasoconstrictors, such as epinephrine, are contraindicated in digital blocks.

Each finger or toe is supplied by four nerves, two each along the ventral and dorsal aspects (Fig. 4-15). The block is performed with a 25-gauge needle. The nerves are approached from the lateral aspect of the finger at the base of the digit. The local anesthetic is injected into the skin and subcutaneous tissue down to the bone. The needle is withdrawn and directed anteriorly over the superior aspect of the bone and more local anesthetic is injected. The same procedure is repeated with the needle directed under the bone. The procedure is then repeated from the medial aspect of

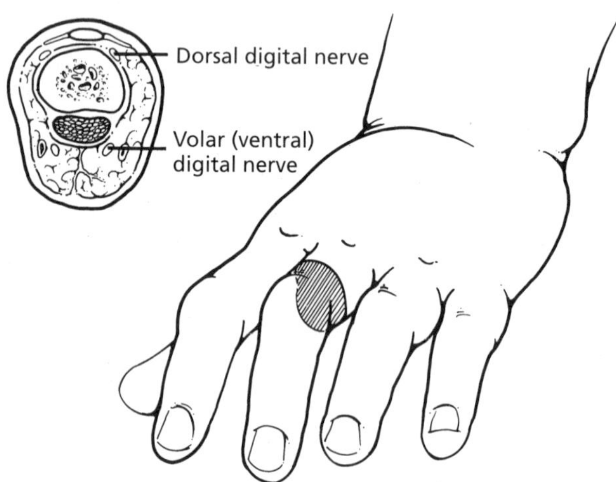

FIG 4-15.
Technique for digital block of either the fingers or toes. Each finger or toe has four nerves, two along the ventral and two along the dorsal aspect of the digit. The needle is inserted from the lateral aspect at the base of the digit. Local anesthetic is injected over the superior and inferior side of the bone. The procedure is then repeated from the medial aspect of the digit.

the digit. The total volume of anesthetic (1% or 2% lidocaine) should not exceed 2 ml per digit.

Ankle Block

Ankle or wrist blocks may also have a place in pediatric anesthesia for superficial and brief procedures that are confined to the hand or foot. Since both blocks require more than one injection, the discomfort associated with the blocks limits their utility in younger patients unless preceded by sedation. For either block, vasoconstrictors are not added to the local anesthetic solution. The typical volume of local anesthetic used in an adult is 5 ml of 0.5% bupivacaine for each of the five nerves of the foot (total of 25 ml). For children 0.1 to 0.15 ml/kg of 0.25% bupivacaine is recommended for each nerve.

The foot is innervated by five separate nerves, each of which must be individually anesthetized (Fig. 4-16). The *saphenous nerve* is the only branch of the femoral nerve with a distribution beyond the knee. It innervates the medial aspect of the ankle and the foot, including the great toe. The saphenous nerve runs anterior to the medial malleolus next to the saphenous vein. It is easily anesthetized by infiltrating local anesthetic around the saphenous vein. The other four nerves that innervate the ankle and foot are branches of the sciatic nerve. The *deep peroneal* (anterior tibial) *nerve* runs parallel to the anterior tibial artery, on the anterior surface of the distal end of the tibia, between the extensor hallucis longus and tibialis anterior tendons. Its sensory distribution includes the first web space of the foot. The nerve is blocked by insertion of a needle lateral to the extensor hallucis longus tendon down to the tibia. The needle is withdrawn 1 to 2 mm, and the local anesthetic solution is injected. Identification of the extensor hallucis longus tendon is facilitated by having the patient extend his or her great toe. The plantar surface of the foot is supplied by the *posterior tibial nerve,* which courses along the medial aspect of the ankle and foot, posterior to the medial malleolus and posterior tibial artery. The nerve is blocked posterior to the pulsation of the posterior tibial artery. The *sural nerve* is a purely sensory

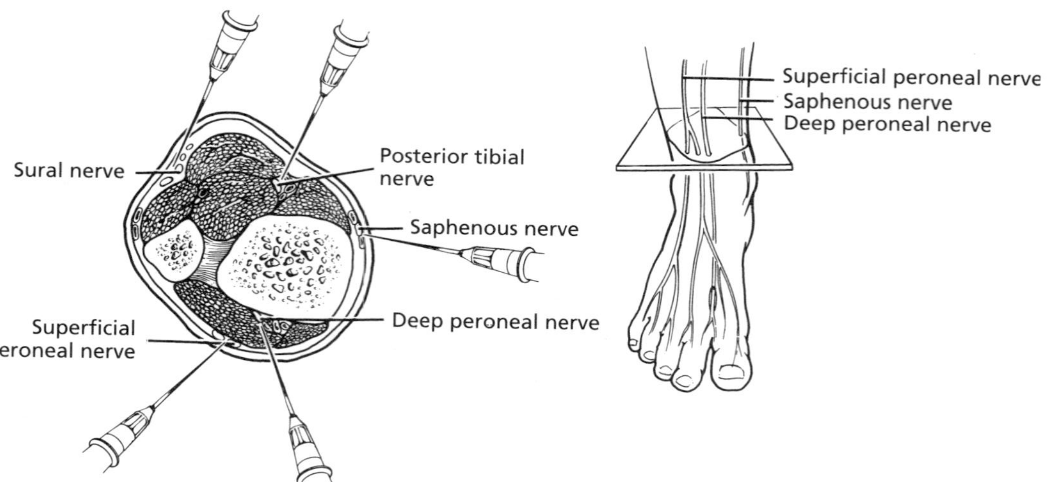

FIG 4-16.
An ankle block includes separately anesthetizing the five nerves of the foot, including the saphenous nerve, the deep peroneal (anterior tibial) nerve, the posterior tibial nerve, the sural nerve, and the superficial peroneal nerve, which innervates the dorsum of the foot.

nerve that supplies the lateral aspect of the foot. It is blocked by infiltration of local anesthetic from the lateral malleolus posterior to the Achilles tendon. The last of the five nerves of the foot and ankle is the *superficial peroneal nerve,* which innervates the dorsum of the foot. It is blocked by superficial infiltration from the lateral malleolus to the extensor hallucis longus tendon.

Wrist Block

The wrist and hand are supplied by three nerves: the ulnar, median, and radial (Fig. 4-17). The ulnar and median nerves are most easily approached from the volar aspect of the wrist, and a lateral approach is used for the radial nerve. As with blocks of the foot and ankle, local anesthetic (0.25% or 0.5% bupivacaine) without vasoconstrictor is used. For all three nerves, a 25-gauge needle is used with the injection of 0.5 ml/year of age (up to 3 ml) of local anesthetic.

The *median nerve* courses between the palmaris longus tendon and the flexor carpi radialis tendon. The tendons are easily identified by having the patient flex the wrist. The needle is inserted between the two tendons at a point 1 to 2 cm proximal to (up the arm from) the first wrist crease. To anesthetize the palmar cutaneous branch, 1 ml of local anesthetic should also be injected as the needle is withdrawn.

The *ulnar nerve* is also approached from the volar aspect of the hand and wrist. This nerve follows the ulnar artery along the medial aspect of the forearm and wrist and lies under the flexor carpi ulnaris tendon. It should be blocked proximal to the pisiform bone (first crease of the wrist) so that both the deep and superficial branches are properly anesthetized. The needle is inserted perpendicular to the skin at the most proximal crease of the wrist, medial to the pulsation of the ulnar artery. If the patient is awake, a paresthesia is sought since the nerve lies under a fascial plane.

The *radial nerve* is approached from the lateral aspect of the wrist (Fig. 4-17). The anatomic snuff box is identified by having the patient extend the thumb. Local anesthetic (1 to 2 ml) is injected subcutaneously for 1 to 2 cm along the course of the exten-

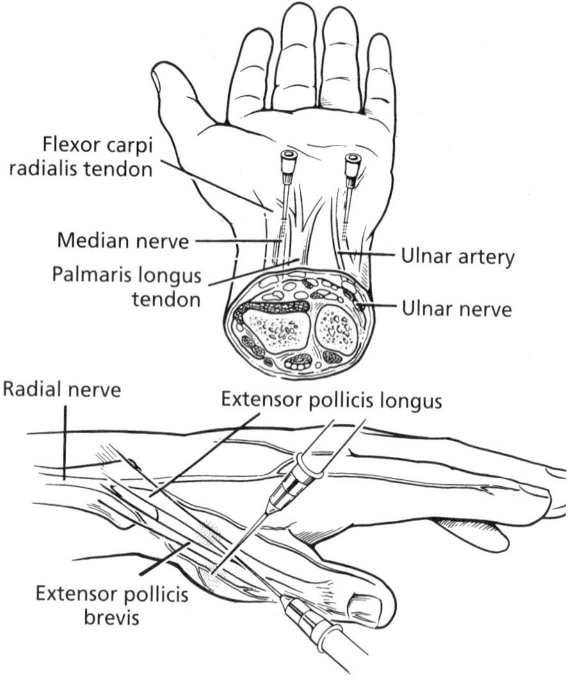

sor pollicis longus starting at the base of the first metacarpal. The needle is then withdrawn and reinserted at a right angle to the initial plane, and another 1 to 3 ml of local anesthetic is injected in a line that crosses the extensor pollicis brevis. This field block should effectively anesthetize the terminal branches of the radial nerve.

Summary

Blockade of the peripheral nervous system has several applications in the practice of pediatric anesthesia, including its use instead of general anesthesia, as an adjunct to general anesthesia, or for postoperative analgesia. The major adverse effect associated with these blocks is local anesthetic toxicity. Attention to dosing

FIG 4-17.

Technique of blockade of the ulnar, median, and radial nerves at the wrist. The ulnar and median nerves are most easily approached from the volar aspect of the wrist, whereas a lateral approach is used for the radial nerve. The median nerve courses between the palmaris longus tendon and the flexor carpi radialis tendon. The ulnar nerve is also approached from the volar aspect of the hand and wrist. The nerve follows the ulnar artery along the medial aspect of the forearm and wrist and lies under the flexor carpi ulnaris tendon. The radial nerve is approached from the lateral aspect of the wrist. The anatomic snuff box is identified by having the patient extend the thumb. Local anesthetic is injected subcutaneously for 1 to 2 cm along the course of the extensor pollicis longus starting at the base of the first metacarpal. The needle is withdrawn and reinserted at a right angle to the initial plane in a line that crosses the extensor pollicis brevis. This field block should effectively anesthetize the terminal branches of the radial nerve.

---

guidelines with limitation of the total dose of local anesthetic is recommended. With such precautions, regional blockade can be a valuable addition to the pain management armamentarium in infants and children. Although these techniques are generally used in the perioperative period, they may also have a role in providing analgesia for pain of other etiologies, such as trauma, burns, and various medical conditions.

References

1. Tobias JD, Haun SE, Helfaer M et al: Use of continuous caudal block to relieve lower-extremity ischemia caused by vasculitis in a child with meningococcemia, *J Pediatr* 115:1019, 1989.
2. Kvalheim L, Reiestad F: Interpleural catheter in the management of postoperative pain, *Anesthesiology* 61:231, 1984.
3. Riegler FX, Vadeboncouer TR, Pelligrino DA: An animal model of interpleural analgesia, *Anesthesiology* 71:744, 1989.

4. McIlvaine WB, Knox RF, Fennessey PV et al: Continuous infusion of bupivacaine via intrapleural catheter for analgesia after thoracotomy in children, *Anesthesiology* 69:261, 1988.
5. Queen JS, Kahana MD, DiFazio CA et al: An evaluation of interpleural analgesia with etidocaine in children, *Anesth Analg* 68:S228, 1989.
6. Tobias JD: Analgesia after thoracotomy in children: a comparison of interpleural, epidural, and intravenous analgesia, *South Med J* 84:1458, 1991.
7. Stromskag KE, Reiestad F, Holmqvist ELO et al: Intrapleural administration of 0.25%, 0.375%, and 0.5% bupivacaine with epinephrine after cholecystectomy, *Anesth Analg* 67:430, 1988.
8. Tobias JD: The anesthetic implications of Ehler-Danlos syndrome, *Anes Rev* 20:133, 1993.
9. Berde CB: Convulsions associated with pediatric regional anesthesia, *Anesth Analg* 75:164, 1992.
10. Agarwal R, Gutlove DP, Lockhart CH: Seizures occurring in pediatric patients receiving continuous infusion of bupivacaine, *Anesth Analg* 75:284, 1992.
11. Reiestad F, McIlvaine WB, Kvalheim L et al: Successful treatment of chronic pancreatitis pain with interpleural analgesia, *Can J Anaesth* 36:713, 1989.
12. Durrani Z, Winnie AP, Ikuta P: Interpleural catheter analgesia for pancreatic pain, *Anesth Analg* 67:479, 1988.
13. Reiestad F, McIlvaine WB, Barnes M et al: Interpleural analgesia in the treatment of severe thoracic postherpetic neuralgia, *Reg Anesth* 15:113, 1990.
14. Fineman SP: Long-term postthoracotomy cancer pain management with interpleural bupivacaine, *Anesth Analg* 68:694, 1989.
15. Reiestad F, McIlvaine WB, Kvalheim L et al: Interpleural analgesia in the treatment of upper extremity reflex sympathetic dystrophy, *Anesth Analg* 69:671, 1989.
16. Perkins G: Interpleural anaesthesia in the management of upper limb ischaemia: a report of three cases, *Anaesth Int Care* 19:575, 1991.

17. Delikan AE, Lee LK, Yong NK: Postoperative local analgesia for thoracotomy with direct bupivacaine intercostal blocks, *Anaesthesia* 28:561, 1973.
18. Fleming JH, Sarafian LB: Kindness pays dividends: the medical benefits of intercostal nerve blocks following thoracotomy, *J Thorac Cardiovasc Surg* 74:273, 1977.
19. Moore DC: Intercostal nerve block for postoperative somatic pain following surgery of thorax and upper abdomen, *Br J Anaesth* 47:284, 1975.
20. Olivet RT, Nauss LA, Payne WS: A technique for continuous intercostal nerve block analgesia following thoracotomy, *J Thorac Surg* 80:308, 1980.
21. Grossbard GD, Love BRT: Femoral nerve block: a simple and safe method of instant analgesia for femoral shaft fractures in children, *Aust NZ J Surg* 49:592, 1979.
22. Tobias JD: Continuous femoral nerve block to provide analgesia following femur fracture in a pediatric ICU population, *Anaesth Int Care* 22:616, 1994.
23. Johnson CM: Continuous femoral nerve blockade for analgesia in children with femoral fractures, *Anesth Int Care* 22:281, 1994.
24. Carrel ED, Eyring EJ: Intravenous regional anesthesia for childhood fractures, *J Trauma* 11:301, 1971.
25. Fitzgerald B: Intravenous regional anesthesia in children, *Br J Anaesth* 48:485, 1976.
26. Amiot JF, Bouju P, Palacci JH et al: Intravenous regional anaesthesia with ketamine, *Anaesthesia* 40:899, 1985.
27. Casey WF, Rice LJ, Hannallah RS et al: A comparison between bupivacaine instillation versus ilioinguinal/iliohypogastric block for postoperative analgesia following inguinal herniorrhaphy in children, *Anesthesiology* 72:637, 1990.
28. Tobias JD, Haun SE, Helfaer M et al: Use of continuous caudal block to relieve ischemia caused by vasculitis in a child with meningococcemia, *J Pediatr* 115:1019, 1989.
29. Anderson CTM, Berde CB, Sethna NF et al: Meningococcal purpura fulminans: treatment of vascular insufficiency in a 2-

year old child with lumbar epidural sympathetic blockade, *Anesthesiology* 71:463, 1989.

30. Parris WCV, Reddy BC, White HW et al: Stellate ganglion blocks in pediatric patients, *Anesth Analg,* 72:552, 1991.
31. Audenaert SM, Vickers H, Burgess RC: Axillary block for vascular insufficiency after repair of radial club hands in an infant, *Anesthesiology* 74:368, 1991.
32. Edwards WT, Burney RG: Use of repeated nerve blocks in management of an infant with Kawasaki's disease, *Anesth Analg* 67:1008, 1988.
33. Johansen K, Murphy T, Pavlin E et al: Digital ischemia complicating pneumococcal sepsis: reversal with sympathetic blockade, *Crit Care Med* 19:114, 1991.
34. Sanchez V, Segedin ER, Moser M et al: Role of lumbar sympathectomy in the Pediatric Intensive Care Unit. *Anesth Analg* 67:794, 1988.

5

THE MANAGEMENT OF PAIN ASSOCIATED WITH MEDICAL ILLNESSES

Brenda C. McClain
Gail E. Rasmussen
Berklee Robins

SICKLE CELL DISEASE AND ASSOCIATED HEMOGLOBINOPATHIES
ONCOLOGIC DISEASES
ACUTE PAIN ASSOCIATED WITH SPECIFIC CLINICAL PROBLEMS
Otitis media
Chest pain
Burns and thermal injury
Trauma-related pain

Various medical illnesses are associated with acute pain in children. These include sickle cell disease, oncologic diseases, and problems such as otitis media, burns, and trauma. Many strategies used to treat acute pain of different etiologies are similar. However, some approaches may vary depending on the etiology of pain. This chapter discusses the options for pain management in relation to acute medical illnesses.

SICKLE CELL DISEASE AND ASSOCIATED HEMOGLOBINOPATHIES

Sickle cell disease affects approximately 8% of Americans of African, Latin, and Mediterranean descent. The two common clinical manifestations of sickle cell disease are chronic hemolytic anemia and recurring painful crisis. The severity and frequency of pain is unpredictable and shows components of acute and chronic pain syndromes. In some African languages, sickle cell disease has various descriptive names, such as "body biting" and "body chewing". The severity is onomatopoeically described in the Ga language as "Chwe-chwe-chwe" to connote the repetitive nature of the painful crisis.

Because there are no outward signs of pathology or accurate detectors of the pain magnitude, caregivers must rely on patient reports, as well as nonspecific clinical signs, to guide supportive therapy. Management of patients with sickle cell disease is complicated by several factors, such as fear of addiction, concern of opioid side effects, and, at times, the patient's sense of hopelessness and learned helplessness. Frustration and hopelessness often set in because there is no known cure for the disease and because the character and frequency of the vasoocclusive crisis (VOC) may increase during adolescence. Healthcare professionals, the majority of whose ancestry is not similar to that of these patients, often have an unfounded fear that the patients are drug seekers and malingerers. Thus, suspicion of the patient's intentions coupled with the unpredictable nature of the disease can result in adversarial relationships between the medical staff and the patient.

About 20% of patients with sickle cell disease have frequent and severe episodes. Most hospitalizations for pain involve this group. About 30% rarely have VOC pain, whereas the remaining 50% have only one severe crisis per year or multiple mild crises that do not require repeated hospitalizations.[1]

There are many causes of pain in sickle cell disease. Bone pain related to VOC is the most frequent. Splenic infarction and cholecystitis can cause visceral pain. Patients with chronic pain complicating sickle cell disease usually have acute episodic pain on top of the chronic pain picture, thereby giving a mixed expression of acute and chronic pain behaviors. There are no concise management guidelines for treating patients with sickle cell disease. The care of patients with sickle cell disease should involve a multidisciplinary approach to address the pathophysiologic, psychologic, and socioeconomic aspects of the disease.

This discussion addresses the pathophysiology of sickle cell hemoglobinopathy followed by a discussion of various pharmacologic and nonpharmacologic techniques for the control of pain. Newer modalities of pain management, such as the application of regional anesthetic blockade, are also discussed.

Sickle cell disease results from the substitution of one amino acid on the beta chain of the hemoglobin molecule. The residue located at position 6 of the beta chain is normally glutamic acid and has a charged sidechain. In sickle cell hemoglobin, the glutamyl residue is replaced by valine and is uncharged, resulting in a hydrophobic bond and an electrically neutral sidechain. In normal red blood cells the sum attractive and repulsive forces between molecules is negative. The valine substitution at position 6 results in a net attractive force that results in sickling in the deoxygenated conformation.[2] The rate of polymerization of deoxyhemoglobin S is dependent on the concentration of sickle hemoglobin.

The other hemoglobinopathies, which can also result in sickling and painful crisis, result from other amino acid substitutions. Substitution of lysine for glutamate at position 6 on the beta chain results in hemoglobin C. Patients with the SC phenotype can have morbidity as great as those with the SS phenotype (Box 5-1).

Fetal hemoglobin is an effective inhibitor of polymerization of deoxyhemoglobin S. Fetal hemoglobin has alpha and gamma

BOX 5-1.
Sickle Cell Hemoglobinopathies in Decreasing Order of VOC

Homozygous state: SS
Sickle cell SC disease
Sickle cell-beta thalassemia
Heterozygote state: AS

VOC, Vasoocclusive crisis.

chains and no beta chains. It can functionally substitute for the defective beta-globin of sickle cell disease. There has recently been renewed interest in the use of agents that induce hemoglobin F production, such as butyrate and hydroxyurea. These agents may be effective in raising the production of fetal hemoglobin, thereby limiting the occurrence of VOC and other manifestations of sickle cell disease. Fetal hemoglobin levels of 20% are required for this protective effect. Trials with these agents have resulted in a twofold to sixteenfold increase in hemoglobin F and a decrease in the number of painful crises.[3,4] Several chemotherapeutic agents have been shown to increase hemoglobin F production; however, the cytotoxicity of these drugs may preclude their long term administration.[5] Erythropoietin, alone or in combination with hydroxyurea, has not had a significant effect on the percentage of hemoglobin F. Larger trials to determine long-term tolerance, efficacy, and adverse effects of these agents are warranted.

VOC results from the sludging of blood flow because of sickling in the microcirculation. This results in focal and/or regional ischemia with tissue hypoxia. The cascade of events may be triggered by dehydration, acidosis, marked temperature changes, or hypoxic insult. Many times no specific inciting event can be identified. Little is known about the epidemiologic features of vasoocclusive episodes or risk factors for their occurrence. Dr. Platt and colleagues investigated the pain rate (the number of episodes of vasoocclusive crisis per year) in a group of patients with sickle cell disease.[6] Patients with an average of three or more episodes per year had a higher mortality rate than those with fewer than three episodes per year. There was no correlation between pain and mortality in patients younger than 20 years of age. The pain rate varied directly with hematocrit and inversely with blood viscosity.

The management of chronic and acute pain in sickle cell disease must address the clinical and pathophysiologic manifestations of the disease. Transfusions are indicated in the management of severe anemia or complications that are unresponsive to other therapies (acute chest syndrome or priapism). During VOC, rehydration, correction of acidosis, treatment of hypoxia or infection, and adequate analgesic administration are the foundation of the therapeutic regimen. The choice of analgesics continues to be controversial. Mild or moderate pain can often be managed on an outpatient basis with nonsteroidal antiinflammatory drugs (NSAIDs) or the combination of NSAIDs with a weak opioid, such as codeine, oxycodone, or propoxyphene (Table 5-1). Although the combination of the opioid and NSAID in a single tablet may make administration easier, tailoring of analgesic therapy is better performed with single agent medications (separate NSAID and opioid tablets) to allow dose escalations if needed and to avoid excessive intake of NSAIDs. Fixed-interval dosing of ibuprofen (e.g., 10 mg/kg every 6 hrs) or other NSAIDs may effectively lower the total opioid requirements, even for outpatient therapy. This should be supplemented with doses of oral opioids, such as oxycodone, as needed.

Oral codeine is approximately two thirds as effective as parenteral codeine and is usually administered in starting doses of 0.8 to 1 mg/kg every 4 hrs. A percentage of codeine is metabolized by demethylation to morphine, accounting for part of its effect. Oxycodone has similar oral efficacy and is usually started in doses of 0.15 mg/kg every 4 to 6 hrs. Like codeine, oxycodone is dependent on metabolism to an active compound (oxymorphone) for its analgesic effect. Propoxyphene has roughly one fifth the analgesic potency of codeine. Any of these weak opioids can be combined with fixed-interval dosing of NSAIDs, such as ibuprofen.

TABLE 5-1. Treatment of Pain Caused by Otitis Media

Generic Name	Brand Name	Dose
Acetaminophen	Tylenol	10 to 20 mg/kg PO or PR q4h
Ibuprofen	Pediaprofen Advil Motrin	10 mg/kg PO q6h
Acetaminophen + codeine elixir	—	Codeine 0.8 to 1.0 mg/kg q4h

PO, Per os; *PR,* per rectum; *q4h,* every four hours; *q6h,* every six hours.

Oral agents are frequently used for outpatient management of mild to moderate pain crisis or once severe pain has ceased after the administration of parenteral opioids. Managing severe pain with the "weak opioids" may be hampered by dose-limiting side effects, including nausea, vomiting, and constipation.

Severe pain is better managed by hospitalization and parenteral opioids, such as morphine, hydromorphone, or methadone. Morphine is the gold standard with which all other opioids are compared and is widely used in the management of severe acute and chronic pain. Morphine is metabolized in the gut wall and liver to morphine-6-glucuronide (M6G) and morphine-3-glucuronide (M3G). M6G has been shown to be a potent agonist at the mu receptors with both analgesic and respiratory depressant effects. Since its half-life is significantly longer than that of the parent compound, it may accumulate with prolonged morphine administration. The half-life of M6G is dependent on renal excretion and therefore may accumulate in patients with renal dysfunction. Hydromorphone is 5 to 7 times more potent than morphine. It may be effective when adverse effects, such as pruritus, occur with morphine. Since it has no active metabolites, it can be used without adjusting the dose in patients with renal insufficiency. The use of methadone is well established in patients requiring long-term opioid analgesics; however, because of its long half-life, it has limited flexibility for the management of acute pain.

A recent survey by Pegelow reveals that meperidine is the most frequently used parenteral opioid.[7] Intramuscular (IM) meperidine has been a popular means of pain control in patients with sickle cell disease. However, repeated intramuscular injections may lead to the formation of infected or sterile abscesses and tissue fibrosis. Additionally, the IM administration of opioids results in erratic and unpredictable serum levels. The intravenous (IV) route is suggested for the management of severe pain that is unresponsive to oral analgesics. The widespread use of meperidine is probably due in part to the misconception that meperidine produces fewer side effects than other opioids.[8] All opioids, including morphine and meperidine, produce equivalent degrees of respiratory depression when administered in equipotent (equianalgesic) doses.

Some of the major disadvantages of meperidine are its central nervous system (CNS) effects, including dysphoria and seizures. The CNS excitation results from the accumulation of the active metabolite, normeperidine. Normeperidine is more potent than meperidine in terms of excitatory effects but less potent as an analgesic. The intensity of excitation is directly related to the accumulation of plasma levels of normeperidine. The Boston Collaborative Group found that feelings of shakiness occur with plasma normeperidine levels of 422 ng/ml (±53). Grand mal seizures were seen with plasma normeperidine levels of 814 ng/ml (±135).[9] Chronic use of meperidine can result in the accumulation of neurologically toxic levels of normeperidine. Since normeperidine is dependent on renal excretion, accumulation may occur in the setting of renal failure.

The method of administration of the opioid is as important as the choice of agent. As with other acute pain problems, the dose of opioid must be titrated to achieve the desired effect. There may be as much as a tenfold variability in the opioid requirements among patients during a VOC. Patient controlled analgesia (PCA) is routinely used for postoperative and severe acute pain from other causes. Because PCA requires the patient to participate in his or her own care, it is believed that PCA can foster an internal locus of control and help decrease the feeling of helplessness in the sickle cell patient. Schechter and colleagues found that higher loading doses are required for adequate analgesia with PCA in this patient population.[10] Shapiro and colleagues reported a retrospective study of patients with sickle cell hemoglobinopathy who used PCA for painful crises.[11] Patients used less than 50% of the available dose for PCA administration.

The initial dosing guidelines for PCA use in painful crises are similar to those recommended for postoperative pain (Chapter 2). However, frequent adjustments in the dose may be required because of interpatient variability and fluctuations in the severity of pain with sickle cell disease. Even when parenteral opioids are used, the addition of fixed-interval NSAIDs can be used to decrease total opioid requirements. Most patients will wean themselves and stop using PCA as their pain subsides. Oral analgesics should be instituted once the severe pain has subsided and the patient is able to take oral medications.

Hypoventilation and CNS depression, with further exacerbation of the VOC, are real concerns with opioid use in patients with sickle cell disease. Therefore careful monitoring of patients with frequent adjustments of the doses is mandatory to ensure patient safety. When properly administered, PCA appears to be the most effective way of controlling acute pain of any etiology. Hourly infusion rates, PCA bolus doses, and maximum doses must be reassessed at regular intervals. Ideally, PCA should be instituted under the guidance of a multidisciplinary pain service in consultation with the primary physician.

Currently, there is no standard approach to the management of acute or chronic pain related to sickle cell disease. Current treatment strategies include the following: (1) the multidisciplinary approach, (2) behavioral regulation, (3) the administration of high dose steroids, (4) the cancer pain management model, (5) IV analgesia, and (6) regional anesthesia and analgesia.

Multidisciplinary approaches for acute and chronic pain management have been developed for adults and are under development for children. No single discipline has the expertise to treat all patients with sickle cell disease who have pain problems. Therefore a team approach of integrated disciplines better addresses most aspects of the patient's pain experience.[12] Multidisciplinary and interdisciplinary pain service centers can be composed of primary care physicians, anesthesiologists, psychologists, surgical subspecialists, and physical therapists. Patients may be seen in consultation or treated as primary service patients under the care of the pain service.

Although opioids remain the mainstay for the treatment of acute painful crisis, adjunctive techniques may offer several benefits. It is possible that hypnosis, relaxation training, cognitive strategies, and biofeedback may reduce the frequency of emergency room visits and hospitalizations by as much as 33% in patients with sickle cell disease.[13,14] Zeltzer and colleagues demonstrated that hypnosis was able to reduce the length of hospital stay and total dose of analgesics in a selected patient population.[14] Cozzi and colleagues reported that the frequency of emergency room visits was not decreased when comparing a six-month period before and after biofeedback training;[15] however, 70% of the patients reported that the training helped them to lessen the intensity of crisis symptoms, including headache and vasoocclusive pain. Self-regulating measures, such as thermal and electromyographic (EMG) biofeedback, as well as hypnosis and cognitive therapy, may be helpful in mild cases of sickle cell related pain. These studies had small study populations, and prospective studies of larger sample size are needed to determine if such therapies are truly effective.

Corticosteroids may be useful as adjuncts to analgesic therapy. Griffin and colleagues recently demonstrated the efficacy of IV high-dose methylprednisolone for pain management in children and adolescents with sickle cell disease.[16] A dose of 15 mg/kg methylprednisolone to a maximum of 1 g was administered on admission with a second dose given 24 hours later. The high-dose steroids decreased the duration of severe pain in children and adolescents. However, more rebound attacks were observed in the patients who received methylprednisolone. No adverse effects were observed. Caution must be exercised when using high-dose corticosteroids because of the associated risks of aseptic necrosis of the femoral head, bacterial infection, and adrenal suppression. Although the shortened course of VOC is an attractive feature of steroid administration, the likelihood of rebound attacks may limit their usefulness.

Brookoff and Polomano suggest the use of a chronic cancer pain model for the management of sickle cell pain in adults.[17] They hypothesized that giving sustained-release preparations or continuous IV infusions would result in lower opioid doses and fewer side effects. The investigators used IV and oral, controlled-release morphine instead of IM meperidine and short-acting oral opioids. This strategy alleviated the "as needed" (p.r.n.) basis of pain management. The investigators found that the mean duration of stay declined by two days in their population, and the use of emergency room department and inpatient services decreased.

The importance of the Brookoff study is that the use of long-term opioids for the management of nonmalignant pain may have profound implications for clinical practice in patients with sickle cell disease. There is increasing experience to suggest that some patients with chronic, nonmalignant pain will respond to opioid therapy as clinicians expect those with cancer pain to respond—with responsible drug use and benefits that are clearly greater than the risks.[18,19] Although the study by Brookoff and Polomano has limitations, the observed outcome suggests that this conclusion may be applicable to some patients with sickle cell disease.

The use of epidural analgesia in the management of sickle cell pain was first cited in the American literature as a case report described by Finer and colleagues in 1988. The case involved a 22-year-old primigravida who presented in active labor and vasoocclusive crisis. The institution of epidural analgesia with local anesthetics appeared to abate vasoocclusive crisis. Postpartum pain during the first 24 hours was managed by a neuraxial fentanyl infusion. The patient was free of pain 48 hours after the discontinuation of the epidural opioid.[20] Yaster and colleagues investigated the use of epidural local anesthetics alone and in combination with fentanyl as a continuous infusion for the management of severe, vasoocclusive sickle cell pain.[21] The initiation of epidural analgesia resulted in improved oxygenation and sustained pain relief for the majority of patients. There was a need for adjustments in both the type of local anesthetic administered and opioid doses. Approximately half of the patients developed tachyphylaxis to lidocaine within 48 to 72 hours after epidural administration. Although the use of regional anesthetic techniques, such as epidural anesthesia, are still relatively anecdotal for patients with sickle cell pain, its use makes physiologic sense. In addition to providing effective analgesia, epidural anesthesia may also induce a sympathetic blockade with peripheral vasodilatation, which may improve regional blood flow and decrease sludging in the microcirculation. It may be speculated that epidural anesthesia not only treats pain, but it may also act as a therapeutic modality by altering regional blood flow.

Other regional anesthetic techniques that may be employed for pain of the lower extremities include continuous femoral nerve blockade and fascia iliac compartment blockade. (The techniques involved for these blocks are discussed further in Chapter 4.) These techniques can be used with intermittent dosing or a continuous infusion. Such techniques may limit opioid requirements, thereby limiting opioid-induced side effects.

Regardless of the regional anesthetic technique, there remains a small possibility of infection as a result of an indwelling catheter. This may be particularly worrisome in the sickle cell patient since intermittent fevers are common during VOC. However, regional procedures with indwelling catheters have been used in patients with temperatures up to 39.5°C without the development of local or systemic related infections. Regional techniques should be considered when conventional, parenteral opioid therapy fails or results in complications.

The enormous health and economic impact of sickle cell disease is estimated to be more than $705 million per year. Such a figure strongly argues for increased attention to this disorder. Fears of addiction have been expressed by both healthcare providers and patient populations. Attitudes about the propensity for addiction among black adolescents may interfere with pain management. The studies to date have not demonstrated a higher risk of addiction among adolescents with sickle cell disease. This prejudice may unnecessarily raise the issue of addiction and could lead to serious lapses in treatment of sickle cell patients, thereby contributing to their dysfunction. Pseudoaddiction may result as an iatrogenic syndrome. Inadequate pain relief results in increased requests for analgesics. The healthcare team is then concerned that the frequent requests for medication indicate that the patient is becoming opioid dependent. Therefore, they continue to prescribe medication on a p.r.n. basis, at an inadequate dose, and by an ineffective schedule. The caretakers assume that this will prevent, or at least delay, the onset of both opioid tolerance and dependence. Subsequently the patient feels angry and isolated and may develop a sense of helplessness. In turn, the healthcare team feels frustrated and avoids the patient. A mutual distrust and an adversarial relationship results. Proper supportive care and analgesic administration prevent such an adversarial situation from developing.

ONCOLOGIC DISEASES

Issues of pain control have become increasingly important in the care of pediatric cancer patients. Increased rates of survival from childhood cancer are attributable to advances in chemotherapeutic and radiation therapy regimens. However, the treatment regimens may be highly toxic and contribute to the pain experienced by the children who receive them. In addition, adverse effects, such as mucositis, dermatitis, radiation burns, and drug induced neuropathy, can magnify the painful effects of the regimens.

These treatment regimens also impact on the patients because of the invasive procedures needed for routine surveillance during and after therapy. Such procedures include frequent venipuncture, lumbar punctures (LP), and bone marrow aspirates and biopsies, which many children find more painful than the underlying condition. The next section of this chapter deals briefly with strategies to deal with therapy related problems, such as mucositis, as well as techniques for sedation during invasive procedures.

Procedural pain is perceived by most children as the number one cause of pain associated with oncologic diseases rather than the malignancy itself. (A full discussion of the pharmacologic agents available to alleviate procedure-related pain and anxiety are outlined in Chapter 8.) Pain related to repeated venipuncture has become less of a problem since many children have permanent central venous-access devices (e.g., Hackman catheter or Port-a-cath) that can be used to obtain blood samples and administer IV medications. However, such devices may not be placed until initial therapy has been instituted; therefore, frequent venipuncture may be necessary. With the advent of EMLA cream (eutetic mixture of local anesthetics), the skin can be anesthetized before the needle sticks. It is important to remember that EMLA cream must be placed on the skin at least one hour before the procedure in order to be effective. It can also be applied to the skin of the lumbar spine to decrease the intensity of the needlestick from an LP and potentially decrease the amount of sedation needed to perform the procedure.

In younger patients, deep sedation may be required for the performance of both LPs and bone marrow aspirates. This type of sedation, no matter where it is performed, requires a person to monitor the child, monitoring equipment (at the minimum a pulse oximeter), available supplemental oxygen, a working suction apparatus, and ready access to resuscitation equipment because of the risk of decreased respiratory effort and ultimately decreased oxygenation. (The agents used for sedation and analgesia during LP and bone marrow aspiration and biopsy are discussed in Chapter 8.)

Because of the frequency of these procedures in certain patients, a sedation log should be kept to include which drugs have been used in the past, the doses required, and the child's response to the specific agents. This gives valuable information in the event that different physicians are called upon at different times to sedate the same patient.

Mucositis is a common side effect from the intensive chemotherapy and radiation regimens used for childhood malignancies. Its incidence is directly related to the intensity of the chemotherapy and occurs in up to 90% of patients receiving bone marrow transplantation. Since the epithelial cells of the gastrointestinal (GI) system are rapidly-dividing cells (like the bone marrow cells), they are readily affected by the chemotherapeutic agents. Although the initial investigation may indicate that mucositis is limited primarily to the oropharynx, the entire GI tract can be affected. Mucositis can cover the whole spectrum from isolated aphthous ulcers to generalized desquamation of the entire enteral mucosa.

In isolated cases, mucositis may be related to secondary infectious processes, such as candidiasis or herpes simplex virus infection. In these cases, palliative therapy with analgesic agents should be combined with specific antiinfectious agents. For candidiasis, this may include oral nystatin or chlorhexidine gluconate swishes. Prophylactic use of chlorhexidine gluconate has been shown to decrease the severity of mucositis by preventing bacterial and candidal superinfection of the damaged mucosa. Although topical therapy is a useful adjunct to the treatment and prevention of mucositis, parenteral opioid therapy is required to control pain in many cases.

In the majority of cases, mucositis is the result of intensive chemotherapy and not an infectious complication. In these cases, palliative therapy is required until there is a recovery of the neutrophil count. A resolution of the problem usually occurs when the absolute neutrophil count reaches 500 to 1000 cells/ml.[3] It has been suggested that the neutrophils either eliminate microfoci of infection within the ulcers, thus allowing them to heal, or that they act directly by stimulating wound healing and reepithelialization. Preliminary data concerning the use of colony-stimulating factors suggest that they may play a role in reducing the severity and limiting the duration of mucositis.

The goal of therapy is to provide analgesia until the normal healing process occurs. This may include the combination of topical medications combined with parenteral analgesic agents. Some topical therapies and their proposed mechanisms and therapeutic effects are outlined in Box 5-2. A suggested approach to the prevention and treatment of mucositis is outlined in Box 5-3. Although topical anesthetics, such as viscous lidocaine or dyclonine mouthwash, can effectively anesthetize the oral mucosa, absorption of local anesthetics can be rapid through the abraded oral mucosa. The risk of systemic toxicity is magnified in the pediatric patient because of his or her smaller size. Therefore topical medications should be used sparingly, if at all, with strict attention to avoid exceeding recommended dosing guidelines. They should be used once a day, perhaps at bedtime. Capsaicin has recently been suggested to ameliorate the pain of mucositis. This agent depletes peripheral nerves of substance P, thereby decreas-

BOX 5-2.
Agents Used in the Treatment of Mucositis

Agent	Mechanism or Therapeutic Effect
Lip balm	Prevents cracking and bleeding of dried lips.
Toothbrush	Removes loose debris. Limit use with thrombocytopenia.
Toothette	Similar to the effect of a toothbrush but with less chance of trauma.
Normal saline rinse	Removes debris.
Sodium bicarbonate	Neutralizes intraoral pH. Loosens debris.
Chlorhexidine rinse	Potent antibacterial action. Decreases secondary infection of abraded mucosa.
Nystatin rinse	Treats secondary candidal infections.
Hydrogen peroxide	Not recommended. Delays healing by breakdown of proteins.
Mylanta	Increases oral pH. Coating action protects mucosa.
Sucralfate suspension	Increases oral pH. Coating action protects mucosa.
Commercial mouthwash	Not recommended. High alcohol content can be painful.
Benadryl elixir	Topical anesthetic action.
Viscous lidocaine	Topical anesthetic action. Repeated doses can lead to toxicity.
Dyclonine mouthwash	Topical anesthetic action. Repeated doses can lead to toxicity.
Oral capsaicin lozenges	Inhibits nociceptive activity of free nerve endings, perhaps related blockade of substance P release.

ing nociceptive input to the CNS. Although the information concerning its use is still relatively preliminary, capsaicin has been incorporated into a lozenge that may have some role in the treatment of mucositis. Severe involvement may lead to dysphagia and inability to take oral medications. In such cases, parenteral opioids may be indicated and should be dosed as described in Chapter 2 for postoperative pain. As in most cases of acute pain,

BOX 5-3.
Suggested Scheme for the Prevention and Treatment of Mucositis

- Get a professional cleaning and evaluation by a dentist.
- Carefully clean the teeth and tongue with a toothette or soft toothbrush.
- Rinse the mouth for 1 minute after meals and at bedtime with a nonirritating solution, such as normal saline.
- Avoid commercial mouthwashes, which may contain alcohol.
- Apply lip balm to prevent cracking and bleeding.
- Rinse three times a day with chlorhexidine rinse.
- If crusting develops, rinse with a half-strength bicarbonate solution.
- Treat other infectious etiologies, such as candida or herpes simplex.
- Avoid repeated use of topical anesthetic solutions or preparations.
- Get oral opioid therapy for mild to moderate cases or parenteral opioid therapy by PCA for severe pain or if unable to ingest oral medications.

regardless of the etiology, PCA seems to be the superior method for providing analgesia.

Acute pain in the pediatric oncology patient may be related to the disease process itself, or it may be the presenting complaint or a manifestation of the terminal stages of the disease. Pain related to the initial presentation of the disease may be treated with oral medications for mild to moderate pain, or it may require parenteral opioids for moderate to severe pain. Problems such as severe bony pain with leukemia usually subside once the underlying disease process is treated. Rarely, the acute pain accompanying the underlying disease cannot be controlled, or more commonly, pain recurs as a manifestation of the terminal stages of the disease. In such cases, the issues surrounding pain management become those of a chronic problem, necessitating the use of a continuous opioid regimen supplemented with additional doses for breakthrough pain. The opioid regimen can consist of oral therapy for many patients, thereby eliminating the need for chronic IV access and, at times, the need for hospitalization. In such cases, the baseline analgesic regimen should include an opioid preparation, taken two or three times a day, that maintains a steady state serum concentration. This can be accomplished with methadone or long-acting preparations of opioids, such as morphine (MS-Contin) or hydromorphone. These agents are administered on a fixed-interval schedule every 8 or 12 hours and supplemented with p.r.n. doses of oral opioids, such as oxycodone, hydrocodone, or immediate release morphine or dilaudid. The latter two are available as liquid preparations. The fentanyl transdermal system has also been used to treat cancer pain. Although not suitable for routine use to control postoperative pain, it may be used instead of long-acting oral preparations of opioids to provide a steady state serum concentration. Even with transdermal fentanyl, breakthrough pain occurs and needs to be treated with supplemental doses of opioids.

Adjuvant therapy may be helpful when dealing with terminal malignancy pain. Oral NSAIDs may provide some degree of analgesia and allow for a decrease in the total opioid dose, thereby limiting opioid-related side effects. Tricyclic antidepressants (TCAs) may be helpful for reducing both chronic and neuropathic pain. This is true even in the patient who is not clinically depressed. These agents alter the concentrations of various neurotransmitters within the CNS, thereby modulating the nociceptive input. The most commonly used TCAs are amitriptyline and nortriptyline, given at small doses at bedtime to avoid the disturbing anticholinergic side effects, such as dry mouth, blurred vision, and sedation.

Neuropathic pain has multiple etiologies and may be the most severe pain associated with childhood malignancy. Unlike acute pain of other etiologies, it may be refractory to even high doses of opioids. Several etiologies of neuropathic pain have been described, such as direct nerve compression from a tumor or metastatic disease, radiation-induced nerve injury, or chemotherapy induced from agents such as vincristine. Tumor compression and radiation effects can lead to pain and dysesthesias that are described as numbness and tingling to severe intractable burning or dysesthetic pain, usually in the extremities.

Anticonvulsants may also be tried as adjuvant therapy for neuropathic pain. They are used at doses lower than those needed for control of clinical seizure activity. Their mechanism of analgesic action is through the alteration of CNS neuronal excitability. The two most commonly used agents are phenytoin and carbamazepine. Serum levels of these two agents must be closely monitored in all patients to avoid toxicity. Both agents can cause alterations in hepatic function and bone marrow suppression.

Corticosteroids may also be helpful in the treatment of neuropathic pain, particularly if there is direct tumor compression of a nerve or nerve root. These agents (e.g., dexamethaxone) are used to decrease tumor swelling and may alleviate some of the intractable pain from direct nerve compression.

Chronic pain remains a major problem, especially in the terminal stages of some pediatric malignancies. The recent availability of hospice care for pediatric patients allows for alternatives in pain management when oral outpatient therapy fails. Hospice care facilities are staffed with healthcare workers who are facile in the management of pain associated with the terminal stages of malignancies. Alternatively, home nursing may be available to allow the patient to stay at home and receive parenteral (IV or subcutaneous) opioids.

ACUTE PAIN ASSOCIATED WITH SPECIFIC CLINICAL PROBLEMS

Otitis Media

Otitis media remains one of the most common infectious problems seen in the pediatric patient. Although the causative bacteria are usually not identified, infections are treated empirically based on epidemiologic data. Before the availability of modern antibiotics, otitis pain was treated symptomatically (compresses, etc.). With the advent of antibiotics, medical treatment has been directed at the underlying infectious etiology. Medical treatment failures may require surgical intervention for myringotomy and tube placement. The differential diagnosis of otitis media is usually not difficult. The difficulty lies in finding an effective antibiotic or determining at what point surgical treatment is appropriate.

The ear is innervated by the auriculotemporal nerve, which is a branch of the third division (mandibular) of the fifth (trigeminal) cranial nerve (V3). The auriculotemporal nerve innervates the anterior surface of the ear, as well as the interior of the auditory canal. The inferior portion of the tympanic membrane is innervated by a branch of the tenth (vagus) cranial nerve. The medial aspect of the tympanic membrane and the mucosa of the eustachian tube are supplied by a branch of the ninth (glossopharyngeal) cranial nerve.[22] The external ear is innervated by the greater auricular nerve, which arises from the cervical plexus.

Otitis media is a moderately painful condition. Increased pressure in the middle ear results from eustachian tube dysfunction. Inflammation and swelling results in occlusion of the eustachian tubes, which are important in pressure equalization. In addition, toxic byproducts of localized infection are also important causes of otalgia.

Treatment is directed at the underlying infection. Pain can be a large component, especially early on in the disease process. Patients receiving antibiotics may have their pain treated with acetaminophen (10 to 15 mg/kg every 4 hrs) or ibuprofen elixir (10 mg/kg every 6 hrs). Another option, if the pain is persistent, is the use of both acetaminophen every 4 hours and ibuprofen every 6 hours. In this way, a dose of an analgesic is administered every 2 to 3 hours. Occasionally, acetaminophen with codeine may be required. The commercially available acetaminophen with codeine elixir contains 120 mg of acetaminophen and 12 mg of codeine per 5 ml (teaspoon). The dose should be based on the codeine content (0.8 to 1 mg/kg every 4 to 6 hrs). Since this contains only 10 mg/kg of acetaminophen, additional acetaminophen up to 20 mg/kg every 4 hrs can be administered.

Patients who have myringotomy and insertion of pressure-equalizing tubes may experience moderate discomfort postoperatively. This procedure usually requires general anesthesia in all but the most cooperative children. It is a brief surgical procedure, frequently lasting less than three minutes. For general anesthesia, the child spontaneously ventilates a mixture of nitrous oxide and oxygen in an increasing concentration of halothane. An IV line is usually not placed. Immediate postoperative pain may be treated with acetaminophen (orally or rectally), ibuprofen, or acetaminophen with codeine elixir (see Table 5-1). Alternatively, acetaminophen with codeine may be administered as part of the premedication.[23] This eliminates the delay in onset of action (15 to 20 minutes) that occurs with oral administration of any medication. Acetaminophen with codeine is superior to acetaminophen alone in controlling postoperative pain after placement of pressure equalization (PE) tubes.[23] It is common for these children to require one or two additional doses of acetaminophen at home after surgery.

Chest Pain

Chest pain is a common complaint among school-age children and adolescents. Chest pain may be caused by pathology in a number of organ systems, and the differentiation is not always simple (Box 5-4). In other cases, a primary cause may be found and the treatment options are clear.

The chest is innervated by nerves that arise from the thoracic spinal segments. Each rib is accompanied by an intercostal nerve in the groove just inferior to it, which supplies the overlying chest wall. The thoracic viscera (heart, pericardium, and pleura) are innervated by sympathetic fibers and spinal nerves from T_1 to T_4, whereas the lower thoracic wall and diaphragm are supplied by T_5 and T_6. The peritoneal surface of the diaphragm is also supplied by the thoracic nerves, as is much of the abdominal viscera, which explains why abdominal GI pain is often referred to the distribution of the thoracic dermatomes.

True cardiac etiologies of chest pain are rare in children but are among the most frightening. Most children and their parents know someone with ischemic coronary artery disease. Reports of otherwise healthy athletes and adolescents who experience sudden cardiac death appear in the newspaper or on television. Cardiac causes of chest pain include myocardial ischemia (due most commonly to the anomalous origin of a coronary artery, cocaine ingestion, or aortic stenosis), myocarditis, pericarditis, myocardial contusion, or

BOX 5-4.
Common Causes of Chest Pain

Cardiac

Myocardial ischemia
Coronary artery vasospasm
Myocarditis
Pericarditis
Palpitations
Arrhythmias

Gastrointestinal

Esophagitis
Gastroesophageal reflux
Achalasia
Esophageal spasm
Gastric distension
Gastritis
Peptic ulcer disease
Constipation

Musculoskeletal

Costochondritis
Muscle spasm or strain
Bone or soft tissue trauma
Herpes zoster
Rib fracture
Fibromyalgia
Cystic fibrosis
Sickle cell disease
Slipping rib syndrome

Pulmonary

Pneumonia
Pleural effusion
Pleuritis
Pneumothorax
Cystic fibrosis (muscle strain from coughing)
Pulmonary embolism
Sickle cell disease (acute chest syndrome)
Chest tube insertion

irritation of the pericardial serosa (pericardial effusion). Palpitations may be reported as chest pain and may be caused by drugs (theophylline or caffeine), mitral valve prolapse, or supraventricular tachycardia caused by an aberrant conduction pathway.

The evaluation to rule out cardiac pathology should include a complete history and physical examination. Positive findings noted on the physical examination (e.g., murmur or abnormal rhythm) should dictate the ensuing work-up. In the vast majority of cases, no etiology is found and reassurance and expectant management are appropriate.

Although it is among the benign causes of chest pain, the GI system is responsible for some of the more common etiologies of chest pain. Pain may originate in the esophagus (e.g., esophagitis caused by ingestion, gastroesophageal reflux, achalasia, esophageal spasm, or hiatal hernia), or it may be referred to the chest from the abdomen. Common causes of abdominal pain with a referred component to the chest include gastric distention, resulting from delayed gastric emptying, constipation, or gastritis caused by viral illness or ingestion of NSAIDs. This may be especially common in patients who are treated with NSAIDs for other types of pain.

There are numerous etiologies of chest pain that are musculoskeletal in origin. These tend to present with more localized and less diffuse pain. Such problems include costochondritis, muscle spasm from overuse, blunt trauma (from sports injury, motor vehicle accidents, or physical abuse), slipping rib syndrome, herpes zoster, fibromyalgia, cystic fibrosis, sickle cell disease, or tumor involvement of the chest wall. Differentiation and treatment of the above etiologies are usually straightforward. This may include rest for overuse or traumatic injuries and the judicious use of NSAIDs. The NSAIDs have become increasingly popular in the treatment of a large number of painful conditions, especially musculoskeletal injuries. Although they are generally safe and effective, their use is associated with an increased incidence of gastritis, which can also lead to moderate pain.

As a class, pulmonary processes represent a common cause of acute chest pain. The underlying cause of the pain (e.g., pneumonia, pleuritis, or cystic fibrosis) is usually readily apparent based on the patient's medical history and a physical examination. Pleuritic chest pain (pain aggravated by deep inspiration) may be due to any process that causes diaphragmatic or pleural irritation, such as pneumonia, pleural effusion, pleuritis, or pneumothorax. Pulmonary embolism (more common in female adolescents who use both tobacco and oral contraceptives) and asthma can also have a significant component of chest pain. Acute chest syndrome in patients with sickle cell disease, prolonged coughing spells in patients with cystic fibrosis or asthma, and hyperventilation are all associated with chest pain. Trauma, whether from automobile accidents or related to a sports injury, may result in rib fractures with or without pneumothorax or pulmonary contusion.

Although the differentiation of the causes of pulmonary chest pain is usually not difficult, management of the pain often is. Ineffective management can result in significant morbidity. In certain conditions, such as flail chest or multiple rib fractures, the associated pulmonary morbidity of chest pain can be high, leading to ineffective respiratory function and hypoxemia or cardiopulmonary failure. At times, the treatment is aimed at the underlying pathology. For example, chest pain associated with pneumothorax may require insertion of a chest tube. Unfortunately, the treatment may cause as much or more pain than the original illness (pleural or intercostal irritation).

The treatment of chest pain depends on its etiology. Cardiac and GI pain are usually managed by treating the underlying problem, whereas musculoskeletal and pulmonary pain may require analgesic agents (Table 5-1). In the case of some causes of pain, adequate and aggressive treatment of pain may reduce morbidities, such as hypoventilation or respiratory failure.

Treatment of musculoskeletal or pulmonary pain must balance improvement in pulmonary function and increases in lung volumes with any side effects caused by the treatment. Mild to moderate pain caused by inflammation may be treated with acetaminophen (10 to 15 mg/kg PO [per os] or PR [per rectum] every 3 to 4 hrs) or NSAIDs such as ibuprofen (10 mg/kg every 6 hrs). Ketorolac (0.5 mg/kg IV every 6 hrs) can be used in patients unable to tolerate oral medications. The use of ketorolac is recommended for a maximum of 3 days. It should only be used in patients who are well-hydrated, who are not at risk for bleeding because of platelet inhibition, and who have normal renal function. It may also be given intramuscularly (IM), but this is not recommended in the pediatric population. Ketorolac is contraindicated in patients allergic to aspirin or other NSAIDs. Patients with chronic or recurrent chest pain caused by cystic fibrosis may benefit from the addition of low-dose TCAs to their pain management regimen. Transcutaneous electrical nerve stimulators (TENS) have also been used in the cystic fibrosis population with some success.

More severe pain may be treated with oral opioids, such as codeine (0.8 to 1.0 mg/kg PO every 4 hrs) in younger children and oxycodone (0.1 to 0.15 mg/kg every 4 hrs) or hydrocodone in older children (Table 5-2). Severe pain, unresponsive to oral opioids, may require hospitalization and IV opioids. PCA, with or without a basal rate, is an effective option in patients over age 6. Adolescents do especially well controlling their own analgesia. This requires some teaching of both the patient and parents concerning the use of this method of drug delivery.

All opioids are respiratory depressants and their beneficial effects must be weighed against the risk of adverse effects. However, severe pain, especially of the chest wall, can have significant deleterious effects on respiratory function, and it can lead to respiratory failure. Other side effects of opioids include pruritus, nausea, vomiting, and constipation. Some patients may be extremely sensitive to the sedative effects (e.g., those with cystic fibrosis) or poorly tolerant of hypoxia (sickle cell). Conversely, these same patients may be tolerant of the analgesic action of opioids and require staggeringly large doses for adequate pain relief. The concomitant use of NSAIDs may be synergistic, allowing a lower opioid dose.

TABLE 5-2. Oral Preparations of Common Analgesic Agents

Generic Name	Trade Name	Formulation	Dosage
Acetaminophen	Tylenol	Elixir (160 mg/5 ml); Tablets (80 mg, 325 mg)	10-20 mg/kg q4h PO
		Suppository (120 mg)	10-20 mg/kg q4h PR
Ibuprofen	Pediaprofen,	Elixir (100 mg/5 ml)	10-15 mg/kg q6h PO
	Advil, Motrin	Tablets (100, 200, 300, 400, 800 mg)	10 mg/kg q6h PO
Ketorolac	Toradol	Injection (15, 30, 60 mg)	0.5 mg q6h IV
Codeine	Tylenol w/ codeine	Elixir (120 mg/12 mg/5 ml)	0.8-1.0 mg/kg q4h PO
	Tylenol #2	Tablets (300 mg/15 mg)	(based on codeine)
	Tylenol #3	Tablets (300 mg/30 mg)	
	Tylenol #4	Tablets (300 mg/60 mg)	
Oxycodone	Percocet	Tablets (325 mg acetaminophen/5 mg)	0.1 mg/kg q4h PO
	Percodan	Tablets (325 mg ASA/5 mg)	(based on oxycodone)
	Tylox	Tablets (500 mg acetaminophen/5 mg)	
Hydrocodone	Lorcet HD	Tablets (500 mg acetaminophen/5 mg)	0.1 mg/kg q4h PO
	Lorcet Plus	Tablets (650 mg acetaminophen/7.5 mg)	(hydrocodone)
	Lortab	Elixir (167 mg acetaminophen/2.5 mg/5 ml)	
		Tablets (500 mg acetaminophen/2.5 mg)	
		Tablets (500 mg acetaminophen/5 mg)	
		Tablets (500 mg acetaminophen/7.5 mg)	
	Vicodin	Tablets (500 mg acetaminophen/5 mg)	
	Vicodin ES	Tablets (750 mg acetaminophen/7.5 mg)	
Hydromorphone	Dilaudid	Suppository (3 mg), Elixir (5 mg/5 ml), Tablets (2, 4, 8 mg)	0.03-0.05 mg/kg q4h

q4h, Every four hours; *q6h,* every six hours; *PO,* per os; *PR,* per rectum; *ASA,* acetylsalicylic acid.

Patients with severe pain, or those with inadequate control because of side effects from opioids, may benefit from epidural analgesia. This requires the availability of an anesthesiologist around the clock to treat problems or adjust dosages. It also requires a nursing staff that has been instructed concerning the care of patients with epidural catheters. In many hospitals, protocol allows epidural anesthesia to be delivered only in monitored care settings, such as the intensive care unit (ICU) or intermediate care unit.

Various combinations of drugs (opioids and local anesthetics) may be used for epidural analgesia (see Chapter 3). Epidural opioids may cause pruritus, nausea, vomiting, and urinary retention. All patients must have IV access in the event that opioid mediated respiratory depression occurs. This is easily treated by the administration of incremental doses of the opioid antagonist, naloxone (2 μg/kg every 2 mins up to 10 μg/kg).

Patients who have chest tubes may benefit from the administration of a local anesthetic agent through the chest tube (see Chapter 4). A long-acting local anesthetic, such as bupivacaine, is usually chosen. The local anesthetic is instilled through the chest tube, which is then clamped for 20 minutes. The patient may be encouraged to assume different positions to facilitate spread of the local anesthetic solution. The chest tube is then returned to suction. This procedure may be repeated every 6 to 8 hours as needed. The chest tube should not be clamped if there is a persistent air leak and risk of tension pneumothorax. The total volume that can be instilled is dependent on the patient's weight, the concentration of the local anesthetic, and the local anesthetic used. (These recommendations are discussed in Chapters 3 and 4.) The maximum allowable dose of bupivacaine is 3 mg/kg, which includes 1.2 ml/kg of the 0.25% solution or 0.6 ml/kg of the 0.5% solution. Because of volume constraints, the efficacy of this technique may be limited in smaller patients. Unfortunately, this treatment modality is limited because of the systemic absorption of the local anesthetic by the vascular pleura and the need for repeated doses, which is labor intensive. If repeated doses are given, careful monitoring for signs of local anesthetic toxicity (perioral paresthesia, change in ECG waveform, or alteration of mental status) is imperative. Confirmation of blood levels of local anesthetics (e.g., lidocaine) can be obtained in many hospital laboratories. The patient must have a patent IV line, and resuscitation equipment must always be available.

Removal of the chest tube can also cause considerable pain. It has recently been demonstrated that the application of EMLA cream around the insertion site for 2 to 3 hours before removal is as effective as an IV bolus of an opioid.

Intercostal nerve blocks provide excellent relief of rib and chest wall pain, but their use is limited by the need for sedation for performance of the block in children and the risk of pneumothorax (see Chapter 4). Although analgesia is usually excellent, the duration is limited by the duration of action of the local anesthetic used, requiring that the block be repeated every 6 to 8 hours. Systemic absorption of the local anesthetic is also a risk, since the intercostal nerve is located in direct proximity to the intercostal artery. This procedure should only be performed by those with experience in performing the block and capable of managing any adverse complications.

Finally, intercostal catheters (see Chapter 4) can be placed percutaneously for the continuous infusion of local anesthetic. Although this avoids the need for repeated procedures, the risk of pneumothorax and systemic absorption of the local anesthetic, as well as the need for sedation for the procedure, limits this modality in children.

Burns and Thermal Injury

Burns and thermal injury are potentially fatal accidents. Among those who survive, many are physically and mentally scarred. Those who do not succumb to asphyxia and acute thermal injury may face a long and painful hospitalization followed by months or years of physical therapy and repeated surgery. With severe injury the initial recovery involves weeks in a burn unit with multiple surgical procedures and painful dressing changes.

Shock, dehydration, smoke inhalation, and carbon monoxide poisoning are all important components of the primary injury. Pain may be physical in nature because of acute burn injury or other coexisting traumatic injuries. It is frequently accompanied by emotional pain in the case of older children who fear disfigurement and are dealing with the loss of friends or family. These concerns are magnified in the case of child abuse victims.

The pain of acute burn injury results from the stimulation of nociceptors at the site of injury. Pain is transmitted via C- and A-delta fibers to the dorsal horn of the spinal cord. The traditional view that third-degree burns are not painful because of destruction of the nociceptors is now known to be false.[24] It is likely that damaged but viable nerve endings at the tissue margins are still functional and may be responsible for pain.[25]

The treatment of an acute burn injury is multifaceted, and pain management must be an integral part of the total care plan. Many of the techniques used are the same as those used to treat acute pain of other etiologies, such as postoperative pain (see Chapter 2). In general, patients have two components to their pain: a static, or baseline, level of pain and a dynamic component that is related to procedures. Assessment of the baseline pain level can be accomplished by calculations based on the percent of body surface area burned and the severity of the burn.[24] Patients may be asked to report their level of discomfort, either verbally or using a pain-scoring system, such as a visual analog scale. Pain treatment is then titrated to achieve the desired effect.

Many of the procedures performed on burn patients take place in the operating room under general anesthesia. These patients are likely to have postoperative pain regardless of whether they had pain preoperatively. The majority of this pain is opioid responsive. However, this may require higher doses of opioids when compared with nonburn patients because of changes in the volume of distribution and the metabolism of opioids.

Pain in the burn unit should be treated with analgesics to control baseline pain, supplemented by additional analgesics or anesthetics, as needed, for procedures such as whirlpool therapy or dressing changes. One of the mainstays of therapy is acetaminophen around the clock. It is helpful in controlling pain, decreasing the total opioid requirements, and treating temperature elevation. NSAIDs may be helpful as well. Unfortunately, their adverse effects on platelet function may limit their usefulness in this setting. In addition, NSAIDs may be nephrotoxic, especially in the setting of hypovolemic patients.

Opioids are the mainstay of pain control in the burn patient. They may be given orally or parenterally, continuously or on demand. Dosages should be adjusted, as needed, for each patient rather than based on any specific dosage guidelines. The proper amount of any opioid is that which provides adequate analgesia without intolerable side effects. A common problem among burn patients is the rapid development of tolerance, requiring increasing doses to achieve adequate analgesia. Metabolism may also be increased, contributing to the need for larger doses.[26] This is not to imply that opioids should be withheld from these patients but to stress that management may be difficult, and repeated assessment of the level of analgesia and the need to titrate doses is imperative.

In select patients, adequate analgesia may be obtained by the administration of local anesthetics and/or opioids via an epidural catheter. Epidural analgesia is most applicable for patients with lower extremity or abdominal injuries. Contraindications include burn wounds at the proposed entry site, coagulopathy, or sepsis, all of which occur frequently in the burn patient.

Some components of burn pain may be neuropathic because of direct nerve injury by either burn or other trauma. Neuropathic pain is characteristically unresponsive to opioid analgesics. Although there is little clinical experience among children, continuous infusions of lidocaine[27] or administration of anticonvulsants (e.g., carbamazepine) or tricyclic antidepressants[28] may be helpful in reducing the total opioid dose and improving pain scores.

Pain associated with procedures such as dressing changes may be difficult to manage. (Guidelines and recommended medications for sedating patients during invasive and noninvasive procedures are reviewed in Chapter 8.) Patients who are intubated may have additional opioids administered, as needed, to limit the hemodynamic response to painful stimuli with little concern for respiratory depression. For patients who are not intubated, significant respiratory depression may occur with the dose of opioid that is required to control the procedural pain. Small amounts of opioids, most commonly 1 to 2 μg/kg fentanyl IV may be titrated and repeated, as needed, every 3 to 5 mins. Ketamine is extremely useful in this setting since it confers sedation and analgesia with minimal respiratory depression. Doses of 0.5 to 1 mg/kg IV may be repeated every 3 to 5 mins as needed. Although ketamine may often leave airway reflexes intact, this should never be taken for granted, and airway management equipment and personnel to properly manage the airway must be immediately available. Increased secretions are a common problem with ketamine usage unless an antisialogogue, such as glycopyrrolate, is given. The dysphoria associated with ketamine can usually be prevented by the coadministration of a benzodiazepine, such as midazolam or lorazepam. Tolerance to ketamine, necessitating an escalation of the dose, may develop after repeated administration.

Propofol has become a recent favorite in selected burn units and ICUs. This short-acting anesthetic agent provides sedation without analgesia in subanesthetic doses. Because of its brief duration of action, it is generally administered by a continuous infusion, except for the briefest of procedures. Although spontaneous respiration may be preserved at lower doses, propofol can cause loss of airway reflexes and apnea in higher doses. Hypotension related to its negative inotropic and vasodilator properties may occur in the hypovolemic patient.

Issues of loss of control by the patient on his or her environment may make coping difficult, especially for school-age children and adolescents. Use of PCA may be helpful in restoring a small amount of control to the patient. These techniques may be used in patients with burn injuries to the hands by allowing the nurse or family member to activate the device when the patient complains of pain. It is imperative that the device is only activated in direct response to a patient's complaint of pain. Self-participation in dressing changes is another method to increase patient involvement.[29] The role of hypnosis[30] and relaxation techniques are inherently appealing, but their use in children is currently limited. The availability of psychologic counseling to deal with the multiple issues of loss and grief is of paramount importance.

Trauma-Related Pain

Accidents are a leading cause of morbidity and mortality among children. Pain can be a major problem in the management of those who survive. In addition to the pain related to the initial injury, many patients will have undergone surgical procedures to investigate for concealed trauma or to repair a primary injury.

The acute pain suffered during trauma is an appropriate response to tissue injury. In the acute setting it may be appropriate not to treat the pain until a complete survey of the patient and his or her injuries has been completed. This can be accomplished in the initial 5 to 10 minutes after admission. The initial investigation should include a history of the patient's underlying medical issues, if any, as well as details about the nature of the traumatic injury. This may be obtained from the patient, parents, or other observers. A physical examination follows, along with laboratory and radiographic studies as indicated.

Pain localized to different parts of the body may be reported and treated differently. Traumatic injuries to the scalp are painful and have the potential for extensive blood loss, which is frequently underestimated. Skull fractures may be present with or without scalp injuries but are generally not reported as painful. The frequent accompaniment of closed head injury in the pediatric patient may lead to an altered mental status. The treatment of pain or combativeness in the patient with a closed head injury may be extremely difficult. In addition to increasing the risk of adverse cardiorespiratory effects from sedative and analgesic agents, the association of a closed head injury mandates repeated physical assessments that may be altered by analgesic agents. If the combative patient requires an imaging procedure, control of the airway and mechanical ventilation may be the safest alternative. This can be discontinued once the imaging procedures are completed.

An epidural hematoma or a subdural hemorrhage may be reported simply as a headache but not necessarily as severe pain. Contusions characteristically are not painful, since the brain parenchyma has no pain sensation. Other causes of head pain are listed in Box 5-5.

Neck pain can have multiple etiologies in the trauma patient (Box 5-6). Cervical tenderness should be viewed as an ominous sign and suggests the possibility of cervical spine injury (cervical vertebral fractures). Immobility of the spine is mandatory until a cervical injury can be ruled out radiographically. Neck pain may also be due to shoulder injury or referred cardiac pain.

Chest pain has multiple etiologies, such as the cardiac (cardiac contusion, traumatic rupture of the aorta, or myocardial ischemia), gastrointestinal (esophageal rupture or referred abdominal pain from trauma to the small or large bowel, liver, spleen, or pancreas), and pulmonary (pulmonary embolism, rib fracture, or pneumothorax with or without tamponade physiology) organ systems. Musculoskeletal injuries to the thorax are particularly common (Box 5-7).

BOX 5-5.
Common Causes of Headache Related to Traumatic Injury

Scalp laceration
Epidural hematoma
Subdural hemorrhage
Skull fracture
Cervical spine injury
Referred facial injury (temporomandibular joint)
Functional headaches (stress, dehydration, etc.)

BOX 5-6.
Common Causes of Neck Pain Related to Traumatic Injury

Cervical spine injury
Tension or stress
Musculoskeletal pain (e.g., whiplash)
Referred cardiac pain

BOX 5-7.
Common Causes of Chest Pain Related to Traumatic Injury

Cardiovascular

Contusion
Ischemia
Aortic tear or dissection
Pericardial tamponade
Hemothorax

Gastrointestinal

Esophageal rupture
Referred abdominal pain

Pulmonary

Pulmonary embolism
Pulmonary contusion
Pneumothorax

Musculoskeletal

Rib fracture
Thoracic vertebral injury

Pain limited to an upper or lower extremity is usually due to bone or soft tissue injury (Box 5-8). However, primary nerve injury is also common, particularly with avulsion injuries. Blood loss may be significant, especially with femur fractures, and is usually hidden. In the case of spinal injury, extremity pain may not be reported despite significant injury to the limb.

Abdominal pain is usually related to injury of the gastrointestinal tract (bowel, pancreatic, splenic, or hepatic injury) or the urinary tract (traumatic rupture of the bladder or urethra, renal or ureter injury) (Box 5-9). Damage to the reproductive organs in female patients may also accompany abdominal trauma. This damage may consist of vascular or soft tissue injury to the abdominal wall. The pain may be reported as vague and diffuse abdominal

BOX 5-8.
Common Causes of Extremity Pain in Traumatic Injury

Muscle or soft tissue injury
Fracture
Compartment syndrome
Acute neuropathic pain (e.g., avulsion or burn)
Arthralgia
Phantom limb pain

BOX 5-9.
Common Causes of Abdominal Pain in Traumatic Injury

Gastrointestinal

Pancreatic injury
Liver hematoma
Splenic rupture
Bowel perforation or peritonitis
Bowel ischemia

Genitourinary

Renal hematoma
Bladder rupture or distension
Urethral tear

Gynecologic

Uterine rupture or hemorrhage
Ovarian injury

discomfort in the case of a perforated viscus or early peritonitis, or it may be more localized if it results from ischemia.

Treatment of the underlying injury is the most important step in the management of the trauma victim's pain. Head injury may require operative decompression or tracheal intubation and hyperventilation to treat increased intracranial pressure, whereas extremity pain may require open or closed reduction of a fracture along with splinting or casting to immobilize the affected limb. Surgical exploration of the abdomen or chest may be required for severe injuries. Initial stabilization and intraoperative anesthetic management of these injuries are beyond the scope of this manual.

In patients who are not at increased risk of bleeding, the use of acetaminophen or NSAIDs, such as ibuprofen, may be adequate to control mild to moderate pain. They may be used either alone or in combination with opioids to reduce the total dose and thereby the adverse effects of opioids. Ketorolac (0.5 mg/kg IV every 6 hrs) may be used when oral administration of NSAIDs is not possible. Because ketorolac is also an NSAID, it is contraindicated in patients who are at risk for bleeding (e.g., head trauma patients), those who are hypovolemic, or those with a history of gastritis or peptic ulcer disease. Although parenteral administration is appropriate when oral or rectal administration is not feasible, there is no evidence to suggest that parenteral administration is more effective than other routes.

Opioids, by various routes, are frequently used in the trauma setting for the control of severe bone or soft tissue pain or in the postoperative setting. They are contraindicated in patients with altered neurologic status or in patients with the possibility of an acute abdominal injury where excessive sedation may interfere with serial physical examinations. If a decision to use them is made, PCA is an excellent option in patients old enough to understand its technique (age 6 or older). Patients with bilateral hand injuries may be physically unable to activate the PCA machine. It is permissible for these patients to ask their parents to push the PCA device for them. Parents and siblings must not be allowed to make the decision as to whether the patient is comfortable or to push the button without a specific request from the patient. This is a potentially fatal complication. Therefore it is imperative that if analgesics (opioids) or anxiolytics (benzodiazepines) are administered, they are prescribed judiciously and titrated carefully to the desired effect. This is especially true for patients who require sedation for a procedure in the emergency room or treatment room. As mentioned previously (see Chapter 1), appropriate monitoring is mandatory.

Chest trauma, postoperative abdominal pain, and lower extremity orthopedic pain may be effectively managed with epidural opioids and/or local anesthetics. Advantages of regional analgesia include superior pain control and improved pulmonary function.[30,31] Disadvantages include the need for an acute pain service and nurses who are able to manage patients with epidural catheters. This may not be available in all hospitals or on all patient care floors.

The adverse effects associated with epidural anesthesia are discussed in Chapter 3. These may include pruritus, urinary retention, respiratory depression, and lower extremity numbness. In fact, the risk of a compartment syndrome has been cited as a relative contraindication to the use of epidural local anesthetics for fear that they may mask the warning signs (progressive increase in pain) of ischemia. However, with dilute concentrations of local anesthetics (0.1% bupivacaine), analgesia can be provided without the fear of providing total anesthesia, thereby masking the signs of a compartment syndrome. Placement of an epidural catheter is absolutely contraindicated in the presence of a coagulopathy (e.g., massive blood transfusion) or with therapeutic anticoagulation (e.g., after microvascular surgery for limb reattachment).

Summary

This chapter has reviewed the pathophysiology and management of acute pain associated with a variety of clinical conditions that may arise in the child. When formulating a plan to alleviate the child's pain, the underlying cause of the pain must be understood in order to customize the treatment to meet the patient's needs. It is imperative that, during the administration of analgesic medications, provisions are made to ensure the child's safety.

References

1. Shapiro BS: The management of pain in sickle cell disease, *Pediatric Clin North Am* 36:1029, 1989.

2. Mohandas N, Evans E: Rheological and adherence properties of sickle cells: potential contribution to hematologic manifestations of the disease, *NY Acad Sci* 565:327, 1989.
3. Goldberg MA, Brugnara C, Dover GJ et al: Treatment of sickle cell anemia with hydroxyurea and erythropoietin, *New Engl J Med* 323:366, 1990.
4. Perrine SP, Ginder GD, Faller DV et al: A short-term trial of butyrate to stimulate fetal globin-gene expression in the beta-globin disorders, *New Engl J Med* 328:81, 1993.
5. Dover GJ, Humphries RK, Moore JG et al: Hydroxyurea induction of hemoglobin F production in patients with sickle cell anemia, *Blood* 67:735, 1986.
6. Platt OS, Thorington BD, Brambilla DJ et al: Pain in sickle cell disease, *New Engl J Med* 325:11, 1991.
7. Pegelow CH: Survey of pain management therapy provided for children with sickle cell disease, *Clin Pediatr* 31:211, 1992.
8. Miller RR, Jick H: Clinical effects of meperidine in hospitalized medical patients, *J Clin Pharmacol* 17:180, 1978.
9. Kaiko RF, Foley KM, Grabinski PY et al: Central nervous system excitatory effects of meperidine in cancer patients, *Ann Neurol* 13:180, 1982.
10. Shapiro BS, Cohen DE, Howe CJ: Patient-controlled analgesia for sickle cell related pain, *J Pain Symptom Manage* 8:22, 1993.
11. Schecter NL, Berrien FB, Katz SM: PCA for adolescents in sickle-cell crisis, *Am J Nursing* 11:719, 1988.
12. Shapiro BS, Cohen DE, Covelman KW et al: Experience of an interdisciplinary pediatric pain service, *Pediatrics* 88:1226, 1991.
13. Thomas JE, Koshy M, Patterson L et al: Management of pain in sickle cell disease using biofeedback therapy: a preliminary study, *Biofeedback & Self Regulation* 9:413, 1984.
14. Zeltzer LK, Kellerman J, Dash J et al: Hypnotically-induced pain control in sickle cell anemia, *Pediatrics* 69:533, 1979.
15. Cozzi L, Tyron WW, Sedlacek K: The effectiveness of biofeedback-assisted relaxation in modifying sickle cell crises, *Biofeedback & Self Regulation* 12:51, 1987.

16. Griffin TC, McIntire D, Buchanan GR: High-dose intravenous methylprednisolone therapy for pain in children and adolescents with sickle cell disease, *New Engl J Med* 330:733, 1994.
17. Brookoff D, Polomano R: Treating sickle cell pain like cancer pain, *Ann Int Med* 116:364, 1992.
18. Ballas SK, Rubin RN, Gabuzda TC: Treating sickle cell pain like cancer pain, *Ann Int Med* 117:263, 1992.
19. Portenoy RK: Response to treating sickle cell pain like cancer pain, *Ann Int Med* 117:264, 1992.
20. Finer P, Blair J, Rowe P: Epidural analgesia in the management of labor pain and sickle cell crisis: a case report, *Anesthesiology* 68:799, 1988.
21. Yaster M, Tobin JR, Billett C: Epidural analgesia in the management of severe vaso-occlusive sickle cell crisis, *Pediatrics* 93:310, 1994.
22. Rareshide E, Amedee RG: Referred Otalgia, *Journal of the Louisiana State Medical Society* 142:7, 1990.
23. Tobias JD, Lowe S, Hersey S: Analgesia following bilateral myringotomy and placement of PE tubes in children: acetaminophen versus acetaminophen with codeine, *Anesth Analg* (in press).
24. Atchison NE, Osgood PF, Carr DB: Pain during dressing change in children: relationship to burn area, depth and analgesic regimens, *Pain* 47:41, 1991.
25. Choinière M, Melzack R, Papillon J: Pain and anesthesia in patients with healed burns: an exploratory study, *J Pain Symptom Manage* 6:437, 1991.
26. Osgood PF, Szyfelbein SK: Management of burn pain in children, *Pediatr Clin North Am* 36:1001, 1989.
27. Jönsson A, Cassuto J, Hanson B: Inhibition of burn pain by intravenous lignocaine infusion, *Lancet* 338:151, 1991.
28. Carr DB, Osgood PF, Szyfebein SK: Treatment of pain in acutely burned children. In: Schechter NL, Berde CB, Yaster M, editors: *Pain in infants, children, and adolescents,* Baltimore, 1993, Williams and Wilkins.

29. Kavanagh C: A new approach to dressing change in the severely burned child and its effect on burn-related psychotherapy, *Heart & Lung* 12:612, 1983.
30. Paterson DR, Questad KA, Boltwood MD: Hypnotherapy as a treatment for pain in patients with burns: research and clinical considerations, *Journal Burn Care Rehab* 8:263, 1987.
31. Luchette FA, Radafshar SM, Kaiser R et al: Prospective evaluation of epidural versus intrapleural catheters for analgesia in chest wall trauma, *J Trauma* 36:865, 1994.
32. Cicala RS, Voeller GR, Fox T et al: Epidural analgesia in thoracic trauma: effects of lumbar morphine and thoracic bupivacaine on pulmonary function, *Crit Care Med* 18:229, 1990.

6

NEONATAL PAIN MANAGEMENT

Brenda C. McClain
Kawal J.S. Anand

PAIN ASSESSMENT IN THE NEONATE
SEDATION DURING INVASIVE PROCEDURES
CENTRAL VENOUS CATHETER PLACEMENT
ENDOTRACHEAL INTUBATION AND MECHANICAL VENTILATION
CIRCUMCISION
SURGICAL PAIN: INTRAOPERATIVE AND POSTOPERATIVE MANAGEMENT
SEDATION DURING EXTRACORPOREAL MEMBRANE OXYGENATION
OPIOID TOLERANCE AND PHYSICAL DEPENDENCE

The issue of adequate pain management remains a controversial topic in neonatal intensive care units (NICUs) throughout the world. This chapter provides a brief review of the prevailing attitudes of practitioners concerning the need to treat neonatal pain. It then discusses a systematic approach to pain management in this patient population for invasive or painful procedures, such as central line placement, mechanical ventilation, endotracheal intubation, circumcision, and extracorporeal membrane oxygenation (ECMO). Methods of postoperative pain management are also discussed. Although nonpharmacologic comfort measures may impact on the physiologic responses to pain and stress, this discussion is limited to pharmacologic approaches, including systemic and regional analgesia.

Many practitioners acknowledge the existence of neonatal pain, but most disagree on the appropriate ways to manage that pain. As a result, many procedures are still performed with minimal or no analgesia. Physicians may even intellectually know that newborns experience pain but believe it inappropriate to treat them.[1-3] Ironically, practitioners have traditionally withheld opioids from neonates because of the fear of adverse effects related to a presumed intolerance to strong opioids secondary to the neonate's physiologic immaturity. However, research suggests that neonates may be more sensitive to the deleterious physiologic effects of pain, and improved clinical outcome can result from aggressive pain management.[4,5] The issues concerning the increased sensitivity to pain in the newborn are discussed further in Chapter 1.

PAIN ASSESSMENT IN THE NEONATE

Perhaps the major problem with treating pain in the neonate is the difficulty in assessing and quantifying pain. Growing concern for the pain experienced by neonates subjected to surgical or intensive care procedures has led to a search for appropriate assessment tools. Several different tools based on behavioral and physiologic responses have been suggested (Box 6-1). Future studies are needed to determine the optimal tool for grading neonatal pain.

The absence of validated and well-accepted methods for pain assessment in neonates implies that a high degree of suspicion is required for the diagnosis of pain and agitation during routine intensive care and invasive procedures. Attentive vigilance is particularly required in caring for neonates who require muscle paralysis for their management. Because the use of muscle relaxants results in the ablation of facial and motor responses, the clinical appearance may falsely indicate the lack of requirement for analgesics or sedatives.

SEDATION DURING INVASIVE PROCEDURES

A variety of invasive procedures are performed in the NICU population. The distress and pain varies significantly depending

BOX 6-1.
Pain Assessment Methods for Neonates & Infants

Behavioral

Motor responses
- Reflex withdrawal to pain
- Cutaneous flexor reflex
- Photogrammetric technique

Facial expressions
- Neonatal Facial Coding System
- Maximally Discriminative Social Movement Coding System

Crying activity
- Spectrographic analysis
- Formant analysis
- Mean Relative Spectral Energy

Complex behavioral responses
- Brazelton Neonatal Behavioral Scale
- Changes in sleep state

Physiologic

Heart rate
Blood pressure
Respiratory rate
Respiratory pattern
Heart rate and respiratory variability
Intracranial pressure
Transcutaneous pO_2
Oxygen saturation
Transcutaneous pO_2 and pCO_2 variability
Palmar sweating
Skin conductance
Skin blood flow by Laser Doppler Flowmetry

Combined and Global

Douleur Enfant Gustave Roussy
Objective Pain Scale
Observer Visual Analogue Scale (VAS)
Postoperative Comfort Score
Neonatal Infant Pain Scale
Premature Infant Pain Profile

on the procedure and its duration. Table 6-1 lists the procedures commonly performed in neonates and lists the percentage of time that these procedures are performed without analgesia. These practices are compared to similar procedures performed in older children in pediatric intensive care units (PICUs). It is evident from these data that neonatal pain is significantly undertreated.

The interventions described in this chapter are designed to diminish the physiologic and behavioral responses to neonatal pain and to ensure the safety and well being of the neonate.

Central Venous Catheter Placement

Critically ill and premature neonates often require long term central vascular access. The administration of medications, nutritional support, and hemodynamic monitoring can be accomplished with surgically or percutaneously inserted, central venous catheters.[6] Although the medical literature is replete with information on the incidence and types of complications encountered with central vascular catheters, the literature addressing the management of pain related to the placement and subsequent care of these catheters is discouragingly limited.

The somatic and visceral pain encountered during the placement of central vascular access can be treated. The skin is densely

TABLE 6-1. 1992 Survey of Analgesic Use in PICUs and NICUs

Procedure	PICUs	NICUs	P value
Intravenous cannulation	13%	7%	0.42
Bladder aspiration	11%	3%	0.25
Bladder catheterization	3%	0%	0.56
Venipuncture	3%	0%	0.55
Arterial line placement	66%	26%	0.001
Bone marrow aspiration	94%	64%	0.01
Central line placement	92%	68%	0.01
Chest tube insertion	95%	60%	0.001
Lumbar puncture	50%	7%	0.001
Paracentesis	77%	27%	0.001

Modified from Bauchner H et al, *J Pediatr* 121:647, 1992.
PICUs, Pediatric intensive care units; *NICUs,* neonatal intensive care units.

populated with afferent nociceptive fibers (free nerve endings) that transmit acute and chronic pain. As might be expected, the more muscular arteries have a better innervation than do less muscular arteries and veins. The central vessels, especially the great veins and arteries close to the heart, are more heavily innervated with afferent and sympathetic fibers that transmit pain and nociception.[7]

One of the simplest measures to prevent pain associated with catheter insertion is local anesthesia of the skin with either topical application or subcutaneous infiltration of a local anesthetic. The mixture of lidocaine and prilocaine forms a eutectic mixture of local anesthetics (EMLA) and is available as a topical cream. Topical application of EMLA effectively interrupts nociceptive input from the epidermis and deeper structures. Prerequisites for the use of EMLA are placement over the appropriate site, application under an occlusive dressing, and 60 minutes of adequate contact time.[8] Although the low, systemic uptake of these local anesthetics limits their serum concentrations, one of the metabolites of prilocaine (o-toluidine) can cause methemoglobinemia. The risk of methemoglobinemia is greater in neonates because of the increased sensitivity of fetal hemoglobin to oxidant stresses and the decreased function of enzymes that convert the methemoglobin back to the ferrous state. Studies on the use of EMLA in neonates are currently underway and will probably demonstrate acceptable plasma levels of the local anesthetic agents. However, the prescribing information states that EMLA Cream should not be used in infants under the age of one month or in those rare patients with congenital or idiopathic methemoglobinemia or in infants under the age of twelve months who are receiving treatment with methemoglobin-inducing agents.

A second option is the intradermal infiltration of local anesthetics to relieve the somatic pain caused by incision or percutaneous puncture.[9] Local anesthetics can safely be used at the time of catheter placement if an adequate volume is used and time-to-skin anesthesia is allowed (Table 6-2).

Regardless of the agent used, the dose should be within recommended ranges to avoid the risk of toxicity. Although several

TABLE 6-2. Local Anesthetics for Skin and Field Infiltration

Solution	Dose Range	Duration of Action
1% lidocaine	2-4 mg/kg	60-120 mins
1% lidocaine w/epi*	2.5-5 mg/kg	90-120 mins
0.25% bupivacaine	1-2 mg/kg	180-300 mins
0.25% bupivacaine w/epi*	1-2.5 mg/kg	180-400 mins

*Epinephrine concentration is 1:200,000 (5 μg/ml). Solutions containing epinephrine tend to be more painful on injection.

concentrations of lidocaine are available, 0.5% provides adequate anesthesia after local infiltration. Volumes should be limited to 0.5 to 0.7 ml/kg (2.5 to 3.5 mg/kg). Because of the immaturity of the neonatal liver and the hepatic metabolism of the amide anesthetics (e.g., lidocaine), there may be a greater risk of toxicity with repeated doses because of the prolonged half-life of these agents. Another problem with the available preparations of lidocaine is a low pH of 4.0, which can cause pain on injection. The addition of bicarbonate (0.1 mEq/ml) to the local anesthetic solution raises the pH to 7.0 and limits the discomfort associated with infiltration. Another option is to use local infiltration after application of EMLA cream.

Vascular cannulation and the subsequent placement of indwelling catheters of large diameter may cause some discomfort since the innervation of larger, central vessels extends from the adventitia to the muscular media and may extend to the regions of the vasa vasorum in the intima. Despite these theoretical concerns, ongoing pain from indwelling catheters is not recognized as a significant problem in older, verbal patients.

In addition to local anesthesia, the administration of parenteral agents is frequently required during central line insertion. Although many of these procedures are performed in the operating room with general anesthesia, they may also be performed in the ICU. In this setting, the administration of parenteral agents combined with topical anesthesia can be used to provide effective analgesia. Although several options exist, agents such as fentanyl (initial dose of 2 to 4 μg/kg) or ketamine (1 to 2 mg/kg), with their short half-lives and negligible effects on cardiovascular function, offer the greatest margin of safety. Other commonly used sedative agents, such as benzodiazepines (e.g., midazolam) or barbiturates, do not possess analgesic properties and cannot be expected to blunt the deleterious physiologic effects of pain.

Regardless of whether the central venous catheter is placed in the NICU or in the operating room, for most infants endotracheal intubation and mechanical ventilation is recommended before the administration of opioids for the placement of central venous access. Once this is done, the major adverse effect, respiratory depression, is eliminated. Additionally, the combination of analgesia and sedation with neuromuscular blocking agents provides for a motionless surgical field, thereby increasing the ease of line placement.

The potential for pain is also present when there is pathology related to central venous catheters. The incidence of catheter-related infections ranges from 0% to 82%.[6, 10,11] The lower infection rates were found in neonates of greater than 1500 grams or those who received catheters placed percutaneously. Additional complications may include catheter occlusion, leakage, dislodgement, and vessel thrombosis. The risk of complications increases with the duration of catheter use.

Thrombi and infectious foci release inflammatory substances, such as bradykinin, prostaglandins, histamine, serotonin, norepinephrine, and substance P, which stimulate nociceptive pathways leading to pain. Although the primary focus during catheter-related infections is control of the bacteremia and its sequelae, the identification and management of infection-related discomfort may be overlooked. The cardinal signs of inflammation include pain, heat, redness, and loss of function. Bradykinin has been implicated in all these effects. In addition, the sympathetic nervous system contributes to the peripheral activation of primary nociceptive afferents. As a result, a complex system exists in the periphery by which neurochemicals contribute to the enhancement of the transmission of nociceptive information.[12]

Steroids and nonsteroidal antiinflammatory drugs (NSAIDs) have been shown to inhibit the initiation of the arachidonic acid cascade and the release of modulators of peripheral nociceptive transmission. Indomethacin has traditionally been used in neonates for the closure of patent ductus arteriosus.[13,14] There remains little or no information concerning the other NSAIDs in the neonatal population. Although these agents can have significant adverse effects that may limit their use in neonates (decreased glomerular filtration rate or platelet dysfunction), their potent, antiinflammatory activity may provide another tool for the control of pain.

Opioids have been shown to mediate antinociception and to produce analgesia associated with inflammation.[15] The effectiveness of opioids results from their agonistic effects at mu, delta, and kappa receptors. Thus, the use of opioids is practical in the management of somatic and visceral pain in response to inflammation from tissue injury, whether it is the result of surgery, infection, or thrombosis. Nociceptive thresholds are lowered in the face of tissue injury; therefore, peripheral afferent nerves are more sensitive to activation. Subsequently, pain results with less stimulation. Dosing of opioids in these circumstances should follow the guidelines discussed below in the management of postsurgical pain. Since these complications produce ongoing or persistent types of pain, "around-the-clock" administration, or the continuous infusion of opioids, is suggested.

Endotracheal Intubation and Mechanical Ventilation

Ventilatory support has increased the clinician's capacities in the care of the critically ill neonate. The survival of extremely premature neonates has been due, in part, to improved technology and a better understanding of the pathophysiology of airway diseases. The newer, unconventional modes of ventilation, such as high frequency techniques and other advances (e.g., intratracheal pulmonary ventilation) are designed to lessen barotrauma, decrease dead space, and improve oxygenation.[16] These advances in respiratory management often require the neonate to remain immobile; therefore, sedation is mandatory.

The act of endotracheal intubation is perhaps one of the greatest physiologic stresses that occurs in the neonatal period. The stimulus of direct laryngoscopy results in increased blood pressure and intracranial pressure. This may be of particular concern in neonates with a history of or predilection for intraventricular hemorrhage. The preemptive administration before endotracheal intubation of agents that decrease cerebral blood flow is strongly recommended. Endotracheal intubation in awake patients is not recommended.

In neonates with stable cardiovascular function, a short-acting barbiturate, such as sodium thiopental (4 to 6 mg/kg) or the benzodiazepine, midazolam (0.05 to 0.2 mg/kg), can be used. Both agents have been shown to diminish the cerebral metabolic rate for oxygen ($CMRO_2$) and cerebral blood flow.[17,18] Current practice is to combine these agents with a short-acting, nondepolarizing muscle relaxant, such as vecuronium (0.1 mg/kg) and atropine (0.01 mg/kg–minimum dose 0.1 mg), to facilitate endotracheal intubation. Atropine is administered before intubation in all neonates to prevent vagal responses, such as bradycardia and bronchoconstriction. Because of the direct negative inotropic properties and peripheral vasodilatory effects of both benzodiazepines and barbiturates, hypotension may be observed with either thiopental or midazolam.[19]

Other options are suggested for patients with compromised cardiovascular function. In adults, etomidate (0.2 to 0.3 mg/kg), a nonbarbiturate induction agent, provides amnesia and analgesia with a stable hemodynamic profile. The use of etomidate in neonates has not been previously studied and deserves investigation. In adult patients, etomidate decreases the $CMRO_2$ and cerebral blood flow with little or no effect on cardiovascular function.[20] Adrenal suppression occurs after prolonged use and, although uncommon, it has been seen with a single dose. This effect may detract from its use in premature neonates in whom the hypothalamic-hypophyseal-adrenal axis may be compromised.

Alternatives in the setting of compromised cardiovascular function are fentanyl (2 to 4 μg/kg) or alfentanil (10 to 15 μg/kg), which provide analgesia with little impact on blood pressure and cardiac output. Caveats in regard to their use include the occurrence of chest wall rigidity and questionable effects on intracranial pressure (see Chapter 7). A third option for patients with compromised cardiovascular function is ketamine (1 to 2 mg/kg). Because of the release of endogenous catecholamines, blood pressure is usually well maintained and pulmonary compliance increases. Ketamine increases blood pressure and systemic vascular resistance. It may be the agent of choice when a decrease in systemic vascular resistance is detrimental (e.g., tetralogy of Fallot or aortic stenosis). Since intracranial pressure may increase after ketamine administration, it is not recommended in patients with compromised intracranial compliance.

After endotracheal intubation the maintenance of indwelling endotracheal tubes and effective mechanical ventilation frequently requires the use of analgesics and/or sedatives. These pharmacologic agents should be combined with nonpharmacologic techniques (Box 6-2). The use of such nonpharmacologic techniques may decrease the need for pharmacologic management of anxiety.

Although several agents have been investigated in older children and adults (see Chapter 7), there are few studies comparing agents for sedation in the neonatal population. The authors generally rely on either benzodiazepines (midazolam or lorazepam) or opioids (fentanyl or morphine). Although neuromuscular block-

BOX 6-2.
Nonpharmacologic Approaches for Pain Management

- Environmental changes and distractions
  - Decreased stimulation
  - Decreased light, noise, handling
  - Swaddling, using a pacifier
  - Changing position
  - Touching, music, soothing voice
  - Holding, rocking, rubbing, fanning
  - Hydrotherapy, sponging
- Physical therapy or occupational therapy
- Transcutaneous electrical nerve stimulation

ing agents may, on occasion, be necessary to allow adequate ventilation, they should not be used as a substitute for sedative or analgesic agents.

Midazolam is a water-soluble, short-acting benzodiazepine with an elimination half-life that varies depending on the gestational age of the patient. As with any benzodiazepine, it possesses no analgesic properties and is not meant as a substitute for opioids during painful procedures. Continuous infusions of midazolam, ranging from 0.05 to 0.1 mg/kg/hr, are effective. Hemodynamic depression is dose-dependent and is more likely when opioids and benzodiazepines are coadministered. Midazolam-induced hypotension has been observed with its administration within 6 hours of a bolus dose of fentanyl or during a fentanyl infusion at 2 μg/kg/hr.[19] To limit its effects on cardiovascular function, bolus doses should be administered over 5 to 10 minutes.

Midazolam is metabolized by the P-450 system of the liver with subsequent renal excretion of the metabolites. One of the metabolites, 1-hydroxymidazolam, retains some activity of the parent compound and may accumulate in patients with renal insufficiency. Studies of the long term effects of the prolonged use of midazolam in critically ill neonates are needed. Because of the short half-life of midazolam and the need for frequent administration, many practitioners prefer to use lorazepam. This may be particularly important when intermittent, on-demand administration is the chosen mode of delivery. Since the elimination half-life of lorazepam is 10 to 20 hours, it is not recommended for brief procedures. However, in patients in whom long term sedation is anticipated, lorazepam is a reasonable choice.

Since lorazepam is frequently used for control of seizures in neonates, there is some pharmacokinetic information concerning its use in neonates. McDermott and colleagues investigated the pharmacokinetics of lorazepam in 10 term neonates.[21] When compared with data in adults and older children, lorazepam has a smaller volume of distribution and a prolonged half-life (mean of 40.2 hrs with a range of 17.9 to 73.0 hrs). Since lorazepam is metabolized by the glucuronyl transferase system, the prolonged half-life is easily explained on the basis of immaturity of this enzyme system. Unlike midazolam, there are no active metabolites. The glucuronyl transferase system starts to normalize at roughly 3 months of age but may not reach adult levels until 3 to 4 years of age. Despite such problems, lorazepam has been used for sedation in the NICU population. Maloley and colleagues reported its successful use in doses ranging from 0.1 to 0.4 mg/kg for sedation in 15 ventilator-dependent infants with a mean gestational age of 34 weeks.[22] The authors noted that the number of doses and the total daily doses needed were highly variable and did not correlate with gestational age. Because of such variability and the obvious wide range of half-life of this and other drugs in the neonatal population, titration of doses (up or down) is frequently necessary, regardless of the agent chosen. A dose of 0.05 mg/kg can be repeated every 5 to 10 minutes up to a maximum total dose of 0.4 mg/kg.

One concern with lorazepam is that the solution contains benzyl alcohol, which in toxic doses causes the "gasping" syndrome manifested by metabolic acidosis, central nervous system (CNS) toxicity, and cardiovascular collapse. Lorazepam contains 2% benzyl alcohol, which is below the dose reported to cause toxicity in neonates (100 mg/kg/day),[22] but it should be used with caution in patients with renal or hepatic compromise. The solution also contains propylene glycol and polyethylene glycol, both of which can displace bilirubin from its protein binding sites. Although the quantities of these agents are very low, lorazepam should be used cautiously in premature neonates with hyperbilirubinemia.

Aside from the benzodiazepines, opioids are frequently used for sedation during mechanical ventilation. Although several opioids are available, either morphine or fentanyl are usually used. Guidelines for the use of opioids for sedation during mechanical ventilation are the same as using these agents for postoperative analgesia and are discussed in detail later in the chapter. Although these agents can be administered by intermittent, on-demand dosing, more effective sedation is usually provided by a continuous infusion. Starting doses include 2 to 4 μg/kg/hr for fentanyl or 10 to 20 μg/kg/hr for morphine. As with benzodiazepines, there is wide variability in the half-life of these agents throughout the neonatal period; therefore, titrating the dose to the desired effect is of paramount importance.

A time honored alternative to the opioids or benzodiazepines is chloral hydrate. Chloral hydrate is rapidly absorbed after rectal or oral administration and metabolized in the liver to the active form, trichloroethanol. One advantage is the limited effect on cardiorespiratory function. Although single doses of 50 to 75 mg/kg are acceptable for nonpainful procedures, such as radiologic imaging, repeated doses in the term or preterm neonate can result in rapid accumulation of the active metabolite and resultant toxicity. More appropriate alternatives exist for ongoing sedation in the neonatal population.

Since neither opioids nor benzodiazepines possess all of the ideal characteristics of the perfect agent for sedation, the search continues for agents that will provide analgesia without respiratory depression. Tramadol is a synthetic opioid of moderate analgesic strength similar to meperidine. It binds weakly to the mu receptor and is reported to have fewer and less severe side effects than other opioids. The (+)-enantiomer is an inhibitor of serotonin uptake having a second mechanism of antinociception.[23] Tramadol may be administered by the oral, intravenous, or neuraxial route and is a promising sedative and analgesic agent. Neonatal studies are underway in several European countries with promising preliminary results.

Circumcision

Circumcision is one of the common elective, surgical procedures performed on male infants, with more than 80% of male neonates undergoing this operation in the United States.[24] The procedure is often performed without anesthesia or analgesia despite evidence that neonates are capable of pain perception, even at relatively immature gestational stages. Neurochemical evidence exists for the stress that can be induced by this procedure. Investigations have shown that the cortisol response to circumcision is beyond that mounted with crying alone. Williamson and Evans demonstrated in 1-to 3-day-old infants that the baseline cortisol level of 9.9 μg/dl rose to 22.9 μg/dl at 30 to 40 minutes when circumcision was performed without a local anesthetic.[25] As a comparison, minor procedures, such as venipuncture, resulted in less than a 30% increase above baseline levels.

The use of local anesthetics in neonatal circumcision was first described by Kirya and Werthmann in 1978.[26] Several options exist for the use of local anesthetics and the techniques of penile block. The shaft of the penis, glans, and foreskin are supplied by the two dorsal penile nerves that arise from the hypogastric and sacral plexi (Fig. 6-1). The nerves travel forward, beneath the symphysis pubis, in the suspensory ligament deep to Buck's fascia.

A penile block is performed by injecting local anesthetic at the 10 and 2 o'clock positions on the dorsal surface at the base of the penis.[27] The nerves lie 3 to 5 mm below the skin's surface (Fig. 6-1). An injection of 1% lidocaine in volumes of up to 0.2 ml/kg/side can be used.[28] In a term neonate, 0.5 ml on each side is usually sufficient. The solution must not contain epinephrine since these are end-arteries. Local anesthetic toxicity is possible because of vascular uptake or direct intravascular injection. Accidental puncture of the dorsal artery or vein has rarely been reported but can lead to hematoma formation or gangrene.[29]

An alternative to the dorsal penile block is the ring block, which involves the subcutaneous injection of a local anesthetic (0.5% or 1.0% lidocaine) around the base of the penis.[30] The dose of lidocaine should not exceed 4 mg/kg. A subcutaneous injection at the level of the prepuce has also been reported. The injection of 0.4 ml of 1% lidocaine into the prepuce at the 10 and 2 o'clock positions at the level of the corona may provide more reliable analgesia than dorsal penile nerve blocks, especially in inexperienced hands.[31,32]

The utilization of local anesthetics has expanded to other methods for pain relief. The caudal space is the distal extension of the epidural space. Caudal epidural blocks are easy to perform on the infant.[33] A loss of resistance is felt with the penetration of the needle through the sacrococcygeal membrane. A short-bevelled,

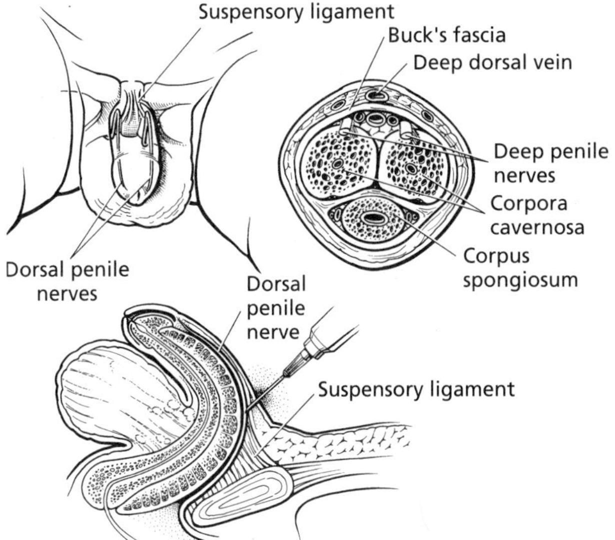

FIG 6-1.
Surface anatomy for performing the dorsal penile nerve block. The dorsal penile nerves are located at 10 and 2 o'clock from the midline. The area around the dorsal penile nerves is vascular. Therefore, careful aspiration for blood before injection of local anesthetics is suggested. Solutions containing epinephrine are contraindicated. The saggital view *(bottom)* demonstrates the injection technique. The injection must be anterior to the suspensory ligament and deep to Buck's fascia for effective blockade.

blunt-tip needle is used and is attached to a saline-filled syringe. After entering the caudal space, the saline syringe is replaced with a syringe containing local anesthetic with 1:200,000 epinephrine (0.5 ml/kg of 0.25% bupivacaine). Caudal blocks can provide safe, effective analgesia; however, some feel that the technique is overkill, and the risks outweigh the benefits.[31] Since caudals are only performed by anesthesiologists, their application for neonatal circumcision is limited. However, this technique is frequently used in the operating room for older patients undergoing circumcision. This may be especially useful as a means of avoiding a general anesthetic in patients with severe, underlying medical compromise. Although bupivacaine (0.5 ml/kg of 0.25%) is usually used, an alternative is 0.5 ml/kg of 3% chloroprocaine. The latter drug provides a denser sensory block with a more rapid onset. Additionally, its short serum half-life (less than 60 seconds) should theoretically decrease the risk of toxicity.

A topical application of local anesthetics may also have some role in the prevention of pain during circumcision. A topical 2% lidocaine solution, used intraoperatively after the removal of the foreskin, has been shown to reduce anesthetic requirements.[34] This technique is not feasible for the majority of neonatal circumcisions since general anesthesia is required to initially render the patient insensitive to the operative incision. Ointments and gels of 2% lidocaine have been used by topical application postoperatively to prevent pain (Fig. 6-2).

The use of EMLA in neonatal circumcision is not approved. Initial studies suggest that EMLA reduces the pain response and may be a useful agent for pain management. A placebo-controlled study of newborn males between 37 and 42 weeks of gestation was conducted, in which EMLA was applied to the outside of the prepuce and covered with an occlusive dressing for 45 to 60 minutes (Fig. 6-3). The infants who had an application of EMLA demonstrated less tachycardia, better oxygen saturation, and decreased facial response to the procedure.[35]

Nonopioid analgesics, such as acetaminophen and NSAIDs, are inadequate in relieving pain during circumcision. Opioid analgesics, although effective, can be associated with significant adverse effects, most notably respiratory depression, in the nonintubated, nonventilated neonate. Because of these problems, their use is not recommended for routine circumcision. Nonpharmacologic

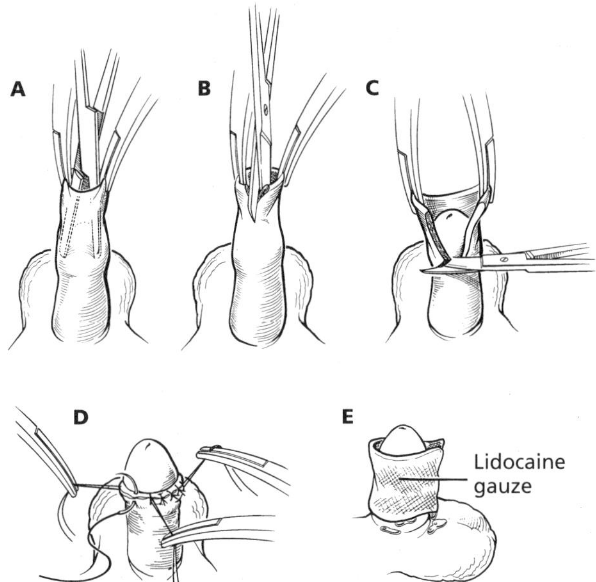

FIG 6-2.

The prepuceal tissue is richly innervated. Mechanosensitive afferent fibers are stimulated during the operative procedure resulting in primary hyperalgesia at the surgical site and secondary hyperalgesia in the surrounding tissue. **A,** Stretching of the prepuce stimulates mechanoreceptors. **B, C,** Incision of the prepuce results in release of prostaglandins and other nociceptive chemicals. **D,** Suture at the level of the glans also initiates A-delta and C fiber nociceptor activities. **E,** Postoperative analgesia can be obtained by the application of a 2% lidocaine gel that is left insitu at the exposed surfaces of the glans.

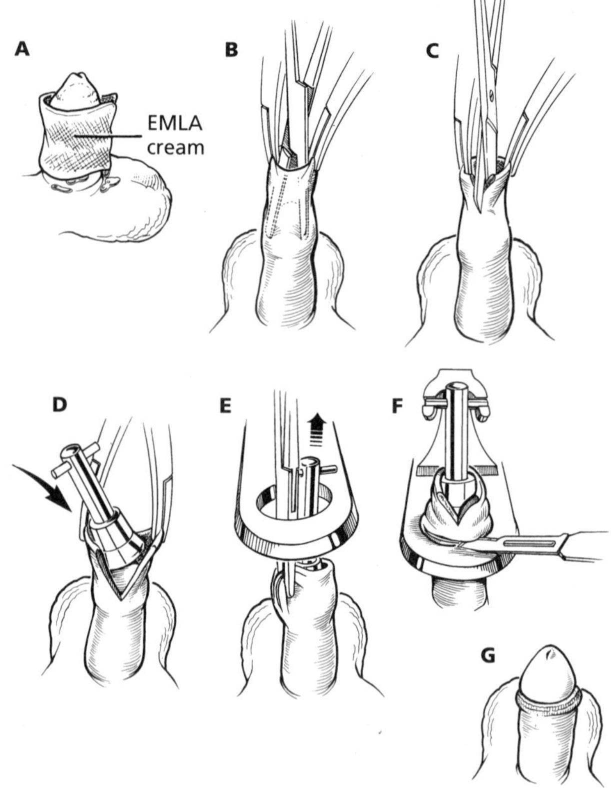

FIG 6-3.

A, EMLA cream is applied under an occlusive dressing for at least 1 hour before the circumcision. **B-G,** Mechanosensitive afferents are stimulated in a fashion similar to circumcision by surgical excision and suture. Preemptive anesthesia and analgesia decrease the stress response and provide comfort.

comfort measures, such as swaddling, pacifiers, and intrauterine sounds (heart beat), can be used as adjuncts for pain reduction.[24]

SURGICAL PAIN: INTRAOPERATIVE AND POSTOPERATIVE MANAGEMENT

In 1985, America was made aware that neonates frequently underwent surgery with minimal, if any, anesthesia when a mother in Silver Springs, Maryland asked why her child had been operated on without anesthesia.[36] It was a common belief at that time that neonates did not experience pain of similar severity as adults. These myths and misconceptions have been replaced with interest in the area of pain assessment and pain management of neonates. Unfortunately, global attention to the subject of neonatal pain has not resulted in an enormous change in postoperative management. It is believed that postoperative pain management although generally improved, continues to be inadequate for the majority of neonates.[37,38] Further studies of institutional practices and perspectives on neonatal pain management are needed.

Studies by Anand and colleagues[4,5] have shown a significant decrease in the stress response of neonates who receive adequate doses of analgesics and anesthetics. These studies have also documented a decreased morbidity in patients who receive adequate analgesia postoperatively. Hormonal and metabolic changes in the term and preterm neonate occur when surgical anesthesia and analgesia are inadequate, resulting in a catabolic state.[39]

Several options exist for the management of postoperative and intraoperative pain in neonates, including opioids and regional anesthetic techniques. The goals of intraoperative management include providing effective analgesia and blunting the deleterious effects of postsurgical stress response. Recent evidence suggests that the commonly used inhalational anesthetic agents may be less effective than synthetic opioids in achieving these goals.[4,5,39] Although fentanyl, in doses of 10 to 20 mg/kg, provides intraoperative analgesia and blunts the stress response without causing hemodynamic compromise, postoperative ventilation is generally required in neonates.

Regardless of which opioids are used for postoperative or intraoperative analgesia and anesthesia, a wide variation in metabolism and clearance can be expected in the neonatal population.[40-43] Decreased clearance has been documented with several different opioids, including morphine, alfentanil, and fentanyl.[40-43] In general, clearance decreases with decreasing gestational age. Another factor that may further decrease clearance is intraabdominal pathology (an abdominal procedure or increased intraabdominal pressure), which is thought to decrease hepatic blood flow, thereby further decreasing opioid clearance. Another factor that may potentiate the effects of opioids in neonates is decreased protein binding, with a resultant increase in the free fraction and an increased permeability of the blood-brain barrier. Since many neonates require postoperative mechanical ventilation, these factors should not limit the use of opioids during major surgical procedures. However, alterations in doses may be required postoperatively to prevent postoperative respiratory depression and an inability to wean from mechanical ventilation.

Regardless of the opioid used, decreases in the infusion rate and bolus doses are required when compared to older infants and children. Lynn and colleagues have demonstrated that morphine at 10 to 20 μg/kg/hr provides effective analgesia in older infants without interfering with weaning from mechanical ventilation.[44] They noted $PaCO_2$s of less than 45 mm Hg with serum morphine concentrations of 10 to 25 ng/ml. Based on the available pharmacokinetic information in neonates,[43] similar blood levels can be achieved with infusion rates of 5 to 10 μg/kg/min following a bolus dose of 50 μg/kg. When used by intermittent, on-demand dosing, the interval should be longer in neonates than in older children (e.g., 0.05 mg/kg every 4 to 6 hrs as opposed to every 2 to 3 hrs).

Although morphine and fentanyl in equipotent doses can be expected to provide equivalent degrees of analgesia and respiratory depression, the synthetic opioids (fentanyl) offer the advantage of hemodynamic stability, decreased pulmonary vascular reactivity, and, perhaps, increased survival after major surgical procedures. Therefore fentanyl has theoretical advantages after major surgical procedures, such as repair of diaphragmatic hernias and congenital cardiac defects. Although doses of 0.5 to 2 μg/kg/hr provide analgesia, higher doses in the range of 8 to 10 μg/kg/hr are needed for its effects on pulmonary reactivity. Doses of 8 to 10 μg/kg/hr cause significant respiratory depression and necessitate ongoing mechanical ventilation. The other synthetic agents, such as sufentanil and alfentanil, offer no advantage over fentanyl and are significantly more expensive. Regardless of the agent chosen, bolus doses equivalent to the hourly rate should be available on an as needed basis to supplement the infusion.

Although morphine and fentanyl are acceptable for neonates, the use of meperidine is not recommended. Although early reports claimed that meperidine causes less respiratory depression than morphine, this is no longer considered to be the case. More importantly, a metabolite, normeperidine, may cause seizures, whereas the parent compound can cause direct myocardial depression.

The mode (continuous or intermittent administration) and route of delivery should also be considered. Continuous infusions of opioids provide a steady state serum concentration and may give more consistent results.[45] Although intravenous administration is usually chosen, alternative routes of delivery are being investigated, including the subcutaneous, transdermal, and intratracheal routes. For the most part, the reports concerning these routes are anecdotal, and their use in neonates is still relatively experimental.

Several studies have suggested that premature infants and neonates may have an increased risk for perioperative morbidity after general anesthesia. Several factors have been proposed that may account for the increase in postoperative morbidity, such as an immaturity of respiratory musculature and central respiratory control. Such immaturity leads to an increased incidence of perioperative apnea and respiratory complications. Additionally, general anesthesia in neonates requires tracheal intubation and mechanical ventilation. As a consequence of these factors, some neonates may require postoperative mechanical ventilation. In an effort to avoid the respiratory depressant effects of opioids, the interest in regional anesthesia in neonates continues to increase. Regional anesthetic techniques may be used instead of general anesthesia, with general anesthesia, or solely for postoperative analgesia.

Spinal anesthesia is frequently used in neonates with severe underlying medical problems as a means of avoiding the need for general anesthesia.[46,47] The most common uses include lower abdominal and lower extremity procedures, such as inguinal herniorrhaphy. Regardless of the technique used (spinal or epidural), larger doses of local anesthetic are required in neonates when compared with adults because of the large size of the epidural and intrathecal spaces in relation to body weight.

Intravenous access is obtained, and the infant is medicated with atropine (0.01 mg/kg). Holding the infant in the sitting position and using a 22-gauge, 1.5 inch, spinal needle is preferred. After sterile preparation and drape, local anesthesia is applied with 0.5% lidocaine. An alternative, which is now preferred, is the preoperative application of EMLA to the site of the lumbar puncture 1 hour before the procedure. Various dosing regimens for spinal anesthesia in neonates have been suggested with doses of tetracaine and bupivacaine ranging from 0.4 to 1.0 mg/kg. The authors generally use 0.7 mg/kg of bupivacaine with epinephrine. After placement of the block, it is imperative not to lift the infants feet or legs above the head; otherwise, a high block will occur. This has been done to place the pad for the electrocautery unit. After placement of the block, the infant can frequently be calmed down by allowing him or her to suck on a pacifier that is dipped in a solution containing glucose (5% or 10% dextrose in water). Because of the success of this technique for routine procedures, such as inguinal herniorrhaphy, it has also been suggested as an acceptable alternative to general anesthesia during more complicated cases, such as repair of gastroschisis.[48] The report by Vane and colleagues includes only four cases. The safety and efficacy of this technique needs further testing. Spinal anesthesia for gastroschisis repair cannot currently be recommended, although the combination of spinal anesthesia with general anesthesia may be a suitable technique.

The disadvantages of spinal anesthesia include a limited duration of surgical anesthesia (60 to 90 minutes) and difficulty in identifying the space in a large percentage of patients, even in experienced hands. Other authors have reported their experience with epidural (caudal or lumbar) anesthesia.[49-51] The advantage of this technique is the ease of identification of the caudal epidural space. The disadvantages of this technique include the need for larger doses of local anesthetics, incomplete motor block with 0.2% or 0.25% bupivacaine, and a longer onset of action. Dosing recommendations vary from author to author ranging from 1.0 to 1.5 ml/kg of 0.2% or 0.25% bupivacaine. It should be noted that the use of 1.5 ml/kg of 0.25% bupivacaine gives a total dose of bupivacaine of 3.75 mg/kg. Webster and colleagues reported their experience with lumbar epidural anesthesia for the same purpose with doses of 1.0 ml/kg of 0.25% bupivacaine.[51] The advantage of lumbar administration over caudal administration is a decrease in the volume required to achieve the same sensory level.

Regardless of whether spinal or epidural anesthesia is chosen, a maximum of 90 minutes of surgical anesthesia can be achieved. Since some surgical procedures may require a more prolonged anesthetic, repeated doses of local anesthetic may be needed. Although this may be accomplished by placement of a catheter in the caudal or lumbar epidural space, repeated doses of bupivacaine carry the risk of toxicity, especially in neonates, because of the immaturity of hepatic function and the resultant, prolonged serum half-life of bupivacaine.[52] Henderson and colleagues[53] were the first to describe the use of chloroprocaine for continuous caudal anesthesia in infants. Because of its short plasma half-life of less than 60 seconds, the risk of toxicity is less than with bupivacaine, even with repeated dosing. In the report of Henderson and colleagues, chloroprocaine levels were measured in 5 patients. The levels were 0.0 μg/ml in 4 patients and 0.5 μg/ml in the fifth at the end of the continuous infusion (2 ml/kg/hr of 3% chloroprocaine).

This technique is useful for more prolonged surgical procedures lasting up to 3 hours in infants as small as 1400 grams.[54,55]

The authors have found a relatively quick onset of complete motor and sensory blockade (5 to 7 mins) with 3% chloroprocaine. Therefore the slow onset and incomplete motor blockade with previous reports of caudal epidural anesthesia in infants may be a problem only with dilute concentrations of bupivacaine (0.2% to 0.25%). Catheter placement is accomplished with the infant in the lateral decubitus position after sterile betadine preparation and local infiltration with 0.2 to 0.3 ml of 1% lidocaine or 3% chloroprocaine. Standard intravenous catheters (22- or 24-gauge) that are advanced through the sacrococcygeal membrane into the epidural space are preferred. After placement, a t-piece, which has been flushed with 3% chloroprocaine, is attached to the catheter and secured in place with a transparent bioocclusive dressing. The initial dose includes up to 2 ml/kg of 3% chloroprocaine (administered in fractionated doses of 0.5 ml/kg at 3 min intervals) followed by a continuous infusion of 3% chloroprocaine. The infusion rate is set in ml/kg/hr to equal the initial bolus dose. Subsequent bolus doses of 0.3 ml/kg are administered if the infants act as if they are in pain or the sensory level regresses to T_6.

As in adults, the use of regional anesthesia in neonates may be associated with cardiorespiratory compromise. This risk may theoretically be greater in infants with residual bronchopulmonary dysplasia since a high thoracic block may lead to loss of chest wall muscle tone and function, thereby compromising respiratory reserve and the ability to effectively cough and clear secretions. An extremely high block may, of course, affect central control of respiratory drive. An additional concern of these techniques is the occurrence of inadequate intraoperative anesthesia. Inadequate anesthesia may occur even in the most experienced hands. Therefore alternative means of anesthesia must be planned. This may include a second attempt at regional anesthesia on another day for an elective procedure or converting to general anesthesia for urgent procedures. Regardless of the choice, the equipment for general anesthesia should be available before the use of regional anesthesia in any patient population.

The second option for continuous regional anesthesia is a continuous spinal technique. Although previously practiced in the adult population, the technique has fallen out of favor after reports of neurotoxicity and resultant cauda equina syndrome.[56] The exact etiology of this syndrome remains to be determined, and to date it has been reported most commonly with the use of microcatheters (28-gauge or less). There is limited information concerning continuous spinal anesthesia in the neonatal population. Payne and Moore reported their use of continuous spinal anesthesia in combination with regional anesthesia in 10 children, the youngest of whom was 2 months of age.[57] The authors placed 28-gauge catheters through 22-gauge needles. The initial and subsequent doses consisted of 0.2 ml/kg of 0.5% bupivacaine (1 mg/kg). The duration of anesthesia after each dose was 59.7 ± 2.1 minutes. Despite the success of this technique, the authors cautioned against its use because of the reports of cauda equina syndrome in the adult population.

Tobias and colleagues reported their experience with continuous spinal anesthesia in two former, preterm infants who were 30 and 32 weeks old.[54] A 24-gauge, epidural catheter was placed through a 20-gauge, 2 inch Crawford needle. The catheter was inserted 2 cm into the intrathecal space and placement was confirmed by aspiration of cerebrospinal fluid (CSF). The initial dose in both cases consisted of 0.6 mg/kg of bupivacaine administered in D_{10} as a 0.5% solution. Subsequent doses of 0.3 mg/kg were administered, as needed, when the sensory level regressed to T_6. This required redosing the catheters on an hourly basis. Until further information of the mechanisms involved in the cauda equina syndrome are determined, this technique will have limited applicability to the neonatal population.

Another alternative when a combination technique is chosen is to use general and epidural anesthesia. Murrell and colleagues[58] combined lumbar epidural blockade with general anesthesia for abdominal procedures in 14 infants aged 1 to 35 days, as well as 6 former preterm infants. They found that the lumbar epidural administration of 0.25% bupivacaine (up to 0.8 ml/kg) with fentanyl (1 to 2 μg/kg) provides excellent intraoperative surgical conditions, limits the requirements for inhalational anesthetic agent, and eliminates the need for intravenous opioids. They successfully extubated all patients at the completion of the surgical procedure. Similar success has been reported by combining caudal epidural anesthesia using a continuous chloroprocaine infusion with general anesthesia in 18 neonates ranging in age from 1 to 28 days and in weight from 2.2 to 4.9 kg.[59] After anesthetic induction and endotracheal intubation, the caudal catheter was placed using the previously described technique. The initial dose of 3% chloroprocaine included either 1.0 or 1.5 ml/kg administered at 3-minute intervals in doses of 0.5 ml/kg. After the initial bolus dose, an infusion was started at a rate that was equivalent to the initial bolus dose (1.0 or 1.5 ml/kg/hr). Maintenance anesthesia consisted of either 0.2% isoflurane (expired concentration) in 40% oxygen and air or 70% nitrous oxide in oxygen. If the level of surgical anesthesia was judged inadequate as demonstrated by an increase in heart rate or blood pressure in response to surgical stimulation, an additional bolus dose of 3% chloroprocaine (0.5 ml/kg) was administered, and the infusion was increased by 0.5 ml/kg/hr. The two patients who initially received a bolus dose of 1.0 ml/kg, followed by an infusion of 1.0 ml/kg/hr, required an additional bolus dose, followed by an increase in the infusion to 1.5 ml/kg/hr. No infant required more than 0.2% isoflurane or 70% nitrous oxide in oxygen. Of the 18 infants, 16 were extubated in the operating room within 10 minutes of the completion of the surgical procedure. As previously discussed, chloroprocaine is preferred in the neonatal population because of the concerns of bupivacaine accumulation with repeated doses. The denser sensory block with chloroprocaine may explain why the intraoperative anesthetic requirements (0.2% isoflurane or 70% nitrous oxide) were lower than those described by Murrell and colleagues (1.0% isoflurane).

Epidural techniques may also be continued into the postoperative period to provide ongoing analgesia. Despite its success in adults and children, there remains limited information concerning the neonatal population. Enthusiasm over this technique is somewhat limited by concerns of bupivacaine toxicity, especially with prolonged use. The infusion rate of bupivacaine should be limited to 0.25 mg/kg/hr. If the maximum infusion rate is reached and analgesia is inadequate, alternatives, such as adding epidural or systemic opioids or abandoning the technique in favor of systemic analgesics, should be considered.[60] A solution of 1% lidocaine may also be administered as a continuous epidural infusion in rates up to 1 mg/kg/hr (0.1 ml/kg/hr).[61] The advantage of this technique is that lidocaine levels are easy to obtain, and monitoring for toxicity is more easily achieved than with bupivacaine. The authors' approach is to use low concentrations of bupivacaine (1/16%) in combination with fentanyl (1 to 2 μg/ml) at 0.2 ml/kg/hr. This technique has proved successful in the neonatal population.

Aside from the choice of local anesthetic, the second decision is the level at which to place the catheter. When the catheter is left in the caudal region, higher doses of local anesthetics (initial bolus and continuous infusion rate) are required to achieve the same level of blockade when compared with lumbar placement. The major advantage of caudal placement is the ease of identifying the caudal epidural space and avoiding the risk of dural puncture. Although caudal placement can be used for postoperative analgesia for lower extremity or urologic procedures, such as repair of bladder exstrophy, more effective analgesia can be obtained for abdominal procedures with placement of the catheter near the dermatomes involved in the surgery. This may involve threading the catheter up from the epidural space or needle insertion at the level involved. Previous reports have demonstrated the feasibility of threading a catheter from the caudal space to the lumbar or even the thoracic region.[62] For this technique, a 24-gauge catheter can be placed through a 22- or 20-gauge needle, which is inserted through the sacrococcygeal membrane into the caudal epidural space. The major problem with this technique is kinking of the catheter or the inability to pass the catheter to the desired level. Confirmation of placement by x-ray examination is difficult since the smaller catheters are not radiopaque and injection of dye is required to identify the location. The advantage of catheter placement near the level of surgery is analgesia with lower requirements for both local anesthetics and opioids.

Although fentanyl, because of its lipophilic nature, requires placement near the involved dermatomes, morphine travels cephalad in the CSF and may be injected in the caudal/lumbar region to provide analgesia after thoracic or even head and neck procedures.[63] Options for neuraxial morphine include both intrathecal and epidural administration.[64,65] Krechel and Helikson described their experience with intrathecal morphine (10 μg/kg) in three infants after repair of esophageal atresia. All three were successfully extubated at the completion of the surgical procedure and had long lasting pain relief (22 to 36 hrs) without supplemental analgesic agents. In addition to thoracic procedures, intrathecal morphine is useful when combined with spinal anesthesia during major intraabdominal procedures. Spinal anesthesia may be used in combination with general anesthesia to decrease the requirements for inhalational agents or parenteral opioids. In this setting, intrathecal morphine is added to the local anesthetic and administered before the procedure. A final option for providing prolonged analgesia is epidural morphine. Although experience in the neonatal population is limited, caudal epidural morphine in doses of 0.03 to 0.05 mg/kg has been shown to provide prolonged postoperative analgesia in infants and children.[65] The morphine can be added to the local anesthetic solution (1 ml/kg of 0.25 or 0.125% bupivacaine) and administered at the completion of the surgical procedure. Regardless of the route chosen for the delivery of opioids, continuous monitoring of cardiorespiratory function is mandatory because of the risk of respiratory depression. Prolonged monitoring (24 hrs) is recommended when intrathecal or epidural morphine is used because of the risk of delayed respiratory depression. Despite the increased risk of respiratory depression in the neonatal population, analgesia should not be withheld in this patient population.

SEDATION DURING EXTRACORPOREAL MEMBRANE OXYGENATION

ECMO continues to gain popularity in the management of acute respiratory failure resulting from meconium aspiration, persistent pulmonary hypertension of the neonate (PPHN), diaphragmatic hernia, or other pulmonary diseases. ECMO can be venoarterial (VA) or venovenous (VV), requiring cannulation of the common carotid and jugular veins in VA ECMO and cannulation of the right atrium and femoral vein in VV ECMO. Neuromuscular blockade and intravenous general anesthesia (10 to 20 μg/kg fentanyl) is administered during placement of the cannulae. However, the partial cardiopulmonary state of ECMO requires anticoagulation with a risk of intraventricular hemorrhage. The ability to perform neurologic exams regularly during ECMO is mandatory, although there is an equal need for sedation to minimize the likelihood of dislodgement of the cannulae. Such problems preclude the use of ongoing neuromuscular blockade. Several options exist for the provision of sedation during ECMO and have included benzodiazepines, opioids, or a combination of the two.

Midazolam infusions have met with limited success as a result of binding of the drug to the oxygenator of the ECMO circuit. Continuous infusions of fentanyl have been complicated by the rapid occurrence of tolerance with the need for steady increases in infusion rates to maintain a consistent level of sedation. Arnold and colleagues observed an escalation from a mean infusion rate of 9.2 μg/kg/hr on day 1 to 21.9 μg/kg/hr on day 6.[66] Fentanyl levels increased with the increased infusion rates, demonstrating that the increased fentanyl requirements were related to a receptor phenomenon and not the result of increased metabolism of the drug.

Immediately after the institution of ECMO, the increased requirements for fentanyl may be due to the adhesion of fentanyl to the ECMO circuit. Fentanyl binds rapidly to the circuit with a resultant decrease in the plasma level by 75% in the first 5 minutes. During this time, frequent bolus doses are needed to maintain a steady state serum concentration and an acceptable level of sedation. Because of its beneficial effects on pulmonary vascular responsiveness and minimal effects on cardiorespiratory function, fentanyl remains the primary agent for sedation during ECMO. When used for this purpose, escalation of doses up to 70 to 80 μg/kg/hr have been necessary.[67]

Alterations in drug pharmacokinetics may also be seen with the discontinuation of ECMO. Dagan and colleagues have documented decreasing morphine levels with increased clearance after cessation of ECMO.[68] Although they were unable to identify the exact cause of this effect, they postulated that alterations in hepatic blood flow may be responsible. A second possibility may relate to increases in pulmonary blood flow after discontinuation of ECMO and some intrinsic clearance of opioids by the pulmonary parenchyma. Although the exact cause remains to be determined, increases in the morphine dose may be required to prevent opioid withdrawal or inadequate sedation after discontinuation of ECMO.

Because of the problems with the development of tolerance and the need to rapidly escalate doses, the search continues for alternative agents for sedation during ECMO. In the pediatric ECMO population, initial results suggest the efficacy of pentobarbital as an alternative to opioids during ECMO. Tobias and colleagues have reported their preliminary experience with pentobarbital infusion rates of 1 to 6 mg/kg/hr.[69] As with fentanyl, tolerance develops and an increased dose is required with time. However, the escalation in dose requirements is less rapid than with fentanyl. Disadvantages of pentobarbital include its cardiovascular effects, such as peripheral vasodilatation and negative inotropism, both of which can decrease blood pressure. These effects can be minimized by administering bolus doses over 5 to 10 minutes. Additionally, the pentobarbital solution is relatively alkaline, making it incompatible with other medications. Despite these problems, it offers an attractive alternative to opioids for sedation during ECMO.

OPIOID TOLERANCE AND PHYSICAL DEPENDENCE

Tolerance is the decreased effectiveness of a drug with its repeated administration or an increase in the dose required to maintain the same clinical effect. It is not due to changes in metabolism but to changes in receptor number and function related to the duration of opioid receptor occupation.[70] Physical dependence requires the continued administration of the drug to avoid signs of withdrawal. The use of opioids for analgesia or sedation may result in physical dependence, but it does not result in psychological dependence (i.e., addiction). Therefore it is inappropriate to describe physiologically dependent infants or children as addicts or to consider them at risk for developing a substance abuse disorder.[70]

Patients who have received sedative agents for more than 5 to 7 days are considered at risk of drug withdrawal. This can be managed with a gradual taper of no more than 10% to 20% per day in order to avoid signs of withdrawal. Slower tapers are often required in premature infants. Excessive yawning, irritability, gut hypermotility, and palmar sweating are symptoms of withdrawal.

The methadone sliding scale is a versatile technique employed by Berde (personal communication) that can be applied in cases of tolerance, weaning from opioids, or as a maintenance regimen. Around-the-clock administration is used. The patient receives one of three doses every 6 hours: 0.025 mg/kg for mild pain, 0.05 mg/kg for moderate pain, or 0.075 mg/kg for severe pain. If there is inadequate relief with the 0.075 mg/kg dose, then the three doses are increased by approximately 20%. If analgesia is adequate with the initial dosing and schedule, and the patient consistently requires only the dose for mild pain for 24 hours, then the dosing scheme is decreased by 20%.

The methadone sliding scale can be employed in the initial phase of an opioid taper. Once the effective dose to avoid signs of withdrawal is obtained, the sliding scale is stopped and the effective dose is continued every 6 hours for the first 24 hours. Thereafter, the dose is reduced no more than 20% per 24 hours. The taper is continued until the patient requires less than 30% of the initially effective dose. Objective measurement of the signs and symptoms of opioid withdrawal should be measured. Assessment tools for neonatal abstinence or irritability facilitate proper titration of opioids with minimal occurrences of relapse.

Another alternative is to switch from intravenous fentanyl to oral methadone to eliminate the need for intravenous access and in many instances allow earlier discharge home. (The guidelines for changing from intravenous fentanyl to oral methadone are outlined in Chapter 7.)

Summary

The neonate has been shown to experience pain in the same way as adults and may even have lower thresholds for pain perception. The documented increase in morbidity from untreated postoperative pain warrants greater vigilance and treatment of pain in the neonatal population. In the busy setting of the NICU, it is not uncommon to view pain management as a lesser concern. Yet, the evidence is mounting that pain management should be a key priority in the everyday care provided to neonates.

References

1. Purcell-Jones G, Dorman F, Sumner E: Paediatric anaesthetists' perceptions of neonatal and infant pain, *Pain* 33:181, 1988.
2. Scanlon JW: Appreciating neonatal pain, *Adv Pediatr* 38:317, 1991.
3. Grunau RVE, Craig KD: Facial activity as a measure of neonatal pain expression, *Adv Pain Res Ther* 15:147, 1990.
4. Anand KJS, Hickey PR: Halothane-morphine compared with high-dose sufentanil for anesthesia and postoperative analgesia in neonatal cardiac surgery, *N Engl J Med* 326:1, 1992.
5. Anand KJS, Hansen DD, Hickey PR: Hormonal-metabolic stress responses in neonates undergoing cardiac surgery, *Anesthesiology* 73:661, 1990.

6. Schiff DE, Staonestreet BS: Central venous catheters in low birth weight infants: incidence of related complications, *J Perinatol* 13:153, 1993.
7. Gray H: In Pick TP, Howden R, editors: *Gray's anatomy,* Philadelphia, 1974, Running Press.
8. Soliman IE, Broadman LM, Hannallah RS et al: Comparison of the analgesic effects of EMLA (eutectic mixture of local anesthetics) to intradermal lidocaine infiltration prior to venous cannulation in unpremedicated children, *Anesthesiology* 68:804, 1988.
9. Bonica JJ, Buckley FP: Regional analgesia with local anesthetics. In Bonica JL, editor: *The management of pain,* Philadelphia, 1990, Lea and Febiger.
10. Hruszkewycz V, Holtrop PC, Batton DG et al: Complications associated with central venous catheters inserted in critically ill neonates, *Infect Control Hosp Epidemiol* 12:544, 1991.
11. Nakamura KT, Yutaka S, Erenberg A: Evaluation of a percutaneously placed 27-gauge central venous catheter in neonates weighing less than 1200 grams, *J Parenter Enteral Nutr* 14:295, 1990.
12. Aimone LD: Neurochemistry and modulation of pain. In Sinatra RS, Hord AH, Ginsberg B, Preble LM, editors: *Acute pain: mechanisms and management,* St. Louis, 1990, Mosby-Yearbook.
13. Ment LR, Oh W, Ehrenfranz RA et al: Low-dose indomethacin and prevention of intraventricular hemorrhage: a multicenter, randomized trial, *Pediatrics* 93:543, 1994.
14. Gal P, Ransom JL, Weaver RL et al: Indomethacin pharmacokinetics in neonates: the value of volume of distribution as a marker of permanent patent ductus arteriosus closure, *Ther Drug Monit* 13:42, 1991.
15. Stein C, Millan MJ, Shippenberg TS et al: Peripheral opioid receptors mediating antinociception in inflammation: evidence for involvement of mu, delta, and kappa receptors, *J Pharmacol Exp Ther* 248:1269, 1989.
16. Wilson JM, Thompson JR, Schnitzer JJ et al: Intratracheal

pulmonary ventilation and congenital diaphragmatic hernia: a report of two cases, *J Pediatr Surg* 28:484, 1993.

17. Nugent M, Artu AA, Michenfelder JD: Cerebral metabolic, vascular, and protective effects of midazolam maleate: comparison to diazepam, *Anesthesiology* 56:172, 1982.
18. Michenfelder JD: Barbiturates for brain resuscitation: yes and no, *Anesthesiology* 57:74, 1982.
19. Jacqz-Aigrain E, Daoud P, Burtin P et al: Pharmacokinetics of midazolam during continuous infusion in critically ill neonates, *Eur J Clin Pharmacol* 42:329, 1992.
20. Harvey SC: Hypnotics and sedatives. In Gilman AG, Goodman LS, Wall TW, Murad F, editors: *The pharmacological basis of therapeutics,* New York, 1985, MacMillan.
21. McDermott C, Kowalczyk A, Schnitzier ER et al: Pharmacokinetics of lorazepam in critically ill neonates with seizures, *J Pediatr* 120:479, 1992.
22. Maloley PA, Gal P, Mize R et al: Lorazepam dosing in neonates: application of objective sedation score (letter), *Ann Phamacother* 24:326, 1990.
23. Sunshine A, Olson NZ, Zihelboim I et al: Analgesic oral efficacy of tramadol hydrochloride in postoperative pain, *Clin Pharmacol Ther* 51:740, 1992.
24. Howard CR, Howard FM, Weitzman ML: Acetaminophen analgesia in neonatal circumcision: the effect on pain, *Pediatrics* 93:641, 1994.
25. Williamson PS, Evans ND: Neonatal cortisol response to circumcision with anesthesia, *Clin Pediatr* 25:412, 1986.
26. Kirya C, Werthmann MW Jr: Neonatal circumcision and penile dorsal nerve block: a painless procedure, *J Pediatr* 92:988,1978.
27. Myron AV, Maguire DP: Pain perception in the neonate: implications for circumcision, *J Prof Nurs* 7:188, 1991.
28. Schoen JE, Fischell AA: Pain in neonatal circumcision, *Clin Pediatr* 30:429, 1991.
29. Andersen KH: A new method of analgesia for relief of circumcision pain, *Anaesthesia* 44:118, 1989.

30. Broadman ML, Hannallah RS, Belman AB et al: Post-circumcision analgesia: a prospective evaluation of subcutaneous ring block of the penis, *Anesthesiology* 67:399, 1987.
31. Martin LVH: Postoperative analgesia after circumcision in children, *Br J Anaesth* 54:1263, 1982.
32. Masciello AL: Anesthesia for neonatal circumcision: local anesthesia is better than dorsal penile nerve block, *Obstet Gynecol* 75:834, 1990.
33. McClain BC: Pediatric caudal anesthesia: an illustrated handbook. Monograph printed by The Medical College of Georgia, 1990.
34. Marchette L, Main R, Redick E et al: Pain reduction interventions during neonatal circumcision, *Nurs Res* 40:241, 1991.
35. Benini F, Johnston CC, Faucher D et al: Topical anesthesia during circumcision in newborn infants, *JAMA* 270:850, 1993.
36. Cunningham N: Ethical perspectives on the perception and treatment of neonatal pain, *J Perinat Neonat Nurs* 4:75, 1990.
37. Tohill J, McMorrow O: Pain relief in neonatal intensive care, *Lancet* 336:569, 1990.
38. Elsbery NL: Pain reduction interventions during neonatal circumcision, *Nurs Res* 41:127, 1992.
39. Anand KJS, Sippell WG, Schofield NM et al: Does halothane anesthesia decrease the metabolic and endocrine stress responses of newborn infants undergoing operation? *Br Med J* 286:668, 1988.
40. Koehntop DE, Rodman JH, Brundage DM et al: Pharmacokinetics of fentanyl in neonates, *Anesth Analg* 65:227, 1986.
41. Davis PJ, Killian A, Stiller RL et al: Pharmacokinetics of alfentanil in newborn premature infants, *Dev Pharmacol Ther* 13:21, 1989.
42. Bhat R, Chari G, Gulati A et al: Pharmacokinetics of a single dose of morphine in preterm infants during the first week of life, *J Pediatr* 117:477, 1990.
43. Lynn AM, Slattery JT: Morphine pharmacokinetics in early infancy, *Anesthesiology* 66:136, 1987.

44. Lynn AM, Opheim KE, Tyler DC: Morphine infusion after pediatric cardiac surgery, *Crit Care Medicine* 12:863,1984.
45. Clancy GT, Anand KJS, Lally P: Neonatal pain management, *Crit Care Nurs Clin North Am* 4:527, 1992.
46. Mahe V, Ecoffey C: Spinal anesthesia with isobaric bupivacaine in infants, *Anesthesiology* 68:601, 1988.
47. Webster AC, McKishnie JD, Kenyon CF et al: Spinal anaesthesia for inguinal hernia repair in high-risk neonates, *Can J Anaesth* 38:281, 1991.
48. Vane DW, Abajian JC, Hong AR: Spinal anesthesia for primary repair of gastroschisis: a new and safe technique for selected patients, *J Pediatr Surg* 29:1234, 1994.
49. Spear RM, Deshpande JK, Maxwell LG: Caudal anesthesia in the awake, high-risk neonate, *Anesthesiology* 69:407, 1988.
50. Spear RM: Dose-response in infants receiving caudal anaesthesia with bupivacaine, *Paediatric Anaesthesia* 1:47, 1991.
51. Webster AC, McKishnie JD, Watson JT et al: Lumbar epidural anaesthesia for inguinal hernia repair in low birth weight infants, *Can J Anaesth* 40:670, 1993.
52. Mazoit JX, Densen DD, Samii K: Pharmacokinetics of bupivacaine following caudal anesthesia in infants, *Anesthesiology* 50:454, 1979.
53. Henderson KH, Sethna NF, Berde CB: Continuous caudal anesthesia with 2-chloroprocaine for premature infants undergoing inguinal hernia repair, *Anesthesiology* 75:A916, 1991.
54. Tobias JD, Lowe S, O'Dell N et al: Continuous regional anesthesia in infants, *Can J Anaesth* 40:1065, 1993.
55. Tobias JD, Hersey S: Continuous caudal anesthesia during inguinal hernia repair in an awake, 1440 gram infant, *Paediatric Anaesthesia* 4:187, 1994.
56. Rigler ML, Drasner K, Krejcie TC et al: Cauda equina syndrome after continuous spinal anesthesia, *Anesth Analg* 72:275, 1991.
57. Payne KA, Moore SW: Subarachnoid microcatheter anesthesia in small children, *Reg Anesth* 19:237, 1994.

58. Murrell D, Gibson PR, Cohen RC: Continuous epidural analgesia in newborn infants undergoing major surgery, *J Pediatr Surg* 28:548, 1993.
59. Tobias JD, Rasmuseen GE, Holcomb GW III et al: Continuous caudal anesthesia with chloroprocaine as an adjunct to general anesthesia in neonates, *Can J Anaesth* (in press).
60. Berde CB: Convulsions associated with pediatric regional anesthesia, *Anesth Analg* 75:164, 1992.
61. Kost-Byerly C, Greenberg RS, Billet CA et al: Continuous lidocaine epidural analgesia in neonates, *Anesthesiology* 81:A1343, 1994.
62. Bosenberg AT, Bland BAR, Schulte-Steinberg O et al: Thoracic epidural anesthesia via the caudal route in infants, *Anesthesiology* 69:265, 1988.
63. Tobias JD, Deshpande JK, Wetzel RC et al: Postoperative analgesia: use of intrathecal morphine in children, *Clin Pediatr* 29:44, 1990.
64. Krechel SE, Helikson MA: Intrathecal morphine for pain control in term infants for oesophageal atresia/tracheoesophageal fistula repair, *Paediatric Anaesthesia* 3:243, 1993.
65. Krane EJ, Tyler DC, Jacobson LE: The dose response of caudal morphine in children, *Anesthesiology* 71:48, 1989.
66. Arnold JH, Truog RD, Scavone JM et al: Changes in the pharmacodynamic response to fentanyl in neonates during continuous infusion, *J Pediatr* 119:639, 1991.
67. Caron E, Maguire DP: Current management of pain, sedation, and narcotic physical dependency of the infant on ECMO, *J Perinat Neonatal Nurs* 4:63, 1990.
68. Tobias JD, Deshpande JK, Pietsch JB et al: Pentobarbital sedation in the pediatric intensive care unit patient, *South Med J* 88:290, 1995.
69. Anand KJS, Arnold JH: Opioid tolerance and dependence in infants and children, *Crit Care Med* 22:334, 1994.
70. Tobias JD, Schleien CL, Haun SE: Methadone as treatment for iatrogenic narcotic dependency in pediatric intensive care unit patients, *Crit Care Med* 18:1292, 1990.

SEDATION IN THE PEDIATRIC INTENSIVE CARE UNIT

7

Joseph D. Tobias

AGENTS FOR SEDATION

INHALATIONAL ANESTHETIC AGENTS
BENZODIAZEPINES
KETAMINE
PROPOFOL
BARBITURATES
OPIOIDS
MISCELLANEOUS AGENTS

Several factors may be responsible for the anxiety and fear experienced by children during their stay in the Pediatric Intensive Care Unit (PICU). These include separation from parents, invasive procedures, disruption of the usual day/night cycle, and the presence of unfamiliar people and machines. Although reassurance and parental presence alleviate some of the distress, pharmacologic intervention is frequently required.

Since no single agent can be effective in all patients, physicians need to be familiar with several different agents. This allows the physician to switch from one agent to another when the first-line drug is either ineffective or leads to adverse effects. The task of providing sedation in the PICU is further complicated by the diverse group of patients with a wide range of medical and post-surgical problems. No "cookbook" is available to provide definite guidelines for sedation and analgesia. Sedative and analgesic agents cannot be dosed on a per-kilogram basis like antibiotics. Dosing recommendations are meant as guidelines for starting doses and the actual amount administered should be titrated to the desired effect.

Aside from interpatient variability in dosing requirements, there is a wide range of indications for analgesic and sedative agents in the PICU. Although analgesia is certainly required for postoperative patients, sedation and analgesia may also be required during the performance of various procedures, to improve the efficacy of mechanical ventilation, and to alleviate the distress associated with acute medical illnesses. Sedation may also be used as a therapeutic tool in the treatment of raised intracranial pressure (ICP) or to prevent pulmonary vasospasm after cardiac surgical procedures.

AGENTS FOR SEDATION

Inhalational Anesthetic Agents

The inhalational anesthetic agents in common clinical use include halothane, enflurane, and isoflurane with the recent addition of sevoflurane and desflurane. Although their use for ICU sedation is limited in the United States, certain centers in Europe have significant experience with these agents (most commonly, isoflurane).[1,2] Although halothane, enflurane, and isoflurane have all been used for sedation in ICU patients, only the last is now commonly used. Problems with halothane include its direct negative inotropic effects, arrythmogenic properties, especially in the setting of increased catecholamines or with the administration of other medications (aminophylline), and, most importantly, hepatitis, thought to be related to an immunologic reaction directed against the oxidative metabolite, trifluoroacetic acid. Problems with enflurane include a similar negative inotropic effect and the release of fluoride during metabolism. Fluoride at increased concentrations (greater than 50 μ-mol/L) may be nephrotoxic with decreases in the glomerular filtration rate and nephrogenic diabetes insipidus.

One advantage of isoflurane is the limited risk of fluoride toxicity, since less than 1% is metabolized and its major cardiovascular action is peripheral vasodilatation, thereby maintaining cardiac output. Because of these properties, isoflurane is usually the only inhalational agent used for ICU sedation.

Advocates of inhalational anesthetic agents for ICU sedation emphasize rapid onset, rapid awakening, and ease of control of the depth of sedation. Although these agents are effective, several logistic problems limit their usefulness outside of the operating room. Effective scavenging is needed to prevent environmental pollution. Although scavenging is commonplace in the operating room, the cost of installation in most ICUs would be prohibitive. Aside from this concern, delivery of the agent requires specialized equipment. Since moving an anesthesia machine into the ICU is not always practical, most ICUs utilize a Servo 900D ventilator with a vaporizer attached to it. This does not overcome the pollution issue, since the exhaust of the ventilation (exhalation port) should not be vented to the environment. Additionally, rules and regulations abound as to who should regulate the inspired concentration of the agent, and in most centers the nursing staff is not permitted to alter the vaporizer setting. Manpower issues become important if only the physician staff are allowed to alter the vaporizer setting.

Despite several beneficial properties, two additional issues limit the utility of inhalational anesthetic agents. Inhalational anesthetic agents are triggering agents for malignant hyperthermia, and cerebral vasodilatation may lead to clinically significant increases in ICP. Cerebral vasodilation is least likely with isoflurane, may be partially prevented by hyperventilation ($Paco_2$ of 25 to 30 torr),[3] and is more likely to occur in patients with altered intracranial compliance. In addition to these physiologic actions, inhalational agents alter the metabolism of several drugs, such as lidocaine, beta adrenergic blocking agents, benzodiazepines, and local anesthetics.[4] This effect is thought to result from alterations in the intrinsic clearance of the drug and not decreases in cardiac output and hepatic blood flow.

Most importantly, there is limited clinical experience with these agents in the pediatric population. Arnold and colleagues[5] administered isoflurane for sedation during mechanical ventilation to 10 patients, ranging from 3 weeks to 19 years of age. Effective sedation was achieved in all patients without adverse effects. The highest fluoride concentration was 26.1 μ-mol/L, and no evidence of renal toxicity was noted. Despite its anecdotal success in children, the concerns of delivery and scavenging with these agents limits their routine use for sedation in the PICU.

Benzodiazepines

Benzodiazepines remain the most commonly used agents for ICU sedation. Their mechanism of action is thought to be in the limbic system through the inhibitory neurotransmitter, γ-amino butyric acid (GABA). Benzodiazepines impair acquisition and encoding of new information (anterograde amnesia) and have no effect on either retention or retrieval of previously stored information (retrograde amnesia).[6] They have no intrinsic analgesic properties;[7] thus, the concomitant administration of an opioid is suggested in situations requiring analgesia.

There are currently three benzodiazepines that are commonly used for sedation. These are diazepam, midazolam, and lorazepam. For many years diazepam was the agent of choice for sedation in the ICU. Although it is effective by both the oral and intravenous routes, it has a low solubility in water and is administered in a solution of propylene glycol, which can cause pain on injection and thrombophlebitis when administered through a peripheral infusion. Most importantly, prolonged sedation may be seen as a result of its long half-life and hypnotically active metabolites (oxazepam and n-demethyldiazepam). Both of the metabolites have elimination half-lives that exceed that of the parent compound.

Midazolam is an imidazobenzodiazepine with a rapid onset of action and a short elimination half-life. Because of its short half-life, effective use requires its administration by continuous infusion. Several investigations have documented the efficacy of midazolam infusions for sedation in the ICU in doses ranging from 0.05 to 0.2 mg/kg/hr after an initial bolus dose of 0.1 mg/kg.[8-10]

Certain medications or underlying conditions may potentiate the effects of midazolam through either alterations in metabolism or decreases in protein binding. Midazolam is metabolized by the P-450 system of the liver with the possibility of drug interactions with agents such as cimetidine. Alterations in protein binding may also alter the effect of midazolam. Heparin increases the free fraction of midazolam by displacing it from protein binding sites. The free fraction is also increased by up to 2.5 to 3 times normal in patients with hepatic and renal dysfunction.[11,12] Adjustments in the loading dose and infusion regimens are recommended in these conditions.

Although most centers use a continuous infusion to provide prolonged sedation, an alternative that has recently been described is the use of a patient-controlled analgesia (PCA) device to deliver the medication.[13] The authors coined the term "patient-controlled anxiolysis" for their new technique.

Although intravenous administration is usually the route chosen in the PICU, several investigators have described novel routes of delivery of midazolam, such as oral, transmucosal (nasal or rectal), sublingual, and subcutaneous.[14-17] Because of limited absorption, an increased dose is required for these alternative routes of delivery. These routes are rarely used for ongoing sedation in the PICU but may have some role for one time sedation (for procedures see Chapter 8).

The major disadvantage of midazolam is the cost. An estimation of cost for a 20 kg patient (0.1 to 0.2 mg/kg/hr) is $80/day. Because of these concerns, the efficacy of lorazepam has recently been evaluated by continuous infusion. The cost of a one-day dose of lorazepam for the same 20 kg patient is roughly $30. Additionally, there are now generic forms of lorazepam and the price can be expected to drop even further. Although midazolam's short half-life necessitates its administration by continuous infusion, lorazepam's duration of action is 4 to 8 hours; therefore, it may be administered by intermittent, on-demand dosing. A second advantage of lorazepam over other benzodiazepines is metabolism by glucuronyl transferase, not the P-450 system. Medications known to alter the P-450 system (anticonvulsants, rifampin, or cimetidine) have no effect on the pharmacokinetics of lorazepam. In patients with advanced liver disease, phase II reactions (glucuronyl transferase) are better preserved than phase I reactions (P-450 system). Additionally, lorazepam has no active metabolites. Therefore its plasma half-life and sedative properties should be less variable than midazolam, even in patients with altered hepatic and renal function.

Although there is little information concerning lorazepam use in children, both intermittent and continuous infusion techniques may be used for sedation. For intermittent administration, starting with 0.05 to 0.1 mg/kg (maximum starting dose of 4 mg) is recommended every 4 to 8 hours. For a continuous infusion, starting with 0.025 mg/kg/hr is recommended (maximum of 2 mg/hr) after an initial loading dose of 0.05 mg/kg (maximum of 4 mg). As with other sedative agents, the infusion rate should be supplemented with p.r.n. (as needed) bolus doses and adjusted accordingly.

Although benzodiazepines are well tolerated with limited effects on cardiorespiratory function,[18] situations may arise which necessitate the administration of a reversal agent. Flumazenil has recently been marketed as a benzodiazepine antagonist. It has been used to reverse midazolam-induced sedation in the ICU. In a recent clinical trial, reversal of sedation was observed in 14 of 15 patients; however, resedation occurred in 7 patients.[19] The latter finding is easily explained, since the half-life of flumazenil is less than that of midazolam. Therefore continued observation of patients is necessary when flumazenil is used to reverse life-threatening adverse effects. Additionally, seizures may occur because of the antagonistic effects of flumazenil at the GABA receptor and are more common in patients chronically receiving benzodiazepines or other medications that lower the seizure threshold.[20] In such situations the use of flumazenil is contraindicated.

As with opioids, the prolonged administration of benzodiazepines may result in physical dependency, and an abstinence syndrome may develop if these agents are abruptly discontinued.[21] This can be prevented by slowly tapering the intravenous administration of the drug (10% to 15% per day) or switching from intravenous midazolam to an orally active agent with a longer half-life, such as lorazepam. The latter approach obviates the need for intravenous access and may allow for earlier hospital discharge with outpatient follow-up once an appropriate oral dose has been determined.[21]

In addition to tolerance and withdrawal symptoms, a relatively distinct phenomenon has been described after midazolam administration.[22] Although this syndrome has been described only with midazolam, it can also occur after the use of other benzodiazepines. Symptoms include poor social interaction, decreased eye contact, decreased interest in the environment, and a choreoathetotic movement disorder with dystonic posturing. Resolution has usually occurred in 2 to 4 weeks without permanent sequelae. The exact etiology remains unknown. All patients also received a fentanyl infusion, and there does seem to be a higher risk in young, female patients.[22]

Ketamine

Ketamine is an intravenous anesthetic agent chemically related to phencyclidine, first introduced into clinical use in 1965. Its amnesic and analgesic state is often referred to as dissociative anesthesia, which has been further characterized as an electrophysiologic break between the limbic and thalamoneocortical systems.[23] The unique property of ketamine that makes it particularly attractive is the provision of both amnesia and analgesia. Metabolism occurs primarily by hepatic n-methylation to norketamine with further metabolism by hydroxylation pathways and subsequent urinary excretion. A hepatic metabolic product, norketamine retains roughly one third of the analgesic and sedative properties of the parent compound. Since ketamine is primarily dependent on hepatic metabolism, doses should be reduced in patients with hepatic dysfunction.

The major advantages of ketamine are its cardiovascular stability and its limited effects on respiratory mechanics. Ketamine produces a dose-related increase in heart rate and blood pressure that are mediated through the sympathetic nervous system and the release of endogenous catecholamines.[24] An important issue in children with congenital heart disease is the possible effect of ketamine on pulmonary vascular resistance (PVR). This issue is somewhat controversial, and mixed reports have been given. Increased PVR has been reported in adults, and avoidance of ketamine has been recommended in patients with pulmonary hypertension.[25] These initial studies were performed in spontaneously breathing patients, and alterations in PVR may have been related to increases in $Paco_2$, not as the result of a direct effect of ketamine on the pulmonary vasculature. Pending further investigations, ketamine should be used cautiously in patients with pulmonary hypertension, especially during spontaneous ventilation.

Respiratory function is well maintained during ketamine administration. Functional residual capacity, minute ventilation, and tidal volume have been reported to be unchanged after ketamine administration,[26] whereas other studies have demonstrated improved pulmonary compliance and decreased bronchospasm.[27] Although ventilation is well maintained, elevations in $Paco_2$ and a shift to the right of the CO_2 response curve may occur.[28] There remains continued controversy concerning ketamine's effects on protective airway reflexes. Although clinical use and experimental studies suggest that these reflexes are maintained,[29] aspiration has been reported after ketamine administration.[30] An additional effect that may impact on airway patency is increased oral secretions. An antisialogogue, such as atropine or glycopyrrolate, is recommended before the administration of ketamine. Because of the above mentioned effects, as with any sedative agent, close monitoring of cardiorespiratory status is recommended.

Ketamine may also increase ICP and should not be used in patients at risk for intracranial hypertension.[31] Alterations in ICP are due to cerebral vasodilatation, mediated through central cholinergic receptors, and not secondary to alterations in cerebral metabolic rate or changes in $Paco_2$.[32]

The adverse effect related to ketamine that receives the most attention is emergence phenomena, or hallucinations. Emergence phenomena are more common in older patients, they are dose-related, and their incidence can be decreased by the preadministration of a benzodiazepine.[33] The administration of a benzodiazepine (lorazepam or midazolam) 5 minutes before the administration of ketamine is effective in preventing emergence phenomena.

Because of its favorable effects on cardiorespiratory function, ketamine may be useful in patients who develop myocardial depression with opioids or benzodiazepines. It is also useful in situations requiring sedation while maintaining spontaneous ventilation, such as the agitated child with severe asthma or during the use of mask continuous positive airway pressure. When used by continuous infusion for sedation, starting with a bolus dose of 1 to 2 mg/kg is recommended, followed by a continuous infusion of 1.0 mg/kg/hr.[34] The infusion should be supplemented with p.r.n. bolus doses and increased as needed.

Propofol

Propofol is a sedative-hypnotic agent and an intravenous anesthetic agent that is chemically unrelated to barbiturates and other commonly used anesthetic induction agents.[35] Because of its rapid onset, quick recovery time after discontinuation, and lack of active metabolites, it has become a popular agent for sedation in the ICU.[36,37] When compared with midazolam for sedation in adult patients, propofol was found to have shorter recovery times, more rapid titration efficiency, and reduced posthypnotic obtundation with faster weaning from mechanical ventilation.[36] An additional benefit is a decrease in the cerebral metabolic rate for oxygen with a subsequent decrease in ICP. The latter effect is similar to that seen with barbiturates.

With the increased use of propofol for ICU sedation and anesthetic induction, certain adverse effects have been noted and may limit its use for ICU sedation. Its cardiovascular effects are similar to those of the barbiturates and include peripheral vasodilatation and negative inotropic properties. Although well tolerated in patients with adequate cardiac reserve, the use of propofol in hemodynamically unstable patients is not recommended. Aside from its negative inotropic properties, propofol may increase central vagal tone leading to bradycardia and even asystole when combined with other medications known to induce bradycardia (fentanyl or succinylcholine).[38]

Of even more concern are reports of unusual neurologic manifestations, such as opisthotonic posturing, myoclonic movements (especially in children), and convulsions.[39-41] More recently, unexplained metabolic acidosis and fatal cardiac failure have been reported in five children with respiratory infections who received propofol.[42] Although the patients in this latter report were receiving higher than recommended doses (up to 13.6 mg/kg/hr), pending further evaluation, its use can no longer be recommended for continuous infusion in the PICU patient.

Additional problems relate to its delivery in a lipid emulsion. Significant pain on injection is commonly seen when propofol is administered through a peripheral infusion. More importantly, anaphylactoid reactions have occasionally been reported.[43] Unlike other medications used for continuous sedation, propofol does not contain preservatives. Laboratory investigation has demonstrated that the lipid emulsion serves as a suitable culture media for bacteria,[44] whereas systemic bacteremia and wound infections have been linked to extrinsically contaminated propofol.[45] Therefore meticulous aseptic technique is required when using propofol, and opened but unused vials should be disposed of promptly and not saved for later use.

Barbiturates

The barbiturates are one of the oldest classes of agents used for sedation in the PICU. As with many of the agents described, their effects on cardiorespiratory function are dose dependent. In healthy patients, sedative doses have minimal effects on respiratory drive and airway protective reflexes, whereas excessive doses can produce apnea and hypotension. The latter effect is related to both peripheral vasodilatation and a direct negative inotropic effect.

Several different agents are available and are most easily classified according to the duration of activity. Short-acting agents, such as methohexital, pentothal, and thiamylal, have a duration of action of 5 to 10 minutes and are usually used by intravenous bolus administration for brief procedures, such as endotracheal intubation. When a more prolonged effect is needed, a continuous infusion is required to maintain constant plasma levels. The longer-acting agents with half-lives of 4 to 12 hours include pentobarbital and phenobarbital.

Regardless of the agent chosen, the barbiturates have beneficial physiologic effects, such as a decrease in the cerebral metabolic rate for oxygen with reductions in cerebral blood flow (CBF) and ICP. The barbiturates are potent anticonvulsants and may be used to treat status epilepticus, which is unresponsive to other agents. It has also been suggested that they may provide some degree of cerebral protection during periods of hypoxemia.

Although most commonly used for their therapeutic effects, these agents are effective when benzodiazepines and opioids, either alone or in combination, fail to provide adequate sedation.[46] One particularly difficult situation is the provision of sedation during extracorporeal membrane oxygenation (ECMO). Although fentanyl is the most commonly used agent, rapid tolerance and the need for dose escalation has been noted so that doses of 30 to 50 μg/kg/hr are not uncommon. Another commonly used agent, midazolam, is generally ineffective because of binding to the oxygenator. In such patients, pentobarbital is an effective alternative to the more conventionally used agents. After a loading dose of 1 to 2 mg/kg, a continuous infusion of 1 to 2 mg/kg/hr is started. Since barbiturates have negative inotropic effects, their use in patients with moderate to severe cardiovascular dysfunction is not recommended. However, their use is well tolerated as long as the bolus dose is administered slowly over 5 to 10 minutes. Another problem with barbiturates is that the solution is relatively alkaline, making it incompatible with other medications and parenteral alimentation solutions, necessitating an intravenous infusion separate from other medications. Despite such problems, pentobarbital may be effective when the usual benzodiazepine/opioid combination fails.

Opioids

Although generally used for analgesia, opioids also possess sedative properties and are often chosen as first line drugs for sedation in the PICU patient, even when true analgesia is not required. Regardless of the specific agent chosen, opioids provide analgesia without amnesia. Additional agents are needed when amnesia is desired (e.g., for the toddler or older child who is receiving neuromuscular blocking agents).

With the use of opioids, as with other sedative agents, choices need to be made concerning the mode of administration, the route of administration, and the agent to be used. When considering the mode of administration, a continuous infusion maintains a steady state serum concentration, thereby providing uninterrupted sedation. The use of p.r.n. bolus dosing without a continuous infusion tends to be less effective, allowing for low serum levels with periods of inadequate sedation or analgesia and high serum levels after bolus doses.

Although the intravenous route is usually chosen for the PICU patient, certain situations may arise that necessitate the use of alternative routes, such as subcutaneous, oral, transdermal, and transmucosal (sublingual, buccal, intranasal, or rectal) administration. (Further discussion of the use of alternative routes of delivery of opioids is included in Chapter 2.)

One alternative approach to opioid delivery is the recent development of transdermal fentanyl. Although its efficacy has been demonstrated in adults,[47] its use in children is still relatively anecdotal.[48] The transdermal delivery system allows the continuous administration of the potent opioid fentanyl at four different doses (25, 50, 75, and 100 μg/hr). After application, steady state serum concentrations are achieved in 8 hours and last for 72 hours with a single patch. Although the dosing choices may limit its use in smaller patients, this mode of delivery is useful in patients with limited intravenous access who require several different medications that are incompatible with the opioid infusion. Such a patient has recently been cared for in our PICU. The patient was a neonate with complex congenital heart disease who required prolonged postoperative mechanical ventilation. The only venous access that could be maintained was a Broviac catheter. Sedation was provided by a continuous infusion of fentanyl at 45 μg/hr. Fungal sepsis necessitated the use of amphotericin, which had to be administered over 4 hours and is not compatible with fentanyl. Therefore the fentanyl infusion had to be interrupted for 4 hours, which resulted in inadequate sedation and agitation. A fentanyl patch was applied and the fentanyl infusion was discontinued. After the course of antifungal therapy, the fentanyl infusion was restarted.

A recent episode of respiratory depression with the fentanyl patch in a child for routine, postoperative analgesia stresses its potential complications. These problems have led the Janssen Pharmaceutical Company to advise against its use in children younger than 12 years of age. It has been used in younger children, but only in special circumstances when options for the route of opioid administration were limited and with close monitoring of cardiorespiratory function.

Subcutaneous administration should also be considered when drug incompatibilities preclude the intravenous route. Although this route has generally been reserved for the terminal cancer patient, Bruera and colleagues have recently described their experience with the use of subcutaneous infusions of opioids in the ICU.[49] Opioids were administered by either intermittent subcutaneous dosing or by continuous infusion to 13 patients for a total of 60 patient days. The infusions were delivered through a 25-gauge butterfly needle inserted under the skin of the subclavicular area or the anterior abdominal wall. The site was changed if erythema, swelling, or leakage was observed or at 7 day intervals. The authors expressed some concern over possible delays in onset of activity or decreased absorption in patients with decreased peripheral perfusion, although they noted no such problems in their patients. Several different opioids may be administered by this route, such as morphine, hydromorphone, and fentanyl. Methadone, on the other hand, causes significant tissue reaction with erythema and is not recommended for subcutaneous administration.

The question of which opioid to use for ICU sedation is somewhat more difficult to answer since several different opioids have been shown to be effective for ICU sedation. In the patient with compromised cardiovascular status or at risk for pulmonary hypertension, such as an infant with a large preoperative systemic to pulmonary shunt, the synthetic opioids (fentanyl and sufentanil) with their cardiovascular stability, beneficial effects on pulmonary vascular resistance, and ability to blunt the sympathetic stress response, may be advantageous.[50,51] Because of their short plasma half-lives, these agents need to be administered by a continuous infusion to maintain plasma concentrations adequate to provide analgesia. When comparing the three synthetic opioids (fentanyl, sufentanil, and alfentanil), there does not seem to be an inherent advantage regarding any of these agents. Fentanyl is usually used since it is the least expensive of the three. One use for sufentanil may be for the patient who has received opioids for a prolonged period of time (weeks to months) and develops tolerance with the need for progressively increased doses. In such patients, it may be necessary to switch to sufentanil (8 to 10 times the potency of fentanyl) to limit the fluid volume required to deliver the sedative agent. When using fentanyl for sedation in the mechanically ventilated patient not previously exposed to opioids, starting with a bolus dose of 2 to 4 μg/kg is recommended, followed by a continuous infusion of 2 to 4 μg/kg/hr. Higher doses (8 to 10 μg/kg/hr) may be needed to prevent pulmonary vasospasm.

Two caveats regarding any synthetic opioids are their effects on ICP and the idiosyncratic occurrence of chest wall rigidity. Recent evidence suggests that synthetic opioids may increase ICP in patients with altered intracranial compliance.[52] Sperry and colleagues also noted a moderate decrease in mean arterial pressure, which, when combined with the increase in ICP, further decreases cerebral perfusion pressure. The mechanisms underlying the effects on ICP have not been determined, but it is postulated that alterations in CBF or decreases in cerebral vascular resistance may lead to changes in ICP. Future studies are needed to define these findings and their clinical implications.

Another deleterious effect that has been described in association with synthetic opioids is chest wall rigidity.[53] Chest wall rigidity is mediated through the central nervous system (CNS) and can be reversed with naloxone or interrupted with neuromuscular blocking agents. Although Pokela and colleagues noted significant decreases in compliance and oxygen saturation in 4 infants receiving alfentanil and concluded that these agents should not be used without concomitant neuromuscular blockade, chest wall rigidity is an idiosyncratic and dose-related effect that does not routinely occur in all patients receiving synthetic opioids. This is especially true in the doses used for sedation in the ICU. In fact, Irazuzta and colleagues demonstrated improved compliance in the majority of patients receiving fentanyl.[54]

Although synthetic opioids maintain stable hemodynamics in patients with compromised cardiovascular function, other alternatives, such as morphine, are acceptable in patients with normal cardiovascular function. Morphine may cause some venodilatation, thereby decreasing blood pressure in hypovolemic patients. However, for the majority of patients, morphine is usually the first choice opioid. Starting doses for sedation during mechanical ventilation include a bolus dose of 50 to 100 μg/kg, followed by a continuous infusion of 20 to 30 μg/kg/hr. Lower doses (50% of the above mentioned guidelines) are recommended for neonates and infants younger than 3 months of age. Because of the immaturity of hepatic function, prolonged serum half-lives may be seen in such patients.

Alternatives to morphine include hydromorphone, meperidine, and methadone. Hydromorphone may be advantageous when adverse effects related to histamine release, such as pruritus, occur with morphine.[55] In such cases, an equipotent dose of hydromorphone should be administered, which can be arrived at by considering the potency ratio of the two opioids with hydromorphone 5 to 7 times as potent as morphine. Certain patients, such as those with severe graft-versus-host disease, may be more prone to pruritus and have problems even with hydromorphone. In these patients, another advantage of fentanyl is that it is associated with little or no histamine release and may thereby limit pruritus.[56]

Meperidine appears to be a relatively poor choice for analgesia because of a relatively high incidence of adverse CNS effects, such as dysphoria, agitation, and seizures.[57] CNS toxicity (including seizures) results from the accumulation of normeperidine, which occurs after hepatic n-methylation of the parent compound. Normeperidine has a long half-life (15 to 20 hrs) and is dependent on renal excretion. High or toxic levels occur more commonly in the setting of renal insufficiency, with the coadministration of drugs, such as phenobarbital, that stimulate hepatic microsomal enzymes, and with large doses (greater than 2 g/day in an adult). The latter issue becomes problematic in the patient who is chronically receiving opioids and needs dose escalations to provide effective analgesia. Because of these considerations, and since meperidine offers no particular advantage over other opioids, morphine or fentanyl is preferred as the initial opioid for intravenous use.

As with any sedative or analgesic agent, prolonged use may result in physical tolerance and withdrawal symptoms if the infusion is abruptly discontinued. Arnold and colleagues described and investigated what they termed "neonatal abstinence syndrome (NAS)" in infants sedated with fentanyl during ECMO.[58] They undertook a retrospective chart review of 37 neonates who required ECMO for respiratory failure and found that the infants at risk for opioid tolerance and withdrawal included those who required ECMO for more than 5 days or received a total dose of fentanyl greater than 1.6 mg/kg. They also demonstrated that plasma concentrations of fentanyl increased as the infusion rate was increased, suggesting that the tolerance was the result of a receptor phenomenon and not related to increased metabolism or clearance.

A subsequent study by Katz and colleagues provides further information concerning opioid tolerance.[59] They prospectively evaluated the incidence of opioid withdrawal in 23 patients (1 week to 22 months of age) after fentanyl was used for sedation during mechanical ventilation. The symptoms of opioid withdrawal were quantified using a scale described by Finnegan and colleagues.[60] Both the total dose of fentanyl and the duration of infusion correlated with the chance of withdrawal, but the maximum fentanyl infusion rate did not. Infants who received fentanyl for 5 days, or a total dose of greater than 1.5 mg/kg, had a 50% incidence of withdrawal, whereas patients who received fentanyl for 9 days, or a total dose of greater than 2.5 mg/kg, had an incidence of withdrawal of 100%. It should be noted that Katz and colleagues tapered the fentanyl infusion quickly so that all infants were theoretically at risk for withdrawal. Such a practice is not recommended in the "at risk" group. A slow taper of the infusion (10% per day) or the use of orally equivalent agents may prevent withdrawal symptoms.

The importance of the NAS is not to limit the use of opioids in infants but rather to emphasize the need to slowly wean the infusion once the acute illness has subsided. Oral methadone has been used to facilitate weaning from intravenous opioid administration.[61] An advantage of methadone is that its oral bioavailability is roughly 75%, thereby allowing oral administration, whereas its serum half-life of 12 to 24 hours allows dosing twice a day. With the switch from intravenous to oral methadone, many patients may be discharged on a tapering schedule that is easily followed by their parents. When switching from intravenous to oral fentanyl, it is important to consider differences in not only potency but also half-life. Although fentanyl is 100 times more potent than methadone, its half-life is 50 times less. Adding the total day's dose of fentanyl and starting with an equivalent amount of oral methadone divided into a twice/day dose is recommended. A 10 kg patient who is receiving an infusion of 10 μg/kg/hr of fentanyl receives 2.4 mg/day of fentanyl. This patient would be started on methadone 1.2 mg orally twice a day. After the second dose, the infusion is decreased by 50%, by 50% again after the third dose, and then discontinued after the fourth dose. Symptoms of opioid withdrawal are treated with intravenous rescue doses of fentanyl and the daily dose of methadone, increased accordingly. If no symptoms are noted, the dose is decreased by 10% to 15% once or twice a week.

Miscellaneous agents

Several other agents or combinations of agents have been used with varying degrees of success for sedation in the ICU. Phenothiazines and butyrophenones are considered the major tranquilizers and are usually used in the treatment of psychiatric disturbances or for their antiemetic properties.

Neither of these classes of agents has found great success as sedatives in the PICU; however, they continue to be used with some regularity in adult ICUs.[62] Of the many agents available, haloperidol appears to be the most frequently chosen of this class. Although not approved by the Food and Drug Administration (FDA) for intravenous administration, there is an abundance of clinical experience with its use by this route. Riker and colleagues published their experience with haloperidol by continuous infusion (range 3 to 25 mg/hr) for sedation in 8 adult ICU patients.[62] The authors cited many benefits of haloperidol, such as a rapid onset, minimal respiratory depression, and no active metabolites. Adverse effects associated with the butyrophenones and phenothiazines include a-adrenergic blockade with hypotension, dystonia and extrapyramidal effects, and, in rare cases, neuroleptic malignant syndrome. Of even greater importance are cardiac events, such as cardiac arrest and ventricular arrhythmias (e.g., torsades de pointes). Although there were no adverse cardiac events related to haloperidol in the study of Riker and colleagues, one patient did develop a prolonged QT interval. Such alterations in repolarization may be particularly dangerous in patients with altered sympathetic function related to fever, pain, or the stresses of an acute illness. One additional adverse effect of these agents is that they lower the seizure threshold.

More commonly, pediatricians and PICU physicians have used the phenothiazines in combination with other agents (e.g., demerol, phenergan, and thorazine [DPT]) for invasive procedures. This practice is no longer recommended since the combination may result in prolonged sedation and the risk of respiratory depression and apnea.[63]

Chloral hydrate, a sedative-hypnotic agent, is still commonly used in children. It is metabolized in the liver to its active form, trichloroethanol, which has a half-life of 8 to 12 hours. Since there is no parenteral formulation, oral or rectal administration is needed. The onset of action may be delayed for up to 20 minutes, making it difficult to control the acutely agitated patient in the PICU. However, it is still a valuable agent for brief, painless procedures such as computed tomography (CT) imaging. Its use is not recommended for infants younger than 3 months of age or patients with hepatic dysfunction.

Clonidine, a centrally acting alpha-2 agonist that decreases central sympathetic outflow, was initially introduced for the treatment of hypertension. Recent work has demonstrated its efficacy as a premedicant for the operating room in adults and children. Beneficial effects include sedation, anxiolysis, decreased anesthetic requirements, cardiovascular stability, and the potentiation of opiate-induced analgesia.[64,65] To date, its use for sedation in the ICU has appeared only in anecdotal case reports.[66]

In addition to their sedative properties, clonidine and other alpha-2 adrenergic agonists possess intrinsic analgesic effects that are thought to be mediated at the spinal level (dorsal horn) through interaction with specific adrenergic receptors. Adrenergic receptors are located on both first and second order neurons. Activation of presynaptic receptors (first order neurons) results in decreased release of the nociceptive transmitter substance P, whereas postsynaptic activation decreases the rate of depolarization of second order neurons. Although the clinical use of these agents is currently limited, their beneficial physiologic properties suggest their potential for future use both as sedatives and analgesics in the PICU patient.

Summary

Because of the diversity of patients and clinical scenarios in the PICU, a cookbook approach to sedation remains impossible. The PICU physician must be facile with several different medications and routes of administration to ensure adequate sedation and analgesia in this diverse patient population (Table 7-1). General principles include the use of a continuous infusion to maintain a steady-state serum concentration of the drug to ensure sedation

TABLE 7-1. Starting Doses for Sedative and Analgesic Agents During Mechanical Ventilation*

Drug	Dosing Range	Comments
Benzodiazepine		
Midazolam	0.05-0.1 mg/kg/hr	Cost issues.
Lorazepam	0.025-0.05 mg/kg/hr	
Diazepam	—	Not recommended because of active metabolites and prolonged effect.
Opioids		
Morphine	0.02-0.04 mg/kg/hr	
Fentanyl	2-4 μg/kg/hr	
Ketamine	1-2 mg/kg/hr	
Barbiturates		
Pentobarbital	1-2 mg/kg/hr	May be useful during ECMO or when opioids and benzodiazepines are ineffective. Solution incompatible with other medications and parenteral alimentation solutions.
Propofol	50-100 μg/kg/min	Not recommended in children younger than 12 years of age.

*The doses listed are suggested starting doses. The infusion should be supplemented with p.r.n. bolus doses, which are equivalent to the hourly rate. The infusion should be increased or decreased as needed to achieve the desired level of sedation. In infants younger than 3 months of age, the starting dose should be half the above listed doses.

and analgesia. The infusion should be supplemented with intermittent, p.r.n. bolus doses which can be administered for breakthrough agitation. These bolus doses should be equivalent to the hourly infusion rate. The baseline infusion rate and the bolus doses should be increased in patients who require frequent bolus doses to maintain sedation.

Although no clear cut guidelines exist, neonates and infants younger than one year of age are generally best sedated with an opioid, whereas benzodiazepines are generally effective in patients older than a year of age. Although fentanyl is frequently chosen as the first-line opioid, morphine is an effective and cost-saving alternative for patients with stable cardiovascular function. Synthetic opioids are recommended for neonates, especially after cardiac surgical procedures and those at risk for pulmonary vasospasm. In this setting the use of synthetic opioids may decrease postoperative morbidity. When considering benzodiazepines, lorazepam offers a cost effective alternative to midazolam and eliminates the concerns regarding active metabolites and interactions with the P-450 system of the liver.

When the above agents fail to be effective or are associated with cardiovascular depression, alternatives include ketamine or pentobarbital. Ketamine may be useful for patients with cardiovascular instability or those with a bronchospastic component to their disease process. Pentobarbital is effective when the combination of benzodiazepines and opioids fails to provide the desired level of sedation. Additionally, pentobarbital may be efficacious during ECMO when commonly used agents, such as midazolam and fentanyl, are ineffective.

References

1. Kong KL, Willatts SM, Prys-Roberts C: Isoflurane compared with midazolam for sedation in the intensive care unit, *Brit Med J* 298:1277, 1989.
2. Breheny FX, Kendall PA: Use of isoflurane for sedation in intensive care, *Crit Care Med* 20:1062, 1992.

3. Drummond JC, Todd MM, Scheller MS et al: A comparison of the direct cerebral vasodilating potencies of halothane and isoflurane in the New Zealand white rabbit, *Anesthesiology* 65:462, 1986.
4. Reilly CS, Wood AJJ, Koshakji RP et al: The effect of halothane on drug disposition: contribution of changes in intrinsic drug metabolizing capacity and hepatic blood flow, *Anesthesiology* 63:70, 1985.
5. Arnold JH, Truog RD, Rice SA: Prolonged administration of isoflurane to pediatric patients during mechanical ventilation, *Anesth Analg* 76:520, 1993.
6. Ghoneim MM, Mewaldt SP: Benzodiazepines and human memory: a review, *Anesthesiology* 72:926, 1990.
7. Rosland JH, Hole K: 1,4-Benzodiazepines antagonize opiate-induced antinociception in mice, *Anesth Analg* 71:242, 1990.
8. Lloyd-Thomas AR, Booker PD: Infusion of midazolam in paediatric patients after cardiac surgery, *Br J Anaesth* 58:1109, 1986.
9. Booker PD, Beechey A, Lloyd-Thomas AR: Sedation of children requiring artificial ventilation using an infusion of midazolam, *Br J Anaesth* 58:1104, 1986.
10. Silvasi DL, Rosen DA, Rosen KR: Continuous intravenous midazolam infusion for sedation in the pediatric intensive care unit, *Anesth Analg* 67:286, 1988.
11. Trouvin JH, Farinotti R, Haberer JP et al: Pharmacokinetics of midazolam in anesthetized cirrhotic patients, *Br J Anaesth* 60:762, 1988.
12. Vinik HR, Reves JG, Greenblatt DJ et al: The pharmacokinetics of midazolam in chronic renal failure patients, *Anesthesiology* 59:390, 1983.
13. Egan KJ, Ready LB, Nessly M et al: Self-administration of midazolam for postoperative anxiety: a double-blinded study, *Pain* 49:3, 1992.
14. Beebe DS, Belani KG, Chang P et al: Effectiveness of preoperative sedation with rectal midazolam, ketamine, or their

combination in young children, *Anesth Analg* 75:880, 1992.

15. McMillian CO, Spahr-Schopfer IA, Sikich N et al: Premedication of children with oral midazolam, *Can J Anaesth* 39:545, 1992.
16. Karl HW, Rosenberger JL, Larach MG et al: Transmucosal administration of midazolam for premedication of pediatric patients: comparison of the nasal and sublingual routes, *Anesthesiology* 78:885, 1993.
17. Theroux MC, West DW, Corddry DH et al: Efficacy of midazolam in facilitating suturing of lacerations in preschool children in the emergency department, *Pediatrics* 91:624, 1993.
18. Fragen RJ, Meyers SN, Barresi V et al: Hemodynamic effects of midazolam in cardiac patients, *Anesthesiology* 51:172, 1979.
19. Breheny FX: Reversal of midazolam sedation with flumazenil, *Crit Care Med* 20:736, 1992.
20. McDuffee A, Tobias JD: Seizure following flumazenil administration in a child, *Pediatr Emerg Care* 11:186, 1995.
21. Tobias JD, Deshpande JK, Gregory DF: Outpatient therapy of iatrogenic drug dependency following prolonged sedation in the pediatric intensive care unit, *Int Care Med* (in press).
22. Bergman I, Steeves M, Bruckart G et al: Reversible neurologic abnormalities associated with prolonged intravenous midazolam and fentanyl administration, *J Pediatr* 119:644, 1991.
23. Corssen G, Miyasaka M, Domino EF: Changing concepts in pain control during surgery: dissociative anesthesia with CI-581, *Anesth Analg* 47:746, 1968.
24. Chernow B, Laker R, Creuss D et al: Plasma, urine, and cerebrospinal fluid catecholamine concentrations during and after ketamine sedation, *Crit Care Med* 10:600, 1982.
25. Gooding JM, Dimick AR, Travakoli M et al: A physiologic analysis of cardiopulmonary responses to ketamine anesthesia in non-cardiac patients, *Anesth Analg* 56:813, 1977.
26. Mankikian B, Cantineau JP, Sartene R et al: Ventilatory and

chest wall mechanics during ketamine anesthesia in humans, *Anesthesiology* 65:492, 1986.

27. Hirshman CA, Downes H, Farbood A et al: Ketamine block of bronchospasm in experimental canine asthma, *Br J Anaesth* 51:713, 1979.
28. Bourke DL, Malit LA, Smith TC: Respiratory interactions of ketamine and morphine, *Anesthesiology* 66:153, 1987.
29. Lanning CF, Harmel MH: Ketamine anesthesia, *Annu Rev Med* 26:137, 1975.
30. Taylor PA, Towey RM: Depression of laryngeal reflexes during ketamine administration, *Br Med J* 2:688, 1971.
31. Shapiro HM, Wyte SR, Harris AB: Ketamine anesthesia in patients with intracranial pathology, *Br J Anaesth* 44:1200, 1972.
32. Oren RE, Rasool NA, Rubinstein EH: Effect of ketamine on cerebral cortical blood flow and metabolism in rabbits, *Stroke* 18:445, 1987.
33. White PR, Way WL, Trevor AJ: Ketamine—its pharmacology and therapeutic uses, *Anesthesiology* 56:119, 1982.
34. Tobias JD, Martin LD, Wetzel RC: Ketamine by continuous infusion for sedation in the pediatric intensive care unit, *Crit Care Med* 18:819, 1990.
35. Sebel PS, Lowdon JD: Propofol: a new intravenous anesthetic, *Anesthesiology* 71:260, 1989.
36. Harris CE, Grounds RM, Murray AM et al: Propofol for long-term sedation in the intensive care unit: a comparison with papaveretum and midazolam, *Anaesthesia* 45:366, 1990.
37. Beller JP, Pottecher T, Lugnier A et al: Prolonged sedation with propofol in ICU patients: recovery and blood concentration changes during periodic interruption in infusion, *Br J Anaesth* 61:583, 1988.
38. Egan TD, Brock-Utne JG: Asystole and anesthesia induction with a fentanyl, propofol, and succinylcholine sequence, *Anesth Analg* 73:818, 1991.
39. Trotter C, Serpell MG: Neurological sequelae in children after prolonged propofol infusions, *Anaesthesia* 47:340, 1992.

40. Saunders PRI, Harris MNE: Opisthotonic posturing and other unusual neurological sequelae after outpatient anesthesia, *Anaesthesia* 47:552, 1992.
41. Collier C, Kelly K: Propofol and convulsions—the evidence mounts, *Anaesth Intensive Care* 19:573, 1991.
42. Parke TJ, Stevens JE, Rice ASC et al: Metabolic acidosis and fatal myocardial failure after propofol infusion in children: five case reports, *Br Med J* 305:613, 1992.
43. Laxenaire MC, Mata-Bermejo E, Moneret-Vautrin DA et al: Life-threatening anaphylactoid reactions to propofol, *Anesthesiology* 77:275, 1992.
44. Sosis MB, Braverman B: Growth of *staphylococcus aureus* in four intravenous anesthetics, *Anesth Analg* 77:766, 1993.
45. Postsurgical infections associated with extrinsically contaimined intravenous anesthetic agent—California, Illinois, Maine, and Michigan, 1990, *MMWR* 39:426, 1990.
46. Tobias JD, Deshpande JK, Pietsch JB et al: Pentobarbital sedation in the pediatric intensive care unit patient, *South Med J* 88:290, 1995.
47. Holley FR, van Steenis C: Postoperative analgesia with fentanyl: pharmacokinetics and pharmacodynamics at constant intravenous and transdermal delivery, *Br J Anaesth* 63:56, 1989.
48. Tobias JD: Transdermal fentanyl: applications and indications in the pediatric patient, *American Journal of Pain Management* 2:30, 1992.
49. Bruera E, Gibney N, Stollery D et al: Use of the subcutaneous route of administration of morphine in the intensive care unit, *J Pain Symptom Management* 6:263, 1991.
50. Hickey PR, Hansen DD, Wessel DL et al: Pulmonary and systemic hemodynamic responses to fentanyl in infants, *Anesth Analg* 64:483, 1985.
51. Hickey PR, Hansen DD, Wessel DL et al: Blunting of stress response in pulmonary circulation of infants by fentanyl, *Anesth Analg* 64:1137, 1985.

52. Sperry RJ, Bailey PL, Reuchman MV et al: Fentanyl and sufentanil increase intracranial pressure in head trauma patients, *Anesthesiology* 77:416, 1992.
53. Pokela ML, Ryhanen PT, Koivisto ME et al: Alfentanil-induced rigidity in newborn infants, *Anesth Analg* 75:252, 1992.
54. Irazuzta J, Pascucci R, Perlman N et al: Effects of fentanyl administration on respiratory system compliance in infants, *Crit Care Med* 21:101, 1993.
55. Rosow CE, Moss J, Philbin DM et al: Histamine release during morphine and fentanyl anesthesia, *Anesthesiology* 56:93, 1982.
56. Tobias JD, Baker DK: Patient-controlled analgesia with fentanyl in children, *Clin Pediatr* 31:177, 1992.
57. Shochet RB, Murray GB: Neuropsychiatric toxicity of meperidine, *J Intensive Care Med* 3:246, 1988.
58. Arnold JH, Truog RD, Orav EJ et al: Tolerance and dependence in neonates sedated with fentanyl during extracorporeal membrane oxygenation, *Anesthesiology* 73:1136, 1990.
59. Katz R, Kelly HW, Hsi A: Prospective study on the occurrence of withdrawal in critically ill children who receive fentanyl by continuous infusion, *Crit Care Med* 22:763, 1994.
60. Finnegan LP, Kron RE, Connaughton JF Jr et al: A scoring system for evaluation and treatment of the neonatal abstinence syndrome: a new clinical and research tool. In Morselli PL, Garattini S, Sereni F, editors: *Basic and therapeutic aspects of perinatal pharmacology,* New York, 1975, Raven.
61. Tobias JD, Schleien CS, Haun SE: Methadone as treatment for iatrogenic narcotic dependency in pediatric intensive care unit patients, *Crit Care Med* 18:1292, 1991.
62. Riker RR, Fraser GL, Cox PM: Continuous infusion of haloperidol controls agitation in critically ill patients, *Crit Care Med* 22:433, 1994.
63. Nahata MC, Clotz MA, Krogg EA: Adverse effects of meperidine, promethazine, and chlorpromazine for sedation in pediatric patients, *Clin Pediatr* 24:558, 1985.

64. Maze MM, Tranquilli W: Alpha-2 agonists: defining the role in clinical anesthesia, *Anesthesiology* 74:581, 1991.
65. De Kock MF, Pichon G, Scholtes JL: Intraoperative clonidine enhances postoperative morphine patient-controlled analgesia, *Can J Anaesth* 39:537, 1992.
66. Bohrer H, Bach A, Layer M et al: Clonidine as a sedative adjunct in intensive care, *Intensive Care Med* 16:265, 1990.

SEDATION FOR IMAGING AND INVASIVE PROCEDURES

8

Sandra Lowe
Shannon Hershey

ENDOTRACHEAL INTUBATION
- Elective intubation (normal airway)

RADIOLOGIC PROCEDURES
- Computerized tomography
- Magnetic resonance imaging

CARDIAC CATHETERIZATION
- Diagnostic cardiac catheterization
- Interventional cardiac catheterization
- Radiofrequency ablation

SEDATION FOR INVASIVE THERAPEUTIC AND DIAGNOSTIC PROCEDURES
- Topical and local anesthesia

AGENTS FOR SEDATION
- Benzodiazepines
- Opioids
- Fentanyl oralet
- Chloral hydrate
- Ketamine
- Barbiturates
- Propofol
- Nitrous oxide
- Combinations of agents
- Regional anesthetic techniques
- Opioid and benzodiazepine reversal agents

NONPHARMACOLOGIC METHODS

Although radiologic imaging and invasive procedures are commonly performed in adults without sedation, stranger anxiety and inherent fears may interfere with a child's ability to cooperate. There are several types of procedures; therefore, the methods of sedation used vary, depending on the specific procedure. The first half of this chapter discusses procedures that involve radiologic imaging and are not inherently painful to the child. Such procedures require a motionless patient for success and can be performed with agents that provide sedation and not necessarily analgesia. The second half of this chapter deals with invasive procedures, which require agents that provide analgesia in addition to amnesia and sedation.

All children old enough to communicate can benefit from information about the procedure if it is presented in an age-appropriate fashion. How a child responds to this preliminary information may offer clues to the amount of pharmacologic intervention that will be required. A cooperative but very anxious child may only require a small dose of an oral anxiolytic for a procedure associated with minimal pain. On the other hand, a hysterical child with a previous bad experience with sedation procedures may require deep sedation or even general anesthesia.

Once the decision is made to sedate a pediatric patient, all healthcare workers involved must understand that, regardless of the intended level of sedation, the drugs administered, or the route of administration, a continuum exists from conscious sedation to general anesthesia. Every sedation attempt carries with it certain risks, such as hypoventilation, apnea, airway obstruction, and cardiopulmonary compromise. These concerns should not limit the use of sedation, but they should emphasize the need to prepare the patient appropriately by following nil per os (NPO) guidelines (Table 8-1) and by having age appropriate airway equipment available.

In 1992 the American Academy of Pediatrics revised its sedation guidelines in an attempt to standardize monitoring practices and encourage high-quality patient care.[1] These guidelines have been extensively discussed previously in this handbook (see Chapter 1). The primary focus of these guidelines is to define conscious

TABLE 8-1. NPO Guidelines for Children

Age	Milk or Solids	Clear Liquids*
Preterm	4	2
Full term to 6 months	6	3
6 months to 12 months	8	4
12 months to 36 months	8	4
More than 36 months	8	4

*Clear liquids may include breast milk, apple juice, Pedialyte, water, or Sprite.

sedation, deep sedation, and general anesthesia and to suggest proper monitoring in each case. In addition, the guidelines suggest which drugs and equipment should be on hand when administering sedative agents.

Proper NPO status must be assured before any elective sedation. This decreases the possibility of aspiration if loss of airway reflexes occurs. Recent liberalization of NPO guidelines by age has made scheduling easier and waiting more comfortable for young patients. Previously, it was common to withhold clear liquids for up to 6 hours before surgery in children under a year of age and for up to 8 hours in older children. More recently, it has been demonstrated that the ingestion of clear liquids may actually promote gastric emptying and raise gastric pH while decreasing hunger, thirst, and irritability in the patient. The guidelines used for fasting are listed in Table 8-1. These guidelines should be reviewed with the parents to ensure that they understand what to do for the child. On the day of the procedure, the parents should be questioned about when the child last ate or drank anything in order to ensure that the patient has had an adequate fast.

Although elective procedures allow for the provision of adequate time for fasting, other procedures may need to be performed on an urgent or even emergent basis. In addition to the child who has just eaten, other conditions, such as pain, trauma, or ongoing abdominal processes, may delay gastric emptying, thereby predisposing the patient to aspiration. Such patients should be considered at risk for aspiration during sedation or general anesthesia. Pharmacologic therapy may be indicated to reduce the morbidity of aspiration.

Most studies on aspiration pneumonitis use the "gold standard" of gastric pH less than 2.5 and a gastric volume greater than 0.4 ml/kg as factors that increase the severity of pulmonary damage after aspiration.[2,3] In the "at risk" population, the prophylactic use of agents aimed at decreasing the acidity or volume of gastric contents may lessen the severity of pulmonary injury if aspiration occurs. Antacids and other prophylactic drugs, such as H_2 receptor-antagonists and metoclopramide, do not reduce the possibility of regurgitation and aspiration. These drugs are used to increase gastric pH, to block histamine-induced secretion of the hydrogen ion by gastric parietal cells, and to increase gastric emptying. These agents can be administered orally (PO) or intravenously (IV) (Table 8-2). The combination of an H_2 antagonist and a motility agent such as metoclopramide is suggested (Table 8-2).

A brief review of the patient's medical history and a physical examination should be performed before sedation (Box 8-1). This

TABLE 8-2. Agents for Aspiration Prophylaxis*

Agent	Dose
H_2 Antagonists	
Ranitidine	1 mg/kg IV (50 mg) 2 mg/kg PO (150 mg)
Cimetidine	5 mg/kg IV (300 mg) 10 mg/kg PO (600 mg)
Motility Agents	
Metoclopramide	0.1 mg/kg PO or IV (10 mg)
Cisapride	0.1 mg/kg PO (10 mg)
Antacids	
Sodium citrate	1 ml/kg PO (30 ml)

*The maximum dose is listed in parentheses.
IV, Intravenous; *PO*, per os (by mouth).

BOX 8-1.
Pertinent Points of Patient History and Physical Examination

Patient's name, age, weight, and gender
Past medical history
  Underlying medical conditions
  Previous anesthetic history or problems
Allergies
Current medications
Family history of anesthetic complications
Dietary history (NPO status)
Pregnancy history
Physical examination
  Baseline vital signs, including room air saturation
  Airway examination
  Cardiorespiratory examination
Laboratory
Summary
  ASA status
  Plan
  Risks discussed

NPO, nil per os (nothing by mouth); *ASA,* American Society of Anesthesiologists.

information should be recorded and included in the patient's permanent record. The information obtained should include previous and ongoing illnesses, drug allergies, family history of anesthetic problems, such as postoperative fevers, which may suggest a family history of malignant hyperthermia, and the patient's current drug regimen. The latter is important since many medications may potentiate the sedative effects of the drugs used. The possibility of pregnancy in a girl of child-bearing age is often overlooked but must be investigated during the evaluation. The physical examination should start with a set of vital signs, including room air oxygen saturation, and it should focus on the airway and the cardiorespiratory system. A brief examination of the airway can be used to determine if the patient may be difficult to intubate. Potential problems should be suspected in patients with micrognathia, limited mouth opening, or limited neck mobility. One of the more useful measures is the Mallampati classification (Fig. 8-1). If the tonsillar pillars and the uvula cannot be visualized (Mallampati grade III or IV), the patient's trachea may be difficult to intubate. Previous anesthetic records should be reviewed to determine if there have been previous airway problems. The possibility of a difficult airway does not preclude the use of sedation, but it may be appropriate to discuss such patients with a pediatric anesthesiologist. Once the history and physical examination are completed, an ASA (American Society of Anesthesiologists) classification can be assigned based on the patient's physical status (Box 8-2). Class III and IV patients may present significant problems when sedated and should also be discussed with a pediatric anesthesiologist.

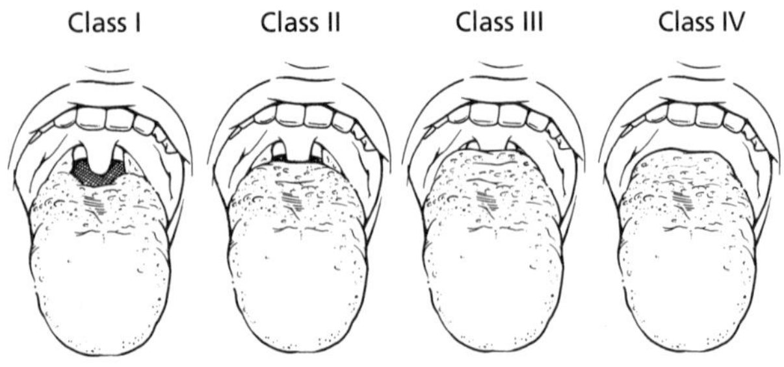

FIG 8-1.
The Mallampati scoring system to evaluate the airway and determine the anticipated difficulties that may occur with endotracheal intubation. In class I patients, the soft palate, fauces, tonsillar pillars (anterior and posterior) and uvula can be seen. In class II, the same structures can be seen except that the tonsillar pillars are blocked by the tongue. In class III, only the base of the uvula can be seen. In class IV, none of the structures can be seen. Class III and IV patients may pose significant problems during endotracheal intubation.

Once the proper preparation has been made and the patient is examined, the practitioner must choose an agent or agents and a route of delivery. There are a wide variety of medications available for the sedation of children (Box 8-3). The practitioner must realize that there is no magic medication or particular dose of a drug

BOX 8-2.
ASA Classification

ASA 1: No Underlying Medical Problems

ASA 2: Mild Systemic Illness

Well controlled asthma
Corrected congenital heart disease

ASA 3: Severe Systemic Illness

Sickle cell disease
Severe asthma-steroid dependence
Uncorrected congenital heart disease

ASA 4: Severe Systemic Illness That Is a Constant Threat to Life

Uncorrected cyanotic congenital heart disease

ASA 5: Patient Who is Unlikely to Survive 24 Hours With or Without Surgery

ASA, American Society of Anesthesiologists

BOX 8-3.
Agents for Sedation and Analgesia During Procedures

Inhalational anesthetic agents
Nitrous oxide
Benzodiazepines
Barbiturates
Propofol
Ketamine
Chloral hydrate
Opioids

that works in all patients. The agents used for sedation should be titrated to achieve the desired effect and cannot be dosed solely on a mg/kg basis like antibiotics.

Proper drug selection involves understanding the procedure (painful vs. nonpainful) and knowing its expected duration. Information concerning the patient, such as the current drug regimen, allergies, and underlying medical conditions that may predispose the patient to cardiorespiratory compromise with the use of sedative and analgesic agents must also be considered. The route of delivery of the sedative drug is also extremely important, particularly in children without IV access. In these situations, nonparenteral administration should be used since many children view starting an IV or administering an intramuscular (IM) injection to be as invasive as the procedure itself. The "needle phobia" of children should never be underestimated, and alternate routes of administration should always be considered. The one drawback to the nonparenteral routes of administration is that the delay in onset of activity makes it difficult to titrate the drug to the desired effect.

The remainder of this chapter focuses on specific clinical scenarios and procedures, including endotracheal intubation, radiologic imaging (computed tomography [CT] scanning, magnetic resonance imaging [MRI]), cardiac catheterization (diagnostic and therapeutic), and invasive diagnostic and therapeutic medical procedures.

ENDOTRACHEAL INTUBATION

Failure to maintain a patent airway for more than a few minutes results in hypoxemia and can lead to permanent central nervous system (CNS) dysfunction or death. More than 85% of all respiratory-related, closed malpractice claims involve a brain damaged or dead patient. The purpose of this section is not to review the techniques used for endotracheal intubation, but to discuss the drugs that can be used to provide sedation and analgesia.

Before sedation is administered, the potential for airway compromise and the capability to ensure endotracheal intubation and ventilation must be noted. If there is any doubt of the chance to successfully instrument the airway, no sedation should be administered. The Mallampati classification of the upper airway is useful in evaluating a child's airway and identifying patients in whom tracheal intubation may be difficult (Fig. 8-1).

Certain basic equipment and monitors are necessary for all endotracheal intubation procedures (Box 8-4). If there is a question that the airway will be difficult to manage, a cricothyrotomy set, jet ventilator, and/or a tracheostomy set may need to be available. The approach to the difficult airway has been outlined by the ASA (Fig. 8-2). It is important to remember that two sets of hands (i.e., at least one helper) are always better than one.

BOX 8-4.
Equipment and Monitors for Endotracheal Intubation

Monitors

Pulse oximeter
Sphygmomanometer (preferably automatic)
Stethoscope
End-tidal CO_2
Electrocardiography

Equipment

Adequate lighting
Oxygen supply
Laryngoscopes
Endotracheal tubes
Stylettes
Oral airways
Resuscitation bag
Masks
Suction (Yankaur and flexible catheters)

Drugs

Neuromuscular blocking agent
Sedative and analgesic agent
Anticholinergic agent

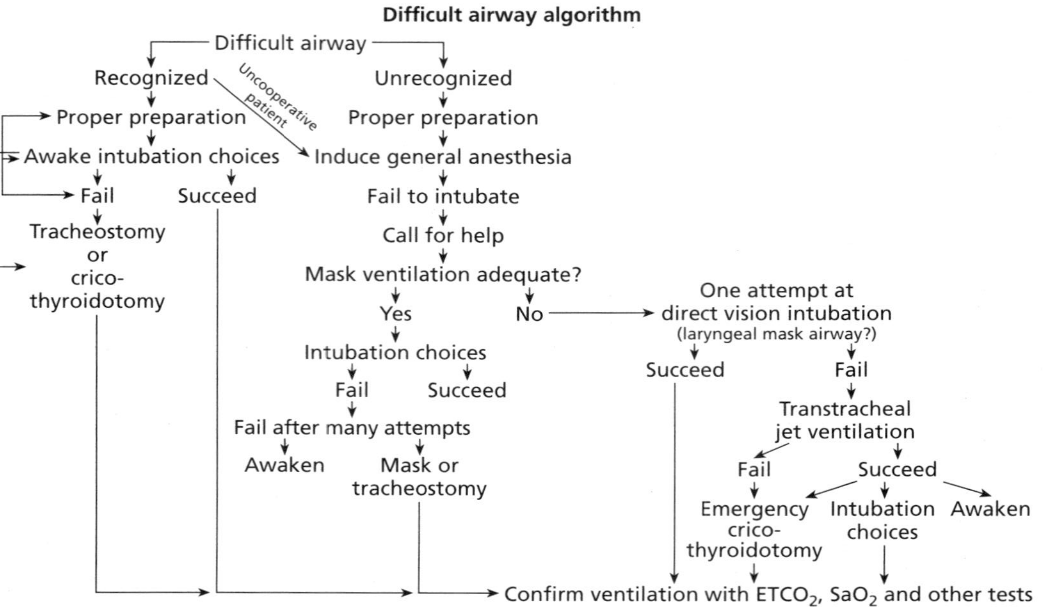
Difficult airway algorithm
Difficult airway
Recognized
Unrecognized
Uncooperative patient
Proper preparation
Proper preparation
Awake intubation choices
Induce general anesthesia
Fail
Succeed
Fail to intubate
Tracheostomy or crico-thyroidotomy
Call for help
Mask ventilation adequate?
Yes
No
One attempt at direct vision intubation
(laryngeal mask airway?)
Intubation choices
Succeed
Fail
Fail
Succeed
Fail after many attempts
Transtracheal jet ventilation
Awaken
Mask or tracheostomy
Fail
Succeed
Emergency crico-thyroidotomy
Intubation choices
Awaken
Confirm ventilation with ETCO2, SaO2 and other tests

FIG 8-2.

The difficult airway algorithm as suggested by the American Society of Anesthesiologists. This guideline should be followed when successful endotracheal intubation cannot be accomplished after the administration of sedative agents and/or neuromuscular blocking agents.

Once the need for intubation has been determined, a plan is developed to accomplish the procedure. Table 8-3 includes suggested medications for endotracheal intubation. These may include a sedative and analgesic agent as well as a neuromuscular blocking drug. If it is recognized that the endotracheal intubation or mask ventilation is going to be difficult (e.g., because of a large tongue, small mandible, or restricted atlantooccipital extension), then the airway may need to be secured while the patient is awake. Consultation with an anesthesiologist is suggested if time permits.

The most important determinant of success of an awake endotracheal intubation is the proper preparation of the patient. It is very difficult to do an awake endotracheal intubation regardless of technique in an uncooperative patient. The procedure should be explained to the patient, and communication should be maintained throughout the procedure. Other helpful adjuncts include an antisialogogue to dry airway secretions, the administration of supplemental oxygen to maintain oxygenation, and topical anesthesia of the airway. The last option may be accomplished by the application of local anesthetic solutions directly to the airway or by the blockade of the innervation of airway structures. This may include glossopharyngeal, superior laryngeal, and inferior laryngeal nerve blockades. The description of such techniques is beyond the scope of this handbook. Because of the risk of adverse effects if performed incorrectly, such techniques should be performed only by physicians specifically trained in this area.

Elective Intubation (Normal Airway)

The most likely scenario for elective intubation involves the patient in whom the airway is considered normal. The success and ease of intubation can be greatly increased with the use of sedation and neuromuscular blocking agents. Several medications can be used to provide amnesia and analgesia before endotracheal intubation (Table 8-3). In the hemodynamically stable patient, an ultrashort-acting barbiturate, such as pentothal (4 to 6 mg/kg), provides satisfactory conditions with a short duration of action. In addition to providing amnesia, the barbiturates decrease the cerebral metabolic rate for oxygen, thereby decreasing cerebral blood flow (CBF) and intracranial pressure (ICP). These agents are considered the drugs of choice to intubate the hemodynamically stable patient with altered intracranial compliance. In the hemodynamically unstable patient, etomidate offers the same cerebral protective effects as the barbiturates without the negative hemodynamic effects. Other agents that may be used include a combination of midazolam and fentanyl, propofol, or ketamine. Keta-

TABLE 8-3. Suggested Medications to Facilitate Intubation

Medication	Dose
Amnestic/Analgesic Agents	
Midazolam	0.05 to 0.1 mg/kg
Pentothal	2 to 6 mg/kg
Propofol	2 to 3 mg/kg
Etomidate	0.2 to 0.3 mg/kg
Fentanyl	2 to 4 μg/kg
Ketamine	0.5 to 2.0 mg/kg
Neuromuscular Blocking Agents	
Succinylcholine	2 mg/kg
Vecuronium	0.1 to 0.3 mg/kg
Rocuronium	0.6 to 1.2 mg/kg
Pancuronium	0.15 mg/kg
Other Agents	
Atropine	0.01 mg/kg (maximum 0.4 mg)
Glycopyrrolate	5 μg/kg (maximum 0.2 mg)
Lidocaine	1 to 2 mg/kg

mine is preferred in a child with trauma or hemodynamic instability because it causes an increase in circulating catecholamines and thereby maintains the blood pressure. However, ketamine increases CBF and ICP and is contraindicated in patients with compromised intracranial compliance.

Neuromuscular blocking agents are useful adjuncts to optimize the conditions for endotracheal intubation. Neuromuscular blocking agents should not be given unless one is confident that the trachea can be intubated. Although these agents produce a motionless patient, they do not possess analgesic or amnestic properties and should not be used without accompanying sedation. Neuromuscular blocking agents may be categorized as depolarizing agents (succinylcholine) or nondepolarizing agents, such as vecuronium or pancuronium. The depolarizing agents, such as succinylcholine, act like acetylcholine and cause depolarization of the skeletal muscle. However, unlike acetylcholine, they are not degraded by acetylcholinesterase and therefore occupy the nicotinic receptors at the neuromuscular junction and prevent further depolarization. Through this mechanism they result in paralysis of skeletal muscle. The advantages of succinylcholine include a rapid onset (30 seconds) and a brief duration of action (3 to 5 minutes). However, the use of succinylcholine is contraindicated in certain conditions (Box 8-5). In such conditions, an exaggerated hyperkalemic re-

BOX 8-5.
Absolute and Relative Contraindications to Succinylcholine

Hyperkalemia
Renal failure
Burns (greater than 15% BSA, more than 48 hours old)
Myopathies (e.g., Duchenne's muscular dystrophy)
Paraplegia
Quadriplegia
Parkinson's disease

BSA, Body surface area.

sponse and cardiac arrest may occur after succinylcholine administration.

The alternatives to succinylcholine are the nondepolarizing agents. These agents act as competitive antagonists to acetylcholine at the neuromuscular junction. There are many nondepolarizing agents available (Table 8-3). They differ in respect to onset of action, duration of action, metabolism, and cardiovascular effects (Table 8-4). The major drawback of these agents is a prolonged onset of action of 60 to 90 seconds. Therefore the airway cannot be secured as quickly as with succinylcholine.

In selected cases, it may be impossible to either ventilate the lungs of a patient via a mask or to intubate the trachea. Therefore an alternative method of ventilation must be immediately available to prevent the patient's death. In the past few years, two alternative ventilation methods have been described that can be instituted quickly and appear to have a low risk to benefit ratio: the laryngeal mask airway (LMA) (Fig. 8-3) and transtracheal jet ventilation (TTJV).

The LMA is a new device that is passed without direct visualization into the oropharynx. At that point, the black line on the tube shaft should be opposite the upper lip. The cuff of the mask is then inflated to provide a seal around the pharynx. When properly placed, the LMA rests over the glottic opening (Fig. 8-3). The top of the LMA connects to the breathing circuit with a standard 15 mm adapter and allows for either spontaneous or controlled ventilation. The LMA is available in five sizes (Table 8-5) that cover all ranges of patient age and size. The LMA can be inserted quickly and works well in approximately 95% of cases. Its use should be considered when intubation and ventilation are not possible before TTJV (Fig. 8-2).

If intubation fails and assisted ventilation cannot be accomplished by mask or LMA, needle cricothyrotomy and jet ventilation are suggested as a means of maintaining oxygenation until a patent airway can be established. For needle cricothyrotomy, a 14- or 16-gauge IV catheter is inserted at a 45 degree angle to the skin, pointing caudad through the cricothyroid membrane. The

TABLE 8-4. Nondepolarizing Neuromuscular Blocking Agents

Agent	Intubating Dose	Onset (secs)	Cardiovascular Effects	Metabolism
Vecuronium	0.1-0.3 mg/kg	60-90	None	70% hepatic/ 30% renal
Rocuronium	0.6-1.2 mg/kg	45-60	None	Hepatic
Pancuronium	0.1-0.15 mg/kg	90-120	Tachycardia	80% renal/ 20% hepatic
Atracurium	0.5 mg/kg	90-120	Histamine release	Hoffman degradation
Mivacurium	0.2-0.3 mg/kg	90-120	Histamine release	Plasma cholinesterase

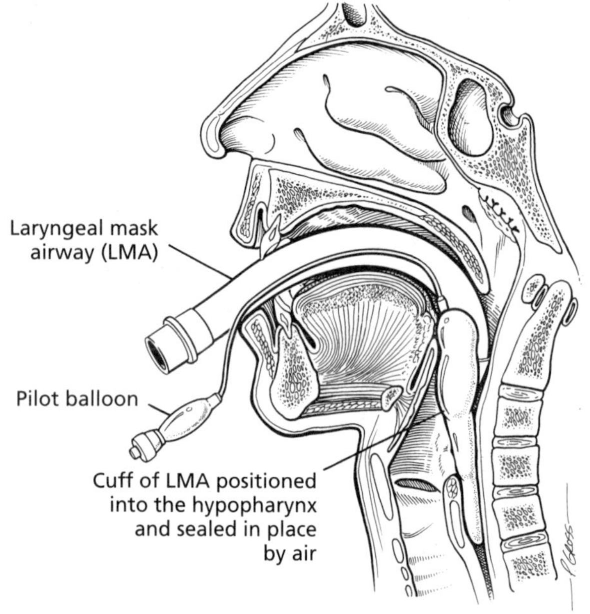

FIG 8-3.
Diagram showing proper position of the laryngeal mask airway after insertion into the oropharynx. After placement, the cuff is inflated to provide a seal over the laryngeal opening. When correctly positioned, the LMA lies with the tip resting against the upper esophageal sphincter, the sides facing the pyriform fossae, and the upper border against the tongue.

cricothyroid membrane lies between the thyroid cartilage (above) and the cricoid (below). The needle is advanced with constant aspiration on the plunger of the syringe. Entry into the trachea is confirmed by aspiration of air into the syringe. The catheter is then advanced off the needle into the trachea. Air is again aspirated through the catheter to confirm placement. The catheter can then

TABLE 8-5. Description of the Different Sizes of the LMA

Mask Size	Patient Weight (kg)	Internal Diameter (mm)	Length (cm)	Cuff Volume (ml)
1	Less than 6.5	5.25	10	2-5
2	6.5-20	7	11.5	7-10
2.5	20-30	8.4	12.5	10-15
3	30-70	10	19	15-20
4	More than 70	12	19	25-30

be connected to a jet ventilating device that has a toggle switch and a pressure regulator. The device is configured to hook into a standard 50 psi wall oxygen outlet. If this is not available, the 15 mm adapter from a 3.0 ET (endotracheal) tube can be removed and inserted into the end of the IV catheter. The 15 mm adapter is then connected to a standard resuscitation bag. Although this will not allow for ventilation, slow, intermittent compression of the bag (10 to 15 times per min) will provide oxygenation. A second option is to attach the barrel of a 3 ml syringe to the IV catheter and to insert the 15 mm adapter from a 7.0 ET tube into the barrel of the syringe. Because of the risks of barotrauma and subcutaneous emphysema with misplacement of the catheter, needle cricothyrotomy should not be performed by inexperienced personnel.

RADIOLOGIC PROCEDURES

Patients scheduled for radiologic procedures requiring sedation or general anesthesia require the same evaluation as any surgical patient. Children and parents require the same explanation of risks and benefits. In other words, the preparation for sedation or general anesthesia is the same regardless of the location in which it is provided. The physician must have a clear understanding of the proposed procedure so that the patient's safety is ensured while providing the conditions necessary to perform the procedures. The success of the study depends on the appropriate planning, understanding, and communication among the child's healthcare providers. It is important to know certain details of the procedure, such as the position of the patient, the geographic relationship of the patient to the physician, and whether an IV line for administering contrast materials and/or sedative medications is needed.

Some procedures may be associated with pain or discomfort. They may require patient immobility for extended periods of time, often in patients that are unable to cooperate. The patients may be hemodynamically unstable or at risk for an allergic reaction to the contrast dye. Finally, invasive radiologic procedures, such as neurovascular embolization, may entail the risk of life threatening complications, such as intracranial hemorrhage, cardiac dysrhythmias, or airway compromise. For these reasons the patient needs not only sedation but also monitoring of cardiopulmonary function.

Monitoring equipment is frequently insufficient or unavailable outside the intensive care unit (ICU) and the operating rooms. Therefore the proposed location for sedating a child should always be evaluated in advance to ascertain the presence of an oxygen supply, suction apparatus, and electrical outlets for equipment. Suction is absolutely necessary for handling patient secretions and also for scavenging gases when a general anesthetic is necessary. Although a centralized oxygen supply is available at most hospitals, it is advisable to have an additional oxygen cylinder and ambu bag. Postponing sedation until appropriate equipment is obtained can be problematic, but it is in the best interest of the patient. To overcome some of these problems, a specialized traveling cart is useful when administering sedation or anesthesia outside the operating room or ICU (Table 8-6).

Most radiology suites are not designed to accommodate the array of monitoring used during sedation. The space is often cramped and accessibility to suction, oxygen, monitoring, and resuscitation equipment may be limited. Additionally, the x-ray equipment often poses logistic problems and may interfere with patient management. For example, the magnetic field induced by MRI makes the use of ferrous materials impossible (Fig. 8-4). It is important for the physician to survey both the patient's needs for

TABLE 8-6. Suggested Mobile Pediatric Equipment Cart

Drawer 1	
Drugs	Atropine, sodium bicarbonate (adult and pediatric), 2% lidocaine, 25% dextrose, phenylephrine, epinephrine (10 and 100 μg/ml), calcium chloride, glycopyrrolate, naloxone, succinylcholine, vecuronium, edrophonium, neostigmine, dexamethasone, dopamine, diphenhydramine, labetolol, esmolol. Controlled drugs not included.
Drawer 2	
Airway	Airways #00 (5), #0 (5), #1 (5), #2 (5), #3 (5), #4 (5) Masks #0 (3), #1 (3), #2 (3), #3 (3) Laryngoscope blades: Miller (0,1,2), Mackintosh (1,2,3), Wis-Hipple 1.5. Nasal trumpets #20 to #36 Magill forceps: Adult and Pediatric
Drawer 3	
Tubes (mmID)	Uncuffed ETTs: 2.5, 3.0, 3.5, 4.0, 4.5, 5.0, Cuffed ETTs: 4.0, 5.0, 5.5, 6.0, 6.5, 7.0
Drawer 4	
Intravenous	Syringes: 10 ml, 6 ml, 3 ml, 1 ml. Needles: 18-, 20-, 22-gauge Butterfly needles: 23 g Intravenous catheters 14-, 16-, 18-, 20-, 22-, 24-gauge Pediatric IV boards, t-connectors, 3-way stopcocks, tape, gauze sponges, alcohol swabs, tubing, tourniquets EMLA cream
Drawer 5	
Monitoring	Precordial stethoscopes, ECG pads, suction catheters (Yankaur and flexible), blood pressure cuffs, pulse oximetry probes, temperature strips, eye pads, corneal lubricant, double stick discs, padding, end-tidal CO_2 sampling tubing, nasal cannulae

ETTs, Endotracheal tubes; *EMLA,* eutetic mixture of local anesthetics; *ECG,* electrocardiogram.

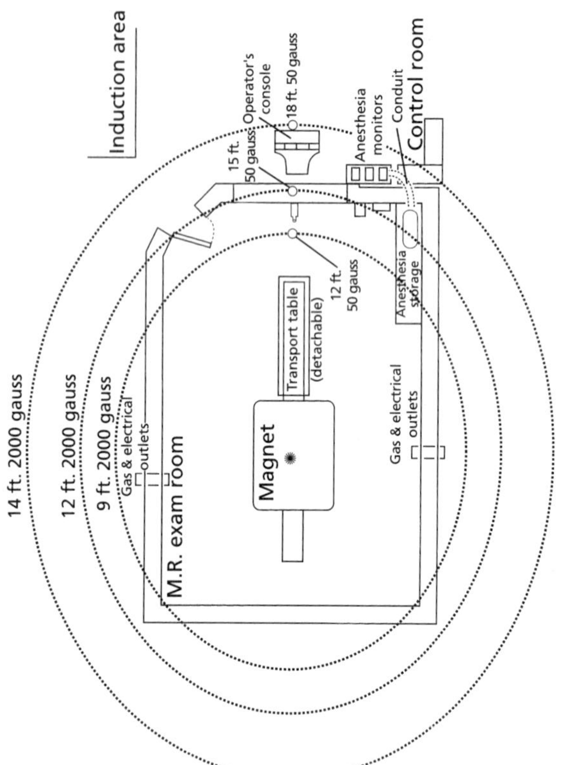

FIG 8-4.
Illustration of standard magnetic resonance (MR) suite including anesthesia induction area, anesthesia storage area, and MR control room. The strength of the magnetic field at various distances from the magnet is illustrated.

the particular procedure and the facilities available. Adequate space for preprocedure evaluations, a parents' waiting room, postsedation recovery, and equipment storage must be identified. The physician must insure that there is enough space to adequately maneuver around the patient. Finally, state and local building codes for areas appropriate for the administration of general anesthesia should be checked.

In order to provide the appropriate level of care for a child, adequate personnel must be available. Physicians routinely depend on other physicians, nurses, and auxiliary personnel to speed patient preparation, transport, and recovery. These people may not be readily available without advanced planning. Certain tasks and responsibilities must be assigned, such as patient scheduling, obtaining preprocedure history, performing physical examinations, ordering laboratory work, and obtaining informed consent. Decisions must be made as to who will observe and monitor patients during their recovery from the sedative medications. This task must be handled by appropriately trained and equipped staff who do not have other concurrent responsibilities. Two areas that are often overlooked when sedation is given outside the traditional operating room environment are the person responsible for postsedation follow-ups and quality assurance. Not only must parents have detailed instructions at discharge, but they should have the same follow-up as surgical candidates. Once these plans are made, one can proceed with sedation.

Computerized Tomography

CT scanning was introduced in the United States in the early 1970s and remains one of the most commonly used radiologic procedures. This procedure involves placement of the patient in the center of a large, rotating, donut-shaped gantry. The gantry projects an x-ray beam onto a set of detectors. Numerous topographic images, horizontal sections of the head or body, are taken and reconstructed by computer to form cross-sectional images. CT is an excellent test for cerebral vascular accidents, hydrocephalus, neoplasms, cerebral degenerative disease, and bony abnormalities of the skull and spine. It is the test of choice for acute abdominal trauma. CT is also commonly used as a guiding tool for stereotactic biopsies.

Contrast media (a hypertonic, hydrogenated solution) is often given IV during the study to identify areas of destruction of the blood-brain barrier, infarcts, neoplasms, and abscesses. The contrast media may be associated with anaphylactic or anaphylactoid reactions. If there is a known history of allergy to contrast or to iodine, the patient should be prophylactically treated with steroids, antihistamines, and H_2 antagonists before the procedure. Emergency resuscitative equipment and medication should be available in the event of a full-blown anaphylactic reaction.

Although CT scanning is painless, the patient must remain motionless during the scan to obtain an adequate study. The time required for a patient to remain motionless has decreased dramatically with newer CT scanners that can provide excellent images in 5 to 10 minutes. Prolonged sedation is infrequently required. Those who cannot cooperate, such as young children, demented patients, and patients with movement disorders may require deep sedation or general anesthesia. Newborns and small infants will often remain still long enough for the procedure if they are swaddled and given a glucose-covered pacifier. Children between 6 months and 6 years of age frequently require some type of sedation for CT scanning (Fig. 8-5).

There is not one drug regimen perfectly suited to each procedure or patient. A wide variety of sedative regimens have been used successfully for CT scanning. A list of suggested medications for radiographic procedures requiring sedation is outlined in Table 8-7. Chloral hydrate (75 to 80 mg/kg per rectum [PR]) and barbiturates (25 to 30 mg/kg pentothal PR) have been especially popular, since many physicians are familiar and comfortable with these agents. Additionally, these agents can be administered via nonparenteral routes. Chloral hydrate is an effective sedative agent that does not possess analgesic properties. Because of its unpalatable nature and ability to cause gastric upset, it may be preferable to administer it PR. Doses of 75 to 80 mg/kg are effective in up to

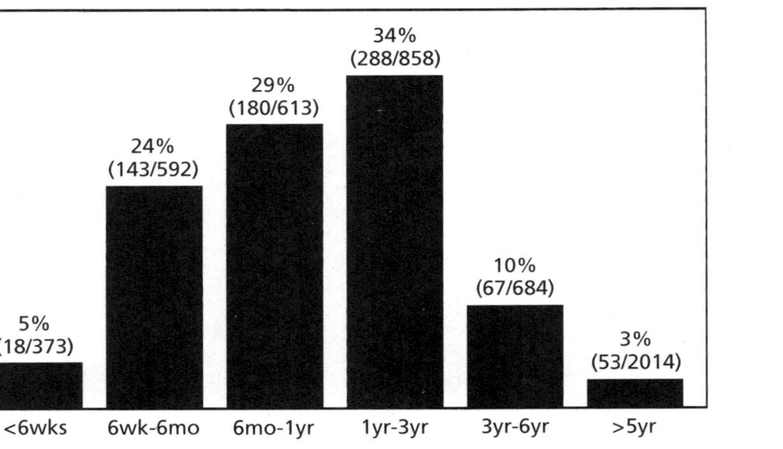

FIG 8-5.
Percentage of children in various age ranges requiring sedation during CT imaging. From Strain J, Harvey L, Foley L et al: Intravenously administered pentobarbital sodium for sedation in pediatric CT, *Radiology* 161:105, 1986.

TABLE 8-7. Drug Strategies for Sedation During Radiographic and Cardiac Catheterization Procedures

I. Conscious Sedation	Monitored with pulse oximeter and NIBP without intravenous access
Chloral hydrate	50-75 mg/kg PO or PR
Midazolam	0.5-1 mg/kg PO or PR
Ketamine	6-10 mg/kg PO
Fentanyl	15 μg/kg transmucosal
Methohexital (10%)	30 mg/kg PR
II. Deep Sedation	Monitored with PCS, pulse oximeter, $ETCO_2$, ECG, NIBP and temperature. Requires intravenous access and supplemental oxygen.
Chloral hydrate	100 mg/kg PO or PR
Midazolam	0.05-0.2 mg/kg IV or IM
Ketamine	4 mg/kg IM or 1 to 2 mg/kg IV
Pentobarbital	3-5 mg/kg IM or IV
Propofol	1-2 mg/kg IV bolus with an infusion of 50 to 200 μg/kg/min.
III. General Anesthesia	Monitored with a PCS, pulse oximeter, $ETCO_2$, ECG, NIBP and temperature. Usually requires an endotracheal tube or LMA.
Inhalational agents	All medications are titrated to effect
Propofol	
Opioids and benzodiazepines	
Ketamine and benzodiazepines	
Muscle relaxants	

NIBP, Noninvasive blood pressure; *PO*, per os; *PR*, per rectum; *PCS*, precordial stethoscope; *ECG*, electrocardiogram; *IV*, intravenously; *IM*, intramuscularly; *LMA*, laryngeal mask airway.

90% of patients. Onset times vary from 15 to 30 minutes. Although most children are awake and responsive within 60 to 90 minutes, sedation may be prolonged and last up to 6 hours. Therefore appropriate monitoring and observation are required until the child is fully awake. If chloral hydrate is ineffective, it may be supplemented with IV midazolam or ketamine. Another alternative to chloral hydrate is oral midazolam.

Regardless of the agents used, there may be problems with oversedation, airway obstruction, and hypoventilation. If not recognized and treated quickly, these may result in patient mortality. Therefore a properly trained caretaker must be assigned to administer and monitor the patient. In a recent national study of sedation and pediatric CT, the radiologist was responsible for the sedation in 47% of the cases, the child's primary care physician was responsible for sedation in 37% of the cases, and an anesthesiologist or anesthetist was responsible for sedation in 4% of the cases. The frequency of reported monitoring in the study was disturbing. With deep sedation, visual inspection alone was the primary monitor. Other monitors, such as electrocardiography (47%), respiratory monitoring (25%), pulse oximetry (20%), and automated blood pressure (15%), were used infrequently. Regardless of the agent used, proper monitoring is mandatory (see Chapter 1).

Once a patient is appropriately sedated, it is important to place him or her in the scanning device in a position that prevents airway obstruction. This is generally accomplished by placing a folded towel or padding beneath the shoulders so that the head is slightly extended at the atlantooccipital junction. The head is held in position with sandbags or padding and the adequacy of air exchange is observed. A pulse oximeter probe can be applied to the toe. For deep sedation and general anesthesia, a blood pressure cuff is applied to an extremity, electrocardiograph leads are placed, and a catheter to sample expired carbon dioxide (CO_2) is taped close to the nares. A useful alternative is to use specialized nasal cannulae that allow for end-tidal CO_2 sampling from one prong and oxygen delivery to the other. CO_2 monitoring is used to demonstrate an adequate respiratory rate and pattern. Although the major concern with sedation is the prevention of hypoxemia, end-tidal CO_2 monitoring alerts the caregiver immediately if there is airway obstruction or apnea. Desaturation measured by pulse oximetry may not occur for 30 to 90 seconds after apnea. Supplemental oxygen should be administered to all patients during sedation. Care must be taken to avoid stimulation of the patient once he or she is sedated (e.g., while applying nasal cannulae and other monitors). All monitors should be turned so that they face the leaded window of the CT scanner. The physician can thus avoid radiation from the scanner while being able to appropriately monitor the patient.

Magnetic Resonance Imaging

MRI has been increasingly used to improve diagnostic capabilities and define plans for therapy for a variety of diseases. MRI examinations are of long duration, usually requiring 30 to 60 minutes of patient immobility. The long, cylindrical configuration of the MRI tunnel may be frightening and claustrophobic to the conscious child or adult. Monitoring equipment may not function properly in proximity to the magnet. The monitor wires may act as conduction loops causing burns to the patient. In addition, ferrous objects brought into the scanning room become dangerous missiles that can potentially injure the patient or attendants. Furthermore, because of the potentially harmful effects of the magnet, MRI is contraindicated in certain patients (Box 8-6).

There is little information about the safety of repeated exposure to magnetic fields; however, short-term exposure appears to be safe. Although this technology is reported to be safe to patients and workers, there is not yet a sufficiently long experience with

BOX 8-6.
Criteria for Exclusion from Magnetic Resonance Imaging

- Temporary or permanent cardiac pacemaker
- Neuroaneurysm or vascular surgical clips (ferrous)
- Unstable vital signs, including severely labile intracranial hypertension
- Automated internal cardiac defibrillator
- Ferromagnetic foreign bodies
- Ferrous endoprosthesis
- Dependence on technology incompatible with magnetic resonance imaging
  - Extracorporeal membrane oxygenator
  - Intraaortic balloon pump
  - Ventricular assist device

MRI. Ongoing studies address the safety of working near these devices on a daily basis.[4] The static magnetic field generated by the magnet extends beyond the boundary set by the Farraday cage that houses the magnet. The engineers who install the magnet mark the strength of the magnetic field on the floor outside the MRI scanner room (Fig. 8-4). The strength of the magnetic field is proportional to the distance from the magnet to the third power. For example, being two feet closer to the magnet increases the magnetic field eightfold.

To safely sedate or anesthetize patients in this technologically hostile environment is a challenge. The most important concern is how to continuously monitor patients even during the scanning procedure. It has been argued that stable patients whose condition is not acute do not require monitoring with special equipment. However, because there is always the potential for an adverse reaction during scanning where access to the patient is limited, appropriate monitoring is crucial. What constitutes appropriate monitoring is dependent on the patient's condition, the depth of sedation, and institutional protocols.

There are unique difficulties with monitoring in the MRI suite. The monitors may interfere with the imaging signals. The MRI is both dependent on the maintenance of the static magnetic field and radio frequency pulses, thus there can be distortion of MR images by unshielded, paramagnetic fields surrounding standard monitors or their cables. The radiofrequency signals of the magnet can induce currents in the ferromagnetic elements of the monitors. This induced current can distort the monitoring signal, making the monitor unstable. There has been a proliferation of individual monitors and monitoring systems specifically designed to be used in the MRI suite without a distortion of signal. These monitors depend on a variety of shielding, nonferromagnetic components, and filters to produce satisfactory output.

The radiofrequency energy from the magnet can produce a rise in temperature and ferromagnetic elements in the monitors sufficient to burn patients. Therefore only equipment that has been tested and recommended for use in the MR scanner by the manufacturer is preferred. Even then, fraying or separation of shielding from the cables can occur with repeated use, providing a source for thermal injuries. All cables should be inspected before use, especially in areas where the cable may be in contact with the patient. If there is a need to keep electrocardiograph wires connected to the patient, meticulous attention should be given to avoid coiling of the wires. Electrocardiograph leads with the shortest distance of wire, including graphite leads that are braided together, may reduce the potential for burn injury.[5] Interference from the magnet can produce an abnormal electrocardiogram (ECG) even in the normal hearts. The ECG changes disappear as soon as the patient is removed from the magnetic field. These are probably not actual biologic effects, but rather alterations of the ECG-detected voltages.

The amplitude of the noise generated from the MR scanner is in the range of 65 and 95 decibels. There have been reported incidences of temporary and permanent hearing loss after MR examination. Magnetic-safe headphones or earplugs are readily available and have been shown to prevent the temporary hearing loss. Protective devices should be used during MR examination.

An automated, noninvasive blood pressure machine with special, extra-long tubing can be used. The added length of the tubing does not significantly affect the accuracy of the measurement. Metallic fittings from the cuff and the tubing can be removed and replaced with nonferrous fittings. The console of the noninvasive blood pressure machine is usually placed outside of the magnetic field. Placing the blood pressure cuff on the lower extremity may limit the length of sampling tube that is required.

The use of a side-stream device to measure end-tidal CO_2 is possible with a very long sampling tube extending out of the MRI scanner room. This allows breath-to-breath monitoring of respirations and rhythm of ventilation. However, when used in this manner, end-tidal CO_2 is not an accurate reflection of arterial CO_2, but serves as a gross monitor. End-tidal CO_2 can also be used in the sedated, nonintubated patient as an earlier warning of apnea or airway obstruction.

Pulse oximetry is perhaps the most important monitor because it provides real time information about the status of the child's circulation and oxygenation. A monitor to detect desaturation is particularly necessary during MR scanning since the patients are completely out of view and in a dark environment, thereby making direct observation impossible. The radiofrequency generated by the MR scanner interferes with the oximeter. Consequently, the majority of currently available "MRI compatible" pulse oximeters function erratically between scanning modes. Even with MRI compatible pulse oximetry, the probe must be placed as close as possible to the edge of the magnet (e.g., on a toe) to ensure as accurate a reading as possible.

Nonferromagnetic monitors, such as plastic precordial stethoscopes and mercury thermometers, are also useful. Anesthesia machines are available with low levels of paramagnetic material and aluminum gas tanks. Such devices can be placed within the confines of the magnetic field and can limit the need for excess lengths of ventilator tubing to connect the patient to a machine that is in another room.

The role of the designated patient observer is unclear. The patient's status as reflected by the various electronic and nonelectronic monitors must be evaluated by a health professional familiar with the monitors and their significance. It is not clear whether this observer needs to be inside the scanner room itself. It is difficult to make any direct observations of a small child who is fully inserted into the scanner. Solid-state television monitors provide some information outside the scanner, but the lack of direct patient contact is still a major limiting factor.

The need for sedation or general anesthesia for children undergoing MR evaluation varies by age of the patient, length of the intended scan, and cooperativeness of the patient. For many patients, conscious sedation is adequate to ensure patient cooperation; however, some children require deep sedation or general anesthesia to provide adequate scanning conditions. Anesthesiologists are not often involved until the patient has been unable to have the scan under standard sedation protocols. There is now considerable experience with a variety of agents and techniques not only to provide adequate scanning conditions but also for quick recovery (Table 8-7).

As with CT scanning, contrast materials are frequently used to enhance the images obtained with MRI. At this time, Imagnabix is the only FDA (Food and Drug Administration) approved, intravenous contrast agent in the United States. Studies of this agent in both adult and pediatric populations have demonstrated a high safety margin when compared with iodinated contrast material. The median lethal dose of Gadalinium (GD-DTPA) (in dogs, mice and rabbits) is approximately 10 μmol/kg, or 100 times the diagnostic dose of 0.1 μmol/kg. Patient tolerance of this drug is also high. The incidence of any type of adverse reaction is approximately 2.4%. Among the reactions temporally related to the administration of this drug are headache, nausea, vomiting, local burning or cool sensation, and hives. Transient elevations of serum iron levels and bilirubin levels, which return to normal within 24 to 48 hours, have also been reported. The safety of GD-DTPA in patients with renal failure has not been clearly established. It has been shown to cross the placenta and appear within the fetal bladder during MR imaging. There are insufficient data to assess the safety of its use in pregnant women. Multiple new ionic and nonionic MR contrast agents are now being developed and may be available in the foreseeable future.

CARDIAC CATHETERIZATION

The cardiac catheterization laboratory is an area in which both sedation and general anesthesia are being used with increasing frequency. Although medications ordered by the cardiologist have been the traditional manner of sedation, there is an increasing reliance on the use of deep sedation or general anesthesia to provide the quiet working conditions and monitoring required for the sickest patients. Procedures in the cardiac catheterization suite vary from purely diagnostic procedures to therapeutic interventions (e.g., radiofrequency ablation or balloon dilatations).

The goals of management of pediatric patients scheduled to undergo diagnostic cardiac catheterization include immobility and sedation while maintaining cardiovascular stability. In some cases the maintenance of spontaneous ventilation is desirable so that the patient's physiology is unaltered and appropriate hemodynamic measurements can be made. Immobility is mandatory during the procedure to avoid cardiac perforation, to minimize radiation exposure, and to obtain technically adequate angiograms.

Diagnostic Cardiac Catheterization

The medications used for sedation and general anesthesia may alter cardiovascular parameters, such as heart rate, blood pressure, or vascular resistance. Therefore it is imperative to consider the underlying cardiac lesion and determine how such changes might affect the child's hemodynamics. It is also important to consider whether such changes will affect the data obtained during the procedure.

The majority of diagnostic, noninterventional procedures are performed with conscious or deep sedation. In infants and young children, this may include an initial dose of chloral hydrate (75 to 100 mg/kg) supplemented with intermittent doses of a benzodiazepine (midazolam 0.05 mg/kg) or an opioid (morphine 0.02 mg/kg or fentanyl 0.5 μg/kg). The application of EMLA (eutetic mixture of local anesthetics) cream to the groin may minimize the need for supplemental, intravenous sedation during vessel cannulation. Alternative agents for patients who cannot be adequately sedated with the above agents include ketamine or propofol. Because of its negative inotropic properties, the latter agent should be used only in patients with stable cardiovascular function. General anesthesia is used when the above techniques fail.

Interventional Cardiac Catheterization

The advent of new dimensions in cardiac catheterization, including the transcatheter treatment of stenotic lesions and septal defects, has further increased the need for deep sedation or general anesthesia. Balloon dilatations have been used in the nonsurgical treatment of pulmonic stenosis, aortic stenosis, and coarctation of the aorta. All of these procedures result in the sudden cessation of flow during the inflation of the balloon and may result in significant disruptions in forward flow. Vascular rupture is a rare, yet very real, concern. Because of the potential for hypotension, malignant arrhythmias, or cardiac arrest during the manipulation, anesthesiologists are increasingly asked to provide deep sedation and/or general anesthesia to these patients. The technical expertise needed to perform such procedures makes it difficult for the cardiologist to be responsible for performing the procedure, monitoring the patient, and supervising the sedation. General anesthesia with endotracheal intubation and controlled ventilation not only ensures the patient's immobility, but it also adds a certain safety factor during a procedure that can lead to significant alterations in cardiorespiratory function.

Sedation is required early in the procedure during patient positioning, draping, and cannulation of the femoral vessels. This is followed by the relatively stable maintenance period of data collection. With balloon dilatations, discomfort occurs with balloon inflation and stretching of the vasculature. Maintenance of sedation has been successfully accomplished with infusions of different agents, such as ketamine or propofol (Table 8-7). These drugs may require adjunct medications, such as a benzodiazepine with ketamine and an opioid with propofol.

Ketamine provides relative cardiorespiratory stability while allowing the maintenance of spontaneous ventilation. However, its effects on pulmonary vascular resistance (PVR) are unclear. Although some studies have suggested a direct effect on the pulmonary vasculature with an increase in PVR, many of these studies were performed in spontaneously breathing patients and did not consider the secondary effects of increases in $PaCO_2$.

Radiofrequency Ablation

Patients with accessory, atrioventricular (AV) connections are at risk for recurrent supraventricular tachycardia (SVT), syncope, and even sudden cardiac death. Catheter ablation of accessory pathways with high-energy, direct-current shocks offers several advantages over other techniques, such as the avoidance of the need for prolonged antiarrhythmic therapy or even surgical procedures (Box 8-7).

Radiofrequency energy is a form of electrical energy generated from a low-power, high-frequency alternating current. Equipment generating radiofrequency energy, called the Bovie device, has been used for electrosurgical cutting since 1929. The radiofrequency current is delivered to the cardiac tissue through a steerable electrode catheter. Good tissue contact of the active electrode, either unipolar or bipolar, is of paramount importance for effective ablation. During the ablation procedure, energy delivery and the coagulation process can be controlled by concurrent monitoring of voltage, current, power, and impedance or catheter tip temperature to avoid overheating and to minimize the risk of cardiac perforation. The actual ablation takes only 10 to 60 seconds,

BOX 8-7.
Advantages of RFA Versus Direct Current Ablation

Less peak voltage (less than 100 V compared with 2000 to 4000 V)
No barotrauma, sparking, or arcing effect
Fewer complications and less morbidity
More discrete and homogeneous lesions (less than 5 mm)
Low arrhythmogenicity
Less depressant effect on left ventricular function
Better energy control and titration
Lower incidence of catheter damage
Allows repeated applications at the same or different locations
No need for synchronization to the QRS
Allows monitoring of the electrocardiogram during ablation
Successfully applicable to all types of supraventricular arrhythmias
Applicable to all areas of the heart
Applicable in adults and children

Modified from Manolis A, Wang P, Estes N: Radiofrequency catheter ablation for cardiac tachyarrhythmias: a review, *Ann Intern Med* 121:452, 1994.
RFA, Radiofrequency ablation.

but correct catheter placement may take several hours. Because of the need to ablate only the specific anomalous tracts, a motionless patient is required.

The results of the radiofrequency ablation (RFA) technique are promising and indicate a bright future for this curative, nonsurgical method. This procedure does have several limitations. It may require extended time (up to 8 hours) with extensive fluoroscopy time (0.5 to 2.5 hours). Because of the extended duration of the procedure, deep sedation or general anesthesia is almost exclusively utilized. In addition to providing the desired conditions for the procedure, the agent used must have limited effects on sinoatrial (SA) and atrioventricular (AV) node function as well as the accessory pathway. It should also not limit the ability of the cardiologist to induce the arrhythmia. Benzodiazepines, propofol, and synthetic opioids do not alter the electrophysiologic function of the heart. However, inhalational anesthetic agents, such as enflurane, halothane, and isoflurane, increase the refractory time of the accessory and normal conduction pathways. Although inhalation agents are the agents of choice for incidental surgery in patients with preexcitation syndromes, they should be avoided during ablation techniques. Our most successful regimen has included general anesthesia with endotracheal intubation and controlled ventilation maintained by an infusion of propofol (50 to 200 μg/kg/min), vecuronium, and a synthetic opioid (alfentanil, sufentanil, or fentanyl).

Routine monitoring should include a continuous electrocardiograph, noninvasive blood pressure, $ETCO_2$, temperature, precordial stethoscope, and oxygen saturation. Once the cannulae are placed, the arterial wave from the cardiac catheterization catheters can be monitored. Resuscitative equipment must always be readily available since these patients have significant underlying dysrhythmias.

SEDATION FOR INVASIVE THERAPEUTIC AND DIAGNOSTIC PROCEDURES

Invasive procedures, such as lumbar puncture, bone marrow aspiration, and central line placement, are a few of the many essential therapeutic and diagnostic procedures that are commonly performed in children (Box 8-8). These procedures vary widely in invasiveness, duration, and level of painful stimuli. Although parenteral sedation is generally not required for brief and minimally painful procedures, such as starting an IV, other procedures can cause a significant amount of distress and require significant sedation. Sedation decreases the distress of the patient and the possibility of psychologic trauma. Moreover, it provides the physician with a cooperative and motionless patient, thereby increasing the chances of a successful procedure and perhaps even limiting the risk of morbidity.

The potential for psychologic trauma exists when a painful procedure is performed on a restrained and awake child in unfamiliar surroundings without parental presence. Surveys of parents and patients with pediatric malignancies have demonstrated that invasive procedures are often perceived as worse than the disease itself. The remainder of this chapter presents strategies for managing the pediatric patient during a painful procedure.

BOX 8-8.
A Partial List of Diagnostic and Therapeutic Procedures in Children

Bone marrow aspiration or biopsy
Lumbar puncture
Central line placement
Skin biopsy
Thoracostomy tube placement
Thoracentesis
Endotracheal intubation
Bronchoscopy
Upper gastrointestinal endoscopy
Sigmoidoscopy
Arterial line placement
Venipuncture
Heelstick
Circumcision
Intravenous cannula placement

Topical and local anesthesia

As important as the use of sedative agents is the proper, topical preparation of the site of the invasive procedure. Regardless of the procedure, a topical application of EMLA cream and subsequent infiltration with local anesthetics can significantly decrease or eliminate the need for parenteral sedation. EMLA cream is a mixture of two local anesthetics (lidocaine and prilocaine) formulated into a cream. It is applied to the skin and covered with an occlusive dressing. After 60 minutes it penetrates intact skin and produces superficial anesthesia of the skin and subcutaneous tissue.[6,7] The depth of penetration is dependent on the duration of contact with the skin. Clinical experience has demonstrated the efficacy of EMLA in various invasive procedures, such as venipuncture, accessing subcutaneous venous reservoirs, lumbar puncture, laser therapy of dermal lesions, and aspiration of joints.[8-10] Additional applications include topical anesthesia before vessel cannulation for cardiac catheterization or before central line placement. EMLA can be used whenever a needle penetrates intact skin. Although it may not provide anesthesia of deeper structures, the use of EMLA cream may allow the painless deep infiltration of a local anesthetic.[11]

If the painful stimulus is eliminated from an invasive procedure, all that may be required is light sedation to provide anxiolysis. After using EMLA for repeated procedures in the pediatric oncology patient, children may no longer require sedation. It may be useful to send the parents home with the EMLA cream and have them apply it over the appropriate sites before coming to the clinic. This avoids any delay in achieving analgesia that may occur since EMLA requires up to 60 minutes to be effective.

Adverse effects related to EMLA cream have been rare. Methemoglobinemia may be induced by prilocaine, particularly in infants.[12] Methemoglobin is hemoglobin in which the iron has been oxidized from the ferrous to the ferric state. It is unable to bind oxygen. Methemoglobin is normally converted back to hemoglobin by the enzyme methemoglobin reductase. Like all hepatic enzyme systems, this enzyme may be deficient in neonates. Additionally, fetal hemoglobin is more susceptible to oxidant stresses and therefore more likely to be converted to methemoglobin. The prescribing information states that EMLA Cream should not be used in infants under the age of one month or in those rare patients with congenital or idiopathic methemoglobinemia or in infants under the age of twelve months who are receiving treatment with methemoglobin-inducing agents.

Lidocaine may be absorbed systemically; however, serum levels of lidocaine are very low with properly applied EMLA cream.[13] EMLA cream should be applied to the smallest possible surface, and it should not be used on mucosal surfaces. Once applied, young children should be under direct observation to prevent accidental ingestion by chewing or sucking on the EMLA cream. If the cream is accidentally rubbed into the eye, corneal anesthesia with the risk of possible injury can result.[14] With these simple precautions, EMLA cream can be an effective, simple, and safe adjunct to painful procedures, particularly if the most painful or distressing portion of the procedure is the initial penetration of the skin with the needle.

TAC is a topically applied mixture of the local anesthetic tetracaine, adrenaline, and cocaine.[15] Its major application has been in the prevention of pain during suturing of lacerations in the emergency room. Formulations can vary from institution to institution. For example, the formulation used at Vanderbilt University Medical Center (0.25% tetracaine, 1:40,000 epinephrine, 5.9% cocaine) is approximately half the concentration of the originally described formulation (0.5% tetracaine, 1:20,000 epinephrine, 11.8% cocaine). Recently, Smith and colleagues[16] reported that a formulation that includes 1% tetracaine, 1:40,000 epinephrine, and 4.0% cocaine has equal efficacy and less potential for toxicity than older formulations.

Despite its efficacy and widespread application, significant adverse effects are associated with the systemic absorption of any of the three drugs. This is especially true if TAC is applied to mucosal surfaces where large amounts of the drug can be quickly absorbed. Death from cocaine toxicity in an infant has been reported when TAC was applied to the oral and nasal mucosa.[17] Seizures after the application of TAC to the oral mucosa for tongue laceration have also been reported.[18]

TAC is effective and safe as long as toxic doses and contact with mucosal surfaces are strictly avoided. The TAC dosage should be based on the patient's weight and the cocaine and tetracaine concentrations of the solution. The dose should be limited to 1 ml/10 kg of Smith's TAC solution. Since both cocaine and epinephrine are vasoconstrictors, TAC should not be applied to areas with limited circulation (pinna of ear, penis, or digits).

Superficial and deep infiltration with local anesthetic solutions can provide effective analgesia during invasive procedures. Regardless of the local anesthetic agent, calculation of the total maximum dose on a mg/kg basis is necessary to avoid toxicity (see Chapters 1 and 3). This is especially important in smaller patients and as the area to be infiltrated increases.

Most practitioners are familiar with the use of lidocaine for topical anesthesia. Problems can arise if higher concentrations (1.0 or 2.0%) are used because toxic doses can be quickly reached and exceeded. Low concentrations (0.5% lidocaine) are effective for the majority of procedures. The total dose should not exceed 5 mg/kg or 1 ml/kg of the 0.5% solution. The injection of lidocaine can be painful. Therefore, the solution should be injected slowly with a 27- or 30-gauge needle. Rapid injection increases the pain associated with infiltration. Pain associated with injection may be related to the low pH of the solution and can be decreased by the addition of 0.1 mEq of sodium bicarbonate to each milliliter of the solution before injection. Alternatively, chloroprocaine, a local anesthetic of the ester class, can be used. Vials of chloroprocaine have a pH close to 7.0, thereby obviating the need of adding sodium bicarbonate. If the drug is carefully and slowly infiltrated after the application of EMLA cream, it is frequently possible to anesthetize the area without causing any discomfort to the patient.

Jet injection devices are also available to administer local anesthetics. These devices rapidly inject 0.35 ml of the local anesthetic 1.5 cm into intact skin. Although not entirely painless, this method can be useful before lumbar puncture or venipuncture and does not require the 60 minute onset time of EMLA cream.

AGENTS FOR SEDATION

Benzodiazepines

Benzodiazepines are anxiolytic, sedative hypnotic agents. They produce antegrade and retrograde amnesia, muscle relaxation, and sedation. However, they have no analgesic properties; therefore, benzodiazepines are frequently used in combination with opioids for painful procedures.

There are three commonly used benzodiazepines—lorazepam, diazepam, and midazolam. Diazepam is the prototype drug of this class and has a long history of use in pediatric sedation. Both lorazepam and diazepam have relatively protracted durations of action and are not useful for the majority of pediatric procedures. An additional problem is that diazepam is not water soluble and the vehicle used as a solvent is propylene glycol, which can cause pain with IV injection.

Midazolam remains the most popular of the benzodiazepines for sedation in children. As noted in Table 8-8, there are multiple options for the route of delivery. It is water soluble; therefore, there is no pain with IV administration. Its elimination half-life is shorter than diazepam, permitting rapid awakening after the procedure. Midazolam has a wide margin of safety; however, respiratory depression can occur, especially when it is administered with other drugs, particularly opioids.[19] Paradoxical excitement or delirium can occur with lower doses of midazolam, particularly in the presence of pain.

TABLE 8-8. Midazolam Dosing Based on Routes of Delivery

Route of Delivery	Dose (mg/kg)
Intravenous	0.05-0.1
Oral	0.5-1.0
Rectal	0.7-1.0
Intranasal	0.2-0.4
Sublingual	0.2-0.4

Aside from its rapid onset and brief duration of action, the major advantages of midazolam are the options for route of delivery. Although IV administration is chosen when access is present, it may also be used by nonparenteral routes in the patient without access, in whom anxiolysis is needed. Oral administration in a dose of 0.5 to 0.7 mg/kg produces anxiolysis in roughly 20 minutes and is currently the preferred agent for premedication in the operating room. The only disadvantage to oral administration is that the IV preparation (5 mg/ml) must be used. It contains the preservative, benzyl alcohol, which tastes bitter; therefore, the medication must be delivered in a solution that hides the bitter taste. One of the more popular alternatives in operating rooms is to dilute the medication in double or quadruple strength Kool-Aid. Mixing the medication in Tylenol elixir is also somewhat effective in hiding the taste.

Because of the problems with oral administration, other nonparenteral routes have been evaluated, such as intranasal and sublingual administration. For intranasal administration, a dose of 0.3 to 0.4 mg/kg is used. The standard 5 mg/ml IV solution is drawn up into a tuberculin syringe, the needle is removed, and the medication is squirted into the patient's nose. This is done while a parent is holding the child in his or her lap. The child may express some discomfort since the benzyl alcohol may burn the nasal mucosa. Sedation occurs in 5 to 10 minutes.

To avoid the problems of discomfort related to the benzyl alcohol, sublingual administration has also be tried. The medication is drawn up in the same manner as for intranasal administration, but it drips in under the tongue. Onset is in 5 to 10 minutes. This works well for the anxious yet cooperative 5-year-old, but is next to impossible for the anxious 2-year-old who won't open his or her mouth.

Opioids

Several opioids have been used for sedation and analgesia during pediatric procedures. Opioids provide analgesia but no amnesia. Therefore they are frequently combined with benzodiazepines, such as midazolam, for procedural sedation. When opioids are combined with other sedative agents, one must always be aware of the potential for respiratory depression.[19] This section briefly addresses the use of opioids and their use in the context of painful procedures.

Morphine and meperidine have significant limitations in this setting. Their duration of action of 2 to 4 hours is longer than most procedures.[20] This may leave the patient at risk for certain adverse effects, such as respiratory depression for a significant period of time after the procedure is completed. This may occur when there is little stimulus to keep the patient awake and when vigilance and monitoring may be more relaxed.

Fentanyl is a potent opioid (100 times that of morphine), with a high lipid solubility, which allows rapid penetration of the blood/brain barrier, accounting for its rapid onset of action. The rapid onset and short duration of action (15 to 20 minutes) makes it an attractive choice in this setting. Although fentanyl is significantly more potent than morphine, the risk of respiratory depression is equivalent with an equipotent amount of drug. It should be noted that fentanyl is available in a 50 μg/ml solution; therefore, careful attention to drug dosing is required to avoid inadvertent overdoses. Dosing guidelines for fentanyl include 0.5 μg/kg up to 25 μg every 3 mins as needed. As with any of the medications used, the dose should be titrated in gradually to achieve the desired effect. There is no set dose that works in all patients and no limit as to how much can be used.

Fentanyl Oralet

Fentanyl is now also available in a transmucosal preparation. The opioid is incorporated into a raspberry flavored lozenge that resembles a lollipop, known as the Fentanyl Oralet. Three sizes are currently available: 200, 300, and 400 μg. This preparation has been most frequently used as a preoperative medication in doses ranging from 10 to 20 μg/kg.[21,22] Onset of analgesia and sedation generally occurs in 10 to 15 minutes. Sedation results from the absorption of fentanyl across the buccal mucosa. If the lozenge is chewed and swallowed, only 5% to 10% is absorbed with limited, if any, effect. Problems include a relatively high incidence of nausea and vomiting. This may be related to the use of higher doses in the initial studies of up to 20 μg/kg. Current recommendations are for lower doses of 8 to 10 μg/kg. Mild to moderate oxygen desaturation has also been noted, thereby emphasizing the need for patient monitoring regardless of the route of administration of sedative and analgesic agents. Although used mainly as a premedicant for the operating room, Conrad and colleagues[23] reported their experience with the Fentanyl Oralet for 93 invasive procedures in 21 children with cancer. The agent provided effective analgesia with five episodes of vomiting and only one episode of mild desaturation.

Schecter and colleagues performed a randomized, placebo-controlled study evaluating the Fentanyl Oralet (15 to 20 μg/kg) in a population of pediatric patients undergoing lumbar puncture and bone marrow aspirates.[24] A significant decrease in pain ratings was reported by both the patients and parents with the administration of oral transmucosal fentanyl citrate. However, 85% of the patients who received the Oralet experienced some adverse effect, such as pruritus (65%), nausea and vomiting (31%), or low oxygen saturation (7%). Future studies are needed to clearly define the role of the Fentanyl Oralet in pediatric sedation. Its major advantage is its nonparenteral route of administration. However, its efficacy may be limited by the high incidence of adverse effects.

Chloral Hydrate

Chloral hydrate remains one of the most popular sedative agents currently used in the pediatric population, especially in infants.[25] After administration it is metabolized to the active compound, trichloroethanol. It has no analgesic properties; therefore, it should not be used to treat pain or during painful procedures. However, it may be useful when only sedation is required (e.g., radiologic imaging). Recommended doses range from 50 to 100 mg/kg administered PO or PR up to a 2 g maximum. The chances of successful sedation can be increased by using the higher spectrum of the dosing range (75 to 80 mg/kg). Since chloral hydrate is somewhat unpalatable and may cause gastrointestinal upset, rectal administration is recommended.

Inadequate sedation may result from erratic or delayed absorption from the gastrointestinal tract with an onset of activity of up to 60 minutes. Prolonged sedation may occasionally be noted because of a half-life of up to 10 hours. Despite a long record of safety with minimal effects on respiratory function in most patients, deaths from respiratory depression have occurred.[26] Like all other sedative agents, respiratory depression can occur with chloral hydrate, and standard monitoring is mandatory. Additionally, the patient should be monitored until he or she is fully awake. More than one patient has been discharged before being fully awake only to be found dead on arrival at home. Anecdotal reports also document the occurrence of ventricular arrhythmias, especially in patients with underlying cardiovascular diseases or when used with other proarrhythmic drugs (e.g., phenothiazines or tricyclic antidepressants). The arrhythmias are postulated to be the result of the active metabolite, trichloroethanol, which is a halogenated hydrocarbon (like halothane).

Ketamine

Ketamine is a dissociative anesthetic chemically related to phencyclidine.[27] Unlike the previously mentioned agents, it provides analgesia and amnesia. Various options for the route of delivery exist, such as oral, rectal, intravenous, and intramuscular (Table 8-9). It is metabolized in the liver and has an active metabo-

TABLE 8-9. Ketamine Dosing Based on Route of Delivery

Route of Delivery	Dose (mg/kg)
Intravenous	0.25-0.5
Intramuscular	2-6
Oral	6-10
Rectal	6-10
Intranasal	6

lite (norketamine), which has an analgesic potency one third that of the parent ketamine. Analgesia with ketamine given via the oral route occurs at a lower plasma level than when ketamine is given IM. This difference may be the result of a higher concentration of norketamine produced from first-pass metabolism in the liver with oral administration.

Ketamine generally preserves airway patency and respiratory function. It has a mild, dose-related, respiratory-depressant effect and shifts the CO_2 response curve to the right. Ketamine produces bronchodilatation as a result of the release of endogenous catecholamines. It can be safely and effectively used to provide sedation and analgesia during invasive procedures (arterial or central line placement) in patients with status asthmaticus. Despite its beneficial effects on airway protective reflexes and respiratory function, prolonged apnea and desaturation may occur. In addition, it can cause an incompetent gag reflex, warranting cautious use in patients with gastroesophageal reflux or full stomachs. Upper airway secretions are also increased and a prophylactic antisialogogue (glycopyrrolate) administration is suggested.

The most frequently mentioned adverse effect related to ketamine is emergence delirium, or hallucinations. These occur more commonly if ketamine is used alone and in older patients. The administration of a benzodiazepine before ketamine use is effective in almost entirely eliminating the chances of emergence delirium. There is no upper age limit for the use of ketamine and it has frequently been used even in adolescents.

Ketamine is contraindicated in patients with increased ICP. The effect of ketamine on patients with seizures is unclear.[28] Ketamine has been used as a therapeutic agent in the treatment of refractory status epilepticus; however, most clinicians view a seizure disorder as a relative contraindication to ketamine.

A ketamine/midazolam/glycopyrrolate combination is extremely useful for a wide variety of painful pediatric procedures, such as bone marrow aspiration or biopsy, percutaneous liver or kidney biopsies, and removal of orthopedic appliances. When intravenous access is in place, a benzodiazepine, such as midazolam (0.05 to 0.1 mg/kg), and glycopyrrolate (5 to 10 μg/kg) are administered 3 to 5 minutes before ketamine. Ketamine is then titrated in incremental doses of 0.5 mg/kg every 3 minutes to achieve the desired level and length of analgesia. Its short duration of action, intense analgesia, and ability to allow spontaneous respiration have made it the agent of choice for most painful procedures. Although short acting, ketamine does not usually produce a state of conscious sedation but rather a state of deep sedation or general anesthesia, and it requires the appropriate monitoring for a deeper level of sedation.

Barbiturates

Barbiturates remain the most commonly used agents for the intravenous induction of anesthesia. Because of their potent respiratory depressant effects, airway management skills and monitoring for deep sedation and general anesthesia are required when using these drugs. The three most commonly used agents, in order of increasing duration of action, are methohexital, thiopental, and pentobarbital. Like benzodiazepines, barbiturates provide amnesia but have no analgesic properties. Consequently, they are generally used alone only for nonpainful procedures (CT, MRI) or in combination with opioids to provide amnesia during painful procedures.

Methohexital, a short-acting oxybarbiturate, has a long history of use PR (20 to 30 mg/kg) as an induction agent in children.[32] Onset of action is 10 to 20 minutes after rectal administration. Methohexital can exacerbate seizures in patients with an underlying seizure disorder.

Thiopental is another short-acting barbiturate and is the most commonly used barbiturate for the intravenous induction of anesthesia. Doses for intravenous administration during endotracheal intubation vary from 2 to 6 mg/kg. Like all barbiturates, thiopental has negative inotropic and vasodilatory properties that can result in hypotension, especially in the setting of hypovolemia or underlying cardiovascular dysfunction. Rapid redistribution accounts for its short duration of action (5 to 10 minutes) after intravenous administration. It decreases the cerebral metabolic rate for oxygen with a reflex cerebral vasoconstriction leading to a decrease in ICP. It remains the agent of choice for intravenous induction and endotracheal intubation in patients with compromised intracranial compliance and normal hemodynamic status. It is a potent anticonvulsant and may be administered by continuous intravenous infusion to control refractory status epilepticus. It can also be administered PR with a "sedation time" of approximately 90 minutes when administered rectally in doses of 25 mg/kg.

Pentobarbital remains a popular choice for sedation during radiologic procedures, such as MRI. Dosing recommendations include 1 to 2 mg/kg IV or 5 to 7 mg/kg IM. The intramuscular administration of this or any medication to children is not recommended. The duration of action (45 to 60 minutes) after a single dose is considerably longer than with either methohexital or thiopental.

Propofol

Propofol is a new sedative and hypnotic agent initially approved by the FDA for the induction and maintenance of general anesthesia.[26] It has a rapid onset and a short duration of action, and it produces dose-dependent levels of sedation varying from conscious sedation to general anesthesia. It can only be administered IV, and because of its short duration, an infusion is generally needed for all but the briefest procedures. It allows faster awakening than midazolam or fentanyl regimens, and it has antiemetic properties. Individual responses vary from patient to patient, but adequate sedation can usually be obtained and maintained with 1 to 2 mg/kg followed by an infusion of 25 to 100 μg/kg/min. Intermittent bolus doses (0.5 to 1 mg/kg) may be used without an infusion for brief procedures.[29]

Like barbiturates, propofol can have significant effects on cardiorespiratory function, including negative inotropic and vasodilatory properties leading to hypotension.[30] Respiratory depression is dose-dependent and the incidence of apnea increases with the dose. CNS effects include opisthotonic posturing, myoclonus, and seizure activity. Because of these concerns, some institutions restrict the use of propofol to anesthesia personnel.

Another drawback with propofol is the high incidence of pain on injection, particularly when injected into the small veins on the dorsum of the hand.[31] Several options have been offered to decrease the incidence of pain, such as the administration of a small dose of fentanyl (0.5 to 1 μg/kg) or lidocaine (0.2 to 0.5 mg/kg) before injection. It may also help to cool the solution before injection.

Nitrous Oxide

Nitrous oxide has many of the characteristics of a desirable sedation agent. It has a rapid onset of action, it is relatively easy and inexpensive to use, and its effects dissipate rapidly once discontinued. Its solubility characteristics allow rapid induction and awakening. (Nitrous oxide is also discussed in Chapter 7.)

Holst reports an astonishing experience of 3 million pediatric dental patients treated with 30% to 60% nitrous oxide without a single serious complication.[33] Griffin and colleagues describe its use with pediatric patients in an emergency room setting for treating burns, lacerations, orthopedic reductions, and freeing penile foreskin trapped in a boy's pants.[34]

Nitrous oxide can be administered by the face or a nasal mask. Another option involves the use of a weighted mouthpiece that falls from the patient, thereby stopping the administration of the agent if the patient becomes too sleepy. Safety issues mandate that nitrous oxide should be administered with a monitor of the inspired oxygen concentration and a fail-safe device that cuts off the nitrous-oxide flow if the oxygen supply fails. Without such a mechanism, the nitrous oxide flow can continue without the addition of oxygen, leading to the delivery of a hypoxic mixture. Alternatively, commercially available tanks are manufactured that contain a 50/50 oxygen and nitrous oxide mixture, thereby limiting the risk of a hypoxic mixture and the need for specialized equipment. A scavenger device attached to the delivery system is also required to remove waste gases and prevent environmental pollution. Repeated exposure of the patient or healthcare workers to nitrous oxide can lead to bone marrow suppression and peripheral neuropathy as a result of its effects on B_{12} metabolism and protein synthesis.

Nitrous oxide diffuses into air filled spaces, increasing the volume of the space, and is therefore contraindicated in bowel obstruction and intrathoracic injuries with the risk of pneumothorax. Nitrous oxide increases ICP and is contraindicated in patients with closed head injury and altered intracranial compliance.

Combinations of Agents

DPT is a combination of meperidine (Demerol), promethazine (Phenergan), and chlorpromazine (Thorazine). It was originally used as an anesthetic induction technique to induce deliberate hypothermia before cardiac surgery. It was later adapted for use during cardiac catheterization.[35] This cocktail produces a state of deep sedation and analgesia and unfortunately remains one of the more common techniques used to sedate children.

The combination of phenothiazines (chlorpromazine and promethazine) and a long-acting opioid act synergistically to produce many undesirable side effects. Phenothiazines lower the pain threshold and may decrease the efficacy of analgesia from the opioid while potentiating the respiratory depression. Phenothiazines lower the seizure threshold. Seizures have been reported after DPT administration to children without risk factors for seizures.[37] Phenothiazines can also cause orthostatic hypotension and dystonic reactions.

Most importantly, the duration of action of DPT can be much longer than the planned procedure, placing the child at risk for cardiorespiratory compromise if there is limited postprocedure monitoring. A sleeptime of 2 to 5 hours with 9 to 15 hours for a "return to baseline" has been reported. Deaths have been reported during and after procedures where DPT has been used, usually from respiratory depression. Although it is an effective drug (i.e., produces a deeply sedated, motionless child) and a familiar combination, the same effect can be produced with a higher margin of safety using other drugs.

Regional Anesthetic Techniques

A complete description of the techniques and applications of regional anesthesia and peripheral nerve blockade are provided in Chapter 4. These techniques should be performed only by anesthesiologists who are familiar with their use and the adverse effects associated with them. One technique that may be readily applicable to prevent procedure-related pain is intravenous regional anesthesia, or the Bier block. It is a simple technique often used in emergency rooms for procedures involving the forearm (primarily laceration closure) and reduction of fractures. As this technique involves high doses (3 to 5 mg/kg) of local anesthetics, such as lidocaine, the potential for toxicity is high and perhaps increased when used by someone who is not an anesthesiologist. An alternative regimen has been described by Julian and colleagues[38] with a low-dose lidocaine technique. A single-bladder blood pressure cuff is placed above the elbow and inflated to 100 mm Hg above systolic blood pressure after partial exsanguination of the arm by elevation. A 1 mg/kg dose of lidocaine is diluted to 0.125% with normal saline and injected into a distal vein in the extremity. Excellent results were achieved in 43 out of 44 patients (one complained of tourniquet pain) ranging in age from 4 to 15 years. With the dose used, cuff failure is a minor inconvenience and not a catastrophic event. The block can be repeated if necessary without reaching toxic levels.

Opioid and Benzodiazepine Reversal Agents

Specific antagonists are available for opioids and benzodiazepines. Naloxone is the familiar opioid antagonist. The starting dose is 1 to 2 μg/kg up to 0.2 mg. The dose can be repeated every 2 to 3 minutes and titrated to effect. Slow injection and careful titration of the dose can maximize reversal of respiratory depression while minimizing analgesia reversal. Naloxone can precipitate full blown withdrawal when given to patients who are opioid dependant. The duration of action of naloxone is shorter than that of opioids, so appropriate monitoring must be continued until the respiratory depressant effects of the opioids have dissipated.

Flumazenil is a competitive antagonist of benzodiazepines that inhibits their activity at gamma amino butyric acid (GABA) receptors.[39] It antagonizes the sedative and, to some extent, the respiratory depressant effects of benzodiazepines. There is no large series in the literature regarding the use of flumazenil in children. Experience in the pediatric population is derived from its use in case reports of benzodiazepine overdoses. Various doses of flumazenil have been reported with most suggesting somewhere around 0.01 mg/kg. The dose may be repeated every 5 minutes to a maximum of 1 mg or until the desired effect is achieved. Flumazenil is available in a 10 ml vial with a concentration of 0.1 mg/ml. Flumazenil has a shorter duration of action than most benzodiazepines,[40] again emphasizing the need for continued monitoring after its administration. Most importantly flumazenil is meant to be used only after acute benzodiazepine administration. As the major adverse effect, seizures have been reported when flumazenil has been administered to patients with a history of chronic benzodiazepine use or to those who have ingested other medications that lower the seizure threshold (tricyclic antidepressant agents). Flumazenil may precipitate ventricular arrhythmias when administered concomitantly with cocaine, methylxanthines, monoamine oxidase inhibitors, chloral hydrate, or tricyclic antidepressants. Despite the efficacy of both naloxone and flumazenil in reversing the sedative and respiratory depressant effects of opioids and benzodiazepines, their availability does not diminish the need for prompt detection of hypoventilation and the ability to intervene by establishing an airway and assisting ventilation.

NONPHARMACOLOGIC METHODS

Nonpharmacologic methods may be used either alone or as an adjunct to pharmacologic treatment. Distraction techniques along with appropriate preparation can significantly influence the amount of sedation required. Preparation can be as simple as informing the child of the intended procedure and the steps involved.

Summary

Before embarking on sedation for procedures, it is mandatory to have the appropriate drugs, equipment, and personnel necessary to resuscitate the child if an adverse reaction occurs. Monitoring of the child is necessary both during and after the procedure. The child is at higher risk for respiratory complications once the stimulus of the procedure is removed.

Knowledge of the procedure, its intended duration, and the patient's underlying medical condition improve one's ability to provide safe and effective sedation. If the procedure is elective, proper NPO status must be assured. If the procedure is urgent, a decision should be made whether to postpone the procedure, to proceed with minimal sedation after aspiration prophylaxis, or to proceed with airway protection (i.e., endotracheal intubation) and general anesthesia. There is a fine line between conscious and deep sedation and a wide interpatient variability exists in response to sedative agents. Therefore sedative drugs must be titrated to achieve the desired effect. There may be up to a tenfold difference between patients in the amount of medication they require for the same procedure. Although drug combinations can be very useful, the incidence of complications increases substantially with the number of drugs used. When possible, a maximum of two drugs (e.g., midazolam and fentanyl), or preferably a single agent (e.g., ketamine), is suggested.

Younger patients may be more prone to life-threatening complications under sedation. Infants are anatomically predisposed to airway obstruction with relatively large tongues and protruding occiputs that push the head forward. The physiologic consequences of obstruction in infants are immediately apparent with rapid and severe desaturation with airway obstruction. Careful attention to head positioning in infants may limit such problems.

When confronted with a child who is about to undergo a painful procedure, two choices should be made: the drug or drugs to be used and the route of administration. For the vast majority of children, some form of amnesia is also preferred. For painful procedures, an analgesic agent is added to limit the distress during the procedure. For the child with intravenous access, the combination of midazolam with fentanyl or ketamine is generally safe and effective.

The child without intravenous access often presents a problem. The vast majority of children consider an intramuscular injection or starting an IV to be as invasive as the procedure itself. The combination of an alternative route for midazolam (e.g., oral) combined with EMLA cream to facilitate placement of an intravenous cannula is an effective means of achieving the desired goal. Other options for the nonintravenous administration of midazolam have been previously discussed. After the placement of intravenous access, ketamine can be titrated in to achieve analgesia during the procedure. Other alternatives to the combination of midazolam and EMLA include oral or nasal ketamine or OTFC. The judicious use of local anesthetics can greatly increase the comfort of the procedure and decrease the amount of sedation required.

Several strategies and drug regimens to facilitate the performance of pediatric procedures have been presented. The overall goal of pain management and sedation during procedures is to make the experience as comfortable and nonthreatening as possible. This is particularly important during the child's first procedure to minimize anticipatory anxiety for subsequent procedures. Psychologic intervention, pharmacologic support, or a combination of the two should be tailored to the particular patient and procedure. With appropriate monitoring, sedative agents can be safely administered by pediatricians, radiologists, emergency room physicians, and other practitioners caring for children. With complicated patients or those with severe underlying medical conditions that may increase the risk of adverse effects, consultation with a pediatric anesthesiologist may be required.

References

1. Guidelines for monitoring and management of pediatric patients during and after sedation for diagnostic and therapeutic procedures, *Pediatrics* 89:1110, 1992.

2. Hall, CC et al: Aspiration pneumonitis: an obstetric hazard, *JAMA* 114:728, 1940.
3. Mendelson CL et al: The aspiration of stomach contents into the lungs during obstetric anesthesia, *Am J Obstet Gynecol* 52:111, 1946.
4. Shellock FG et al: Biological effects and safety aspects of MRI: magnetic resonance imaging 5:243, 1989.
5. Kanal E, Sellock F, Talagala L: Siphon considerations in MRI, *Radiology* 176:593, 1990.
6. Ehrenstrom G, Reiz SLA.: EMLA®-an eutectic mixture of local anesthetics for topical anesthesia, *Acta Anaesthesiol Scand* 26:596, 1982.
7. Hallen B, Olsson GL, Uppfeld TA: Pain-free venipuncture: effect of timing of application of local anesthetic cream, *Anaesthesia* 39:969, 1984.
8. Kapelushnik J, Koren G, Soth H et al: Evaluating the efficacy of EMLA® in alleviating pain associated with lumbar puncture: comparison of open and double-blinded protocols in children, *Pain* 42:31, 1990.
9. Halprin DL, Korin G, Altias D et al: Topical skin anesthesia for venous, subcutaneous drug reservoir and lumbar punctures in children, *Pediatrics* 84:281, 1989.
10. Tan OT, Stafford TJ: EMLA® for laser treatment of port wine stains in children, *Lasers Surg Med* 12:543, 1992.
11. Taddio A, Robiax I, Kran G: Effect of lidocaine-prilocaine cream on pain from subcutaneous injection, *Clin Pharm* 11:347, 1992.
12. Frayling IM, Addison GM, Chattergie K et al: Methaemoglobinemia in children treated with prilocaine-lidocaine cream, *BMJ* 301:153, 1990.
13. Manner T, Kanto J, Iisalo E et al: Reduction of pain at venous cannulation in children with a eutectic mixture of lidocaine and prilocaine (EMLA® cream): comparison with placebo cream and no local premedication, *Acta Anaesthesiol Scand* 31:735, 1987.
14. James IG: EMLA® complications, *Br J Anaesth* 65:295, 1990.

15. Bonadio WA: TAC: a review, *Pediatr Emerg Care* 5:1541, 1987.
16. Smith SM, Barry RC: A comparison of three formulations of TAC (tetracaine, adrenaline, cocaine) for anesthesia of minor lacerations in children, *Pediatr Emerg Care* 6:266, 1990.
17. Dailey RH: Fatality secondary to misuse of TAC solution, *Ann Emerg Med* 17:159, 1988.
18. Daya MR, Burton BT, Schluss MR et al: Recurrent seizures following mucosal application of TAC, *Ann Emerg Med* 17:646, 1988.
19. Yaster M, Nichols DG, Deshpande JK et al: Midazolam-fentanyl intravenous sedation in children: case report of a respiratory arrest, *Pediatrics* 86:463, 1990.
20. Dahlstrom B, Bovine P, Feychting H et al: Morphine kinetics in children, *Clin Pharmacol Ther* 26:354, 1979.
21. Ashburn MA, Streisand JB, Turver SD et al: Oral transmucosal fentanyl citrate for premedication in pediatric outpatients, *Can J Anaesth* 37:857, 1990.
22. Streisand JB, Stanley TH, Hague B et al: Oral transmucosal fentanyl citrate premedication in children, *Anesth Analg* 69:28, 1989.
23. Conrad DL, Rosenblum M, Wiesman SJ et al. Safety and efficacy of oral transmucosal fentanyl citrate (OTFC) for procedures in children, *Anesthesiology* 75:A954, 1991.
24. Schechter NL, Weisman SJ, Rosenblum M et al: The use of transmucosal fentanyl citrate for painful procedures in children, *Pediatrics* 95:335, 1995.
25. Cook BA, Bass JW, Nomique S et al: Sedation of children for technical procedures: current standard of practice, *Clin Peds* 31:137, 1992.
26. Jastak JT, Pallasch T: Death after chloral hydrate sedation: report of a case, *J Am Dent Assoc* 116:345, 1988.
27. White PF, Way WL, Trevor AJ: Ketamine—its pharmacology and therapeutic uses, *Anesthesiology* 56:119, 1982.

28. Myslobodshy MS, Golovchinsky V, Minty M. Ketamine: convulsant or anticonvulsant? *Pharmacol Biochem Behav* 4:27, 1981.
29. Smith I, White PF, Nathanson M et al: Propofol: an update on its clinical use, *Anesthesiology* 81(4):1005-1043, 1994.
30. Short SM, Aun CST: Haemodynamics of propofol in children, *Anaesthesia* 46:783, 1991.
31. Klement W, Arndt JO: Pain an injection of propofol: effects of concentration and delivery, *Br J Anaesth* 67:281, 1991.
32. Khalil SN, Nuutinen LS, Rawal N et al: Sigmoidorectal methohexital as an inducing agent for general anesthesia in children, *Anesth Analg* 67:5113, 1988.
33. Holst JJ: Use of nitrous-oxide-oxygen analgesia in dentistry, *Int Dent J* 12:47, 1962.
34. Griffin GC, Campbell VD, Joni R: Nitrous oxide-oxygen sedation for minor surgery: experience in a pediatric setting, *JAMA* 245:2411, 1981.
35. Smith C, Rowe RD, Vead P: Sedation for children for cardiac catheterization with an ataractic mixture, *Can Anaes Soc* 5:35, 1958.
36. Reier CE, Johnston RE: Respiratory depression: narcotic vs narcotic-tranquilizer combinations, *Anesth Analg* 49:119, 1976.
37. Snodgrass WR, Dodge WF: "Lytic DPT cocktail: time for rational and safe alternatives, *Pediatr Clin North Am* 36:1285, 1989.
38. Juliano PJ, Mayer JM, Cummings RJ et al: Low dose lidocaine intravenous regional anesthesia for forearm fractures in children, *J Pediatr Orth* 12:633, 1992.
39. Sugarman JM, Paul RF: Flumazenil: a review, *Peds Emerg Care* 10:37, 1994.
40. Koltz U, Ziegler G, Riemann W: Pharmacokinetics of the selective benzodiazepine antagonist Ro 15-1788, *Man Eur J Clin Pharmacol* 27:115, 1985.

APPENDIXES

Christi Capers
David F. Gregory

I EMERGENCY MEDICATIONS
II VANDERBILT UNIVERSITY MEDICAL CENTER SEDATION POLICY
III DRUG TABLE
IV GENERIC AND TRADE NAMES

APPENDIX I. Emergency Medications

Drug	Dose/kg	Comments
Adenosine	0.05 mg/kg	Rapid (IVP)
Atropine	0.02 mg/kg	Maximum dose = 1 mg Minimum dose = 0.1 mg
Bicarbonate (4.2%)	1 mEq/kg	Use in patients under 3 months
Bicarbonate (8.4%)	1 mEq/kg	Infuse slowly
Bretylium	5 mg/kg	Dilute to 10 mg/ml for IVP
Calcium chloride (10%)	20 mg/kg (0.2 ml/kg)	Will precipitate if given with bicarbonate
Dextrose (50%)	0.5 g/kg (1 ml/kg)	
Epinephrine (1:10,000)	0.01 mg/kg (0.1 ml/kg)	Repeat dose = 0.1 mg/kg (1 ml/kg)
Epinephrine (1:1000)	0.1 mg/kg (0.1 ml/kg)	First dose for ETT administration
Fentanyl (50 μg/ml)	2 μg/kg	Dose range = 2-4 μg/kg
Lidocaine (20 mg/ml)	1 mg/kg	
Midazolam (1 mg/ml)	1 mg/kg	
Naloxone (400 μg/ml)	2-4 μg/kg	Titrate to desired effect up to 10 μg/kg
Pancuronium (1 mg/ml)	0.1 mg/kg	Intubation medication
Succinylcholine (20 mg/ml)	1 mg/kg	Intubation medication
Thiopental (25 mg/ml)	2-6 mg/kg	Intubation medication

IVP, Intravenous push; *ETT,* endotracheal tube.

Pediatric Drips for Emergency Medications

Drug	Dose (μg/kg/min)
Dobutamine	2.5-20
Dopamine	2.5-20
Epinephrine	0.1-1
Isoproterenol	0.1-1
Amrinone	5-20
Nitroglycerin	0.25-20
Nitroprusside	0.1-10
Norepinephrine	0.1-2
Phenylephrine	0.1-0.5
Lidocaine	20-50

Drip calculation based on intravenous infusion—"Rule of Six"

$$6 \times \frac{\text{desired dose } (\mu\text{g/kg/min})}{\text{desired rate (ml/hr)}} \times \text{wt (kg)} = \frac{\text{mg drug}}{\text{100 ml fluid}}$$

APPENDIX II

Vanderbilt University Medical Center Sedation Policy*

I. SUBJECT Conscious sedation of patients at Vanderbilt University Medical Center (VUMC)

II. PURPOSE To define specific levels of sedation and to describe the guidelines for the administration and management of conscious sedation.

III. POLICY All patients requiring sedation for any diagnostic, therapeutic, or imaging study or procedure will be managed to provide for continuity of care and safety in practice. Sedation will be administered by qualified individuals, as defined in this policy, equipped with the appropriate medications, equipment, supplies, knowledge, and support staff.

IV. SPECIAL INSTRUCTIONS

A. Scope

This policy applies to all patients who require conscious sedation for any diagnostic procedure, thera-

*Policy provided courtesy of the VUMC Office of Quality Improvement

peutic procedure, or imaging study in either the inpatient or outpatient setting at VUMC. It does not include patients being managed emergently in settings such as intensive care units or the emergency department where full physiologic monitoring and respiratory support are in place. It does not include the use of medications administered in dosages that are observed not to impair consciousness.

B. Level of Sedation

Attending physicians generally decide if their patients need conscious sedation. Consultation with radiology or anesthesia, for example, may serve to identify those patients requiring more than conscious sedation for the intervention. If an attending physician believes there is a reasonable expectation, based upon the procedure to be performed, that impaired oxygenation or circulation may occur, then general anesthesia should be employed.

Procedures that require a greater level of sedation beyond conscious, as defined above, may be performed only when supervised by an anesthesiologist, a certified registered nurse anesthetist under the supervision of an anesthesiologist, or another practitioner with designated clinical privileges in the provision of deep sedation and anesthesia.

C. Equipment

The following equipment will be available and in good working order for use in every location where the intervention and conscious sedation take place:

1. An emergency cart with supplemental equipment to handle both adult and pediatric emergencies. (Refer to the Vanderbilt University Par Level List for specific units and departments.) The cart should be checked daily by a designated individual and maintained as per VUMC policy.

2. Oral suction equipment and a variety of suction catheter sizes for adult and pediatric patients.
3. A portable cardiac monitor and defibrillator with cardioversion capability.
4. A pulse oximeter suitable for monitoring every sedated adult and pediatric patient.
5. Oxygen with a positive pressure delivery system capable of delivering greater than 90% O_2.
6. Sphygmomanometer or automated blood pressure monitor with adult and/or pediatric cuff sizes.

D. Personnel

The following guidelines apply when conscious sedation is employed. Unless otherwise agreed upon by the physicians involved in the patient's care, the physician performing the procedure is responsible for the patient during the procedure.

1. The physician supervising the procedure must be present at the procedure or within the procedure area during the entire period of sedation. Training in pediatric and/or adult advanced life support is strongly encouraged.
2. A registered or licensed practical nurse, respiratory therapist, or other appropriately qualified professional* must be present to monitor and document the patient's physiologic parameters and to assist in any supportive or resuscitative measures. This person should be trained in basic life support and anesthesia recovery principles.

E. Procedure

The following general guidelines apply to all levels of conscious sedation as defined in this policy:

*An assistant appropriately trained in monitoring techniques in basic life support must be present to assist the physician and to monitor and document physiologic parameters during the procedure.

1. Informed written consent for conscious sedation, as well as the procedure, must be obtained and documented in the patient's record before sedation as defined in these guidelines.
2. Before sedation, a health evaluation is performed and documented by the physician or their designee. A clinic note performed the same day or within recent days is sufficient for this purpose. Patients referred from outside VUMC, who have not been examined by a VUMC physician, require documentation of their physician's examination at the time of the study. This may be further supplemented by the physician performing the study, requiring conscious sedation. This health evaluation should include:
   a. Age and weight (when appropriate)
   b. Medical history, including drug allergies, current medications, relevant diseases, physical abnormalities, pregnancy status, adverse drug reactions or previous complications associated with sedation or anesthesia, and any relevant family history
   c. Review of systems with specific mention of any airway or respiratory problems
   d. History of specific drug, dosage, and time of any medications taken on the day of the procedure
   e. History of food or fluid intake within the past 8 hours
   f. Vital signs, including heart rate, blood pressure, respiratory rate, level of consciousness, and temperature (when appropriate)

   NOTE: For hospitalized patients the current hospital record may be adequate documentation of presedation health; however, a brief note should state that the chart was reviewed and significant findings should be noted.

3. Conscious sedation orders for patients must be written and are the responsibility of the physician or anesthesiologist responsible for the patient in the particular area where conscious sedation is being administered. Prescriptions or orders from areas outside the area where conscious sedation is administered will not be accepted.
4. All medication will be administered by the physician or licensed nursing staff. Medications administered by IVP may only be administered by the physician or registered nurse.
5. Attending physicians or their designee will maintain a time-based record, which includes the name, route, site, time, dosage, and patient effects of any drugs administered during the procedure. This document will be placed in the patient's record.
6. The patient's vital signs and oxygen saturation will be monitored by the physician or licensed nursing staff throughout the procedure and documented in the record at intervals until discharge or transfer to an inpatient unit.

   Suggested time intervals:

   a. Pediatrics—Every 5 minutes after administration of analgesics or anesthetics until discharge criteria are met or the patient is transferred to an inpatient unit.
   b. Adults—Every 5 minutes after administration of analgesics or anesthetics × 15 minutes then every 15 minutes until discharge criteria are met or the patient is transferred to an inpatient unit.

   NOTE: In circumstances where monitoring the blood pressure may be counterproductive to the sedated state, blood pressure monitoring may be omitted during the procedure providing the patient is stable, has not entered a level of deep sedation, and other vital signs, as indicated above, are being continuously monitored and documented.

7. After the procedure, the patient must be observed in a facility appropriately staffed and equipped with functioning suction apparatus, oxygen apparatus and a ventilation bag or mask until discharge or transfer criteria is met.
8. If the patient is being discharged after completion of the procedure, the attending physician or designee will identify a person responsible for the patient and provide verbal and written instructions to the responsible person accompanying the patient. Information should include limitations of activity, anticipated changes in behavior, dietary precautions, caution not to operate a vehicle or other machinery for twenty-four hours, and a physician or facility phone number available twenty four hours a day in case of emergency.
9. If transferring the patient to a patient care unit, the following procedures should be observed:
   a. The patient must be able to be transferred safely to an area where vital signs, airway patency, and level of consciousness can continue to be monitored by appropriately trained staff.
   b. The patient should be accompanied by the appropriate level of staff and resuscitative equipment depending upon the patient's level of sedation.
   c. A verbal report must be given by the clinical staff to the nurse assuming responsibility for the patient care on the nursing unit.

10. Specific discharge criteria must be met and documented before discharging a patient after sedation.
    a. The patient's vital signs are stable and within the preprocedure range.
    b. The patient has returned to his or her presedation level of consciousness.
    c. The patient has written instructions for postprocedure care including
        (1) Restrictions (i.e., diet, activity)
        (2) Use of prescribed medications
        (3) Follow-up care
        (4) Conditions requiring contact with a physician
        (5) Contacting the physician for postprocedure problems

F. Emergency Assist System

Recognizing that not all facilities affiliated with VUMC have equal access to the VUMC hospital based cardiopulmonary resuscitation (CPR) response system, (e.g., the Village, Medical Center South, Sports Medicine, Dayani Center, and Health Plus) special policies that address CPR response must be developed for these geographically isolated sites. An emergency assist system should be established and ready access to ambulance service must be planned for the emergency protocols for these areas. These emergency assist plans should be submitted to the CPR Committee for review and approval. The VUH Emergency Department is the targeted receiving facility in all back-up emergency protocols.

V. SPECIAL CONSIDERATIONS FOR MONITORING DURING MAGNETIC RESONANCE IMAGING

The special technologic problems associated with monitoring patients in a magnetic resonance imaging scanner—specifically, the powerful magnetic field and the generation of radiofrequency—necessitate the use of special equipment to provide continuous patient monitoring throughout the scanning procedure. Pulse oximeters capable of continuous function even during scanning are now available and should be used in any sedated or restrained pediatric patient. Thermal injuries can result if appropriate precautions are not taken; coiling the oximeter wire should be avoided, and the probe should be placed as far from the magnetic coil as possible to diminish the possibility of injury. Electrocardiogram monitoring during magnetic resonance imaging has been associated with thermal injury, and it should be used with caution in this setting.

VI. DEFINED LEVELS OF SEDATION

A. Conscious sedation refers to the physical state of patients in which they are able to continuously maintain a patent airway independently, to exhibit appropriate responses to verbal stimuli, and to maintain appropriate protective reflexes.

B. Deep sedation refers to a state of depressed consciousness or unconsciousness from which patients are not easily aroused, which may be accompanied by a partial loss of certain protective reflexes but does not compromise oxygenation or circulation. Such sedation may be prescribed by an attending physician; however, it also requires continuous supervision by a certified registered nurse anesthetist (CRNA) under supervision of an anesthesiologist or another physician or dentist with designated clinical privileges in the provision of deep sedation and/or anesthesia.

C. General anesthesia refers to a controlled state of unconsciousness which is accompanied by a loss of vital protective reflexes including the ability to maintain an airway and to respond purposefully to physical or verbal stimulation. Patients receiving this modality will be managed by an anesthesiologist or a CRNA under the direction of a physician anesthesiologist.

APPENDIX III. Drug Table

Drug	Dose	Comments	Dosage Forms
Acetaminophen (APAP) (Tylenol, Panadol)	PO, PR: 10-15 mg/kg/dose q 4-6 hrs p.r.n. Max dose: 4 g/24 hrs	May cause hepatotoxicity in overdose situation. Should not be given to patients with G-6-PD deficiency	Tabs: 160, 325, 500, 650 mg Chewable Tabs: 80, 160 mg Liquid: 48 mg/ml 60 mg/0.6 ml 100 mg/ml 120 mg/5 ml 160 mg/ml 160 mg/5 ml 167 mg/5 ml 325 mg/5 ml Suppositories: 120, 125, 325, 650 mg
Acetaminophen with codeine (Tylenol with codeine)	PO: 0.5-1 mg/kg/dose q 4-6 hrs p.r.n. Max dose: 120 mg/24 hrs (Dose based on the codeine component)		Caps/Tabs: #2 325 mg APAP/15 mg codeine #3 325 mg APAP/30 mg codeine

PO, Per os; *PR,* per rectum; *p.r.n.,* as needed; *IV,* intravenously; *IM,* intramuscularly; *SQ,* subcutaneously; *NS,* normal saline; *GE,* gastroesophageal; *ET,* endotracheal; *q,* every; *TTS,* transdermal therapeutic system; *GI,* gastrointestinal; *IVP,* intravenous push; *MAOI,* monoamine oxidase inhibitor; *PDA,* patent ductus arteriosus; *NSAID,* nonsteroidal antiinflammatory drug; *ICP,* intracranial pressure; *M6G,* morphine-6-glucuronide; *CNS,* central nervous system; *qhs,* at bedtime.

Continued

APPENDIX III. Drug Table—cont'd

Drug	Dose	Comments	Dosage Forms
Acetaminophen with codeine—cont'd			#4 325 mg APAP/60 mg codeine Liquid: 120 mg APAP/12 mg codeine/5 ml
Alfentanil (Alfenta)	Anesthesia <45 minutes IV: initial dose 8-50 μg/kg Infusion: 0.5-1 μg/kg/min Anesthesia >45 minutes IV: Initial dose 50-250 μg/kg Infusion: 0.5-3 μg/kg/min	Rapid infusion may result in skeletal muscle and chest wall rigidity. Inject slowly over 3-5 minutes.	Inj: 500 μg/ml
Amitriptyline (Elavil)	Chronic pain management PO: 0.1 mg/kg/dose qhs Advance over 2-3 weeks to 0.5-2 mg/kg qhs	Tricyclics lower the seizure threshold. May cause tardive dyskinesia. Use with caution in patients with seizure disorders, cardiovascular disorders, glaucoma, or hyperthyroidism.	Tabs: 10, 25, 50, 75, 100, 150 mg Inj: 10 mg/ml
Aspirin (Various manufacturers)	Analgesia/Antipyretic PO: 10-15 mg/kg/dose q 4-6	Use of aspirin in children with febrile illnesses has	Tabs: 81, 165, 325, 500, 650, 975 mg

	hrs Max dose: 4 g/24 hrs Antiinflammatory PO: 60-90 mg/kg/day q 6-8 hrs	been associated with the development of Reye's syndrome. Therapeutic serum concentrations: Analgesia/antipyretic: 30-50 mg/L Antiinflammatory: 250-300 mg/L	Suppositories: 120, 200, 300, 600 mg
Atropine (Various manufacturers)	Preanesthesia PO, IM, IV, SQ 0.01 mg/kg/dose Max dose: 0.4 mg/dose Min dose: 0.1 mg/dose Bradycardia IV: 0.01-0.03 mg/kg/dose q 5 minutes Max dose: 2 mg Min dose: 0.1 mg/dose Bronchospasm Nebulization: 0.05 mg/kg/dose in 2.5 ml of NS q 6-8 hrs p.r.n.	Administer by rapid undiluted injection. May give SQ, IM, or IV. For treatment of bradycardia may give diluted solution (1-2 ml NS) via ET tube.	Inj: 0.05 mg/ml 0.1 mg/ml 0.3 mg/ml 0.4 mg/ml 0.5 mg/ml 0.8 mg/ml 1 mg/ml

Continued

APPENDIX III. Drug Table—cont'd

Drug	Dose	Comments	Dosage Forms
Bethanechol (Urecholine)	Abdominal distention/ urinary retention PO: 0.6 mg/kg/day q 6-8 hrs SQ: 0.15-0.2 mg/kg/24 hrs q 6-8 hrs GE reflux: 0.4 mg/kg/24 hrs q 6 hrs DO NOT give IM or IV	Contraindicated in patients with hyperthyroidism, peptic ulcers, asthma, and seizure disorders. Use cautiously in patients with preexisting cardiac dysfunction.	Tabs: 5, 10, 25, 50 mg Inj: 5 mg/ml
Bisacodyl (Dulcolax)	PO: 0.3 mg/kg/24 hrs alternatively may give 5-10 mg (children 3-12 years old) or 5-15 mg qd (children >12 years old) PR: <2 yrs old 5 mg 2-11 yrs old 5-10 mg >11 yrs 10 mg	Swallow tablets whole and do not chew. Take tablets at least 1 hour after milk or antacids	Tabs: 5 mg Suppositories: 5, 10 mg Enema: 10 mg/30 ml
Bretylium (Bretylol)	IV: 5 mg/kg/dose, repeat q 10-20 min p.r.n.	Transient hypertension may occur with an increase in	Inj: 50 mg/ml

	Maintenance dose: IV: 5 mg/kg/dose q 6-8 hrs	frequency of arrhythmias from the initial release of norepinephrine. Dosage adjustment in renal failure is required. Effects of catecholamines are enhanced and digoxin toxicity may be heightened. For ventricular tachycardia associated with bipivacaine: bretylium 5 mg/kg (up to 3 g), phenytoin 10-20 mg/kg (up to 1 g), magnesium 50-100 mg/kg (up to 2 g).	
Bupivacaine (Marcaine, Sensorcaine)	Dose varies depending on the patient's weight and site of block	Bupivacaine is contraindicated in obstetrics as cervical block anesthesia because administration has resulted in fetal bradycardia and death. Not recommended for Bier block.	Inj: 0.25% 0.5% 0.75% 0.25% (with epinephrine 1:200,000) 0.5% (with epinephrine 1:200,000) 0.75% (with epinephrine (1:200,000)

Continued

APPENDIX III. Drug Table—cont'd

Drug	Dose	Comments	Dosage Forms
Buprenorphine (Buprenex)	IV: 3 μg/kg/dose	Relatively long acting opioid analgesic effective in the acute treatment of moderate to severe pain.	Inj: 0.324 mg (equivalent to 0.3 mg Buprenorphine)/ml
Butorphanol (Stadol)	IV: 20-30 μg/kg	Opioid agonist/antagonist. Antagonist activity approximately 1/40th that of naloxone. Larger doses (30-60 μg/kg) appear to have ceiling effects on the degree of respiratory depression. Dosage adjustment required in renal or liver dysfunction.	Inj: 1 mg/ml 2 mg/ml Nasal spray: 10 mg/ml
Cascara sagrada (Various manufacturers)	PO Infants: 0.5-1.5 ml/day p.r.n. Ages 2-11: 1-3 ml/day p.r.n. Ages 12 and older: 5 ml/day p.r.n.	Should not be used regularly for more than 1 week	Tab: 325 mg Liquid: Aromatic fluid extract

Chloral hydrate (Noctec, Aquachloral)	PO, PR: 50-75 mg/kg/dose Occasionally may require up to 100 mg/kg/dose. Max dose: 2 g/24 hrs	Metabolized in liver to the active metabolite trichloroethanol. The range of half-life in neonates (9-60 hours) may result in drug accumulation. The liquid is irritating to mucous membranes; therefore, dilute in water or fruit juice.	Caps: 250, 500 mg Liquid: 250, 500 mg/5 ml Suppositories: 324, 500, 628 mg
Chloroprocaine (Nesacaine)	Inj: 8-10 mg/kg (max dose) Infiltration and peripheral nerve block: 1%-2% solution Brachial plexus, intraorbital, mandibular, pudendal block: 2% solution Digital, paracervical block 1% solution	Not recommended for subarachnoid administration.	Inj: 1%, 2%, 3%
Chlorpromazine (Thorazine)	>6 months PO: 0.5-1 mg/kg/dose q 4-6 hrs		Tabs: 10, 25, 50, 100, 200 mg Extended Release Tabs: 30,

Continued

APPENDIX III. Drug Table—cont'd

Drug	Dose	Comments	Dosage Forms
Chlorpromazine—cont'd	IM/IV: 0.5-1 mg/kg/dose q 6-8 hrs Max dose: (<5 yrs) 40 mg/day (5-12 yrs) 75 mg/day		75, 150, 200, 300 mg Suppositories: 25, 100 mg Inj: 25 mg/ml
Choline magnesium trisalicylate* (trilisate)	PO: 10-15 mg/kg/dose q 6-8 hrs (Based on total salicylate content)	Use of salicylates in children with febrile illnesses has been associated with the development of Reye's syndrome. Limited effects on platelet function.	Tabs: 500, 750, 1000 mg (total salicylate) Liquid: 500 mg/5 ml (total salicylate)
Cimetidine (Tagamet)	Neonates: PO, IV, IM: 5-10 mg/kg/day q 8-12 hrs Infants: PO, IV, IM: 10-20 mg/kg/day q 6-12 hrs Children: PO, IV, IM: 20-40 mg/kg/day q 6 hrs	Inhibits the cytochrome P-450 system. Rapid IV administration may cause hypotension or arrhythmias. CNS side effects (confusion, hallucinations, somnolence) occur more frequently with	Tabs: 200, 300, 400, 800 mg Liquid: 300 mg/5 ml 150 mg/ml 300 mg in 50 ml NS

		cimetidine than other H_2 antagonists.	
Cisapride (Propulsid)	PO: 0.1-0.2 mg/kg/dose q 6 hrs	Acceleration of gastric emptying may affect the rate of absorption of other drugs. Diarrhea and abdominal pain are the most common side effects.	Tab: 10 mg Liquid: 1 mg/ml (Formulation on file)
Clomipramine (Anafranil)	Initially PO: 25 mg/daily Max dose: 3 mg/kg/day (or 200 mg, whichever is smaller)	Administer in divided doses to reduce GI side effects. Hyperthermia has occurred. The incidence of sexual dysfunction in males is greatly increased in patients on Clomipramine. Has potent anticholinergic side effects.	Caps: 25, 50, 75 mg
Clonidine (Catapres)	PO: 5-10 µg/kg/day q 8-12 hrs, increase to 5-25 µg/kg/day q 6 hrs Max dose: 0.9 mg/day	Abrupt discontinuation may result in hypertension. Reduce the dose gradually over 2-4 days. Change	Tabs: 0.1, 0.2, 0.3 mg Patch: Catapres-TTS-1 (0.1 mg/24 hrs)

*all products contain choline and magnesium salicylate in varying amounts

Continued

APPENDIX III. Drug Table—cont'd

Drug	Dose	Comments	Dosage Forms
Clonidine—cont'd		patch every 7 days.	Catapres-TTS-2 (0.2 mg/24 hrs) Catapres-TTS-3 (0.3 mg/24 hrs)
Cocaine (Cocaine)	Topically: Use lowest effective dose, not greater than 1 mg/kg Concentrations greater than 4% are not used because of the potential for systemic toxicities	Rapidly absorbed from all sites of application. Use cautiously in patients with hypertension or cardiovascular disease. Do not use epinephrine with cocaine.	Tab: 135 mg Topical Solution: 40 mg/ml 100 mg/ml Powder: 5, 25 g
Codeine (Various manufacturers)	Analgesia PO, IM, SQ: 0.5-1 mg/kg/dose Max dose: 60 mg/dose	May need to give 30% larger dose orally than parenterally. This drug may cause a significant histamine release. Not recommended for IV administration.	Tabs: 15, 30, 60 mg Inj: 30, 60 mg Liquid: 10, 15, 60 mg/5 ml
Dextrose	See glucose		

Dezocine (Dalgan)	IM/IV: 0.03-0.1 mg/kg/dose SQ: not recommended, associated with inflammation, irritation, and venous thrombosis in animals	Opioid agonist-antagonist with the same adverse reactions as the opioid class (sedation, nausea, vomiting, dry mouth, constipation). Equipotent to morphine.	Inj: 5 mg/ml 10 mg/ml 15 mg/ml
Diazepam (Valium)	Conscious sedation PO: 0.2-0.3 mg/kg/hr before procedure IM/IV: 0.04-0.3 mg/kg/dose q 2-4 hrs	May cause respiratory depression and hypotension. Avoid rapid IVP. Give 1-2 mg/min to maximum of 5 mg/min.	Extended Release Cap: 15 mg Tabs: 2, 5, 10 mg Inj: 5 mg/ml
Diclofenac (Voltaren)	Adults: 100-200 mg/day q 12-24 hrs Children: 2-3 mg/kg/day q 12-24 hrs	NSAID. Prominent adverse reactions are gastro-intestinal in nature.	Enteric coated tabs: 25, 50, 75 mg
Diphenhydramine (Benadryl)	PO, IM, IV: 1 mg/kg/dose (Max 50 mg) q 6 hrs Max dose: 300 mg/24 hrs	May cause sedation or paradoxical excitement. Anticholinergic side effects.	Caps: 25, 50 mg Tabs: 25, 50 mg Liquid: 12.5 mg/5 ml Inj: 10 mg/vial 50 mg/vial Cream: 2% Lotion: 1%

Continued

APPENDIX III. Drug Table—cont'd

Drug	Dose	Comments	Dosage Forms
Doxacurium (Nuromax)	Children: 2-12 yrs old IV: Initially 0.03-0.05 mg/kg/dose followed by 0.005-0.01 mg/kg 30-45 minutes later >12 yrs old: Initially 0.025-0.05 mg/kg/dose followed by 0.005-0.01 mg/kg 1-1.5 hours later	Long-acting, nondepolarizing, neuromuscular blocker. May be given by rapid IV injection undiluted.	Inj: 1 mg/ml
Doxepin (Adapin, Sinequan)	>12 years old PO: Initially 75 mg/day qhs Range 75-100 mg/day qhs	Tricyclics lower the seizure threshold and may cause tardive dyskinesia. Use with caution in patients with seizure disorders, cardiovascular disorders, glaucoma, and hyperthyroidism.	Caps: 10, 25, 50, 75, 100 mg
Droperidol (Inapsine)	Antiemetic IV: 0.025-0.05 mg/kg or 1.25-2.5 mg/dose	Hypotension and tachycardia are common side effects. Extrapyramidal symptoms have occurred in	Inj: 2.5 mg/ml

		approximately 1% of patients.	
Etidocaine (Duranest)	1% solution Peripheral nerve block Caudal Central nerve block Lumbar peridural 1-1.5% solution Intraabdominal/pelvic surgery Lower limb surgery Caesarean section 1.5% solution Maxillary infiltration Inferior alveolar nerve block		Inj: 1% 1% (with epinephrine 1:200,000) 1.5% (with epinephrine 1:200,000)
Etomidate (Amidate)	Dose for induction: 0.2-0.3 mg/kg over 30-60 seconds	Most frequent adverse reaction is transient skeletal muscle movements (up to 32%).	Inj: 2 mg/ml
Eutectic mixture of local anesthetics (EMLA)	Apply 2.5 g/site for 60 minutes before procedure For more painful	Apply 1-2 hours before procedure.	Topical: 5%

Continued

APPENDIX III. Drug Table—cont'd

Drug	Dose	Comments	Dosage Forms
Eutectic mixture—cont'd	procedures: Apply 2 g/100 cm^2 for 2 hrs		
Fentanyl (Sublimaze)	Sedation/Analgesia IV: 1-5 μg/kg/dose q 30-60 minutes Infusion: 1-5 μg/kg/hr Patch: 25, 50, 75, 100 μg/hr Oralet: 8-12 μg/kg	Rapid onset of action with a duration of action of 0.5-2 hours. Available in a patch and transmucosal (Oralet) formulation.	Inj: 50 μg/ml Patch: 25, 50, 75, 100 μg/hr Oralet: 200, 300, 400 μg
Flumazenil (Romazicon)	IV: 0.01 mg/kg/dose Max dose: 2 mg	Flumazenil use has been associated with the occurrence of seizures, most frequently in patients on long-term benzodiazepine therapy or with tricyclic antidepressant overdose.	Inj: 0.1 mg/ml
Fluoxetine (Prozac)	For patients <18 years old, dose and safety have not been established. PO: 6-17 years old, reports	Use cautiously in patients with liver failure and do not use concomitantly with a MAOI. Discontinue	Caps: 10, 20 mg Liquid: 20 mg/5 ml

	of 20 mg/day q am For patients >18 years old, initiate with 20 mg/day q am and increase to a max of 80 mg/day (divided morning and noon)	MAOI therapy at least 14 days before initiation of fluoxetine therapy.	
Glucose (Various manufacturers)	Emergency: 0.5 gm/kg	Dextrose 5% is an isotonic solution. Long term peripheral administration of dextrose should not exceed 12.5%.	Inj: 2.5, 5, 10, 25, 30, 40, 50, 60, 70%
Glycopyrrolate (Robinul)	PO: 10-40 μg/kg/dose q 6-8 hrs IV: 1-4 μg/kg/dose q 6-8 hrs	Oral absorption is approximately 10%; therefore, the oral dose is 10 times the IV dose.	Tabs: 1, 2 mg Suspension: 1 mg/5 ml (Formulation on file) Inj: 0.2 mg/ml
Haloperidol (Haldol)	PO: 3-12 yrs old Initially 0.05 mg/kg/day in 2-3 divided doses and increase by 0.25-0.5 mg/day Max dose: 0.15 mg/kg/day	May cause hypotension and seizures. Extrapyramidal symptoms can occur.	Tabs: 0.5, 1, 2, 5, 10, 20 mg Liquid: 2 mg/ml Inj: 5 mg/ml 50 mg/ml 100 mg/ml

Continued

APPENDIX III. Drug Table—cont'd

Drug	Dose	Comments	Dosage Forms
Haloperidol—cont'd	IM: 6-12 yrs old 1-3 mg/dose		
Hydrocodone with acetaminophen (Vicodin, Lortab)	PO: 0.15 mg/kg/dose q 6 hrs (Dose based on the hydrocodone component.)	Opioid analgesic, which may cause respiratory depression.	Cap: 5 mg hydrocodone/500 mg acetaminophen Tab: 2.5 mg hydrocodone/500 mg acetaminophen Liquid: 2.5 mg hydrocodone/120 mg acetaminophen/5 ml
Hydromorphone (Dilaudid)	PO: 0.03-0.08 mg/kg/dose q 4-6 hrs p.r.n. Max dose: 5 mg/dose IV: 0.015 mg/kg/dose q 4-6 hrs p.r.n.	Side effects appear to be less prominent with hydromorphone than with morphine Oral doses are approximately two times greater than IV doses.	Tabs: 1, 2, 3, 4 mg Suppositories: 3 mg Inj: 1 mg/ml 2 mg/ml 3 mg/ml 4 mg/ml
Hydroxyzine (Atarax, Vistaril)	PO: 2 mg/kg/day divided q 6-8 hrs	IV administration is not recommended.	Caps: 25, 50, 100 mg Tabs: 10, 25, 50, 100 mg

	IM: 0.5-1 mg/kg/dose q 4-6 hrs p.r.n.		Liquid: 10 mg/5 ml, 25 mg/5 ml Inj: 25 mg/ml, 50 mg/ml
Ibuprofen (Motrin, Advil)	Antipyretic PO: 10 mg/kg/dose q 6-8 hrs Max dose: 40 mg/kg/day	Use cautiously in patients with aspirin hypersensitivity. This drug decreases platelet aggregation which may precipitate bleeding.	Liquid: 100 mg/5 ml Tabs: 200, 300, 400, 600, 800 mg
Imipramine (Tofranil)	PO: 0.2-0.4 mg/kg qhs Max dose: 1-5 mg/kg/dose qhs IM: >12 yrs old, may give up to 100 mg/day	Tricyclics lower the seizure threshold. May cause tardive dyskinesia. Use with caution in patients with seizure disorders, cardiovascular disorders, glaucoma, or hyperthyroidism.	Tabs: 10, 25, 50 mg Inj: 25 mg/2 ml
Indomethacin (Indocin)	PO: 1-2 mg/kg/day q 6-12 hrs Max dose: 4 mg/kg/day (150-200 mg/day)	Use cautiously in patients with aspirin hypersensitivity. This drug decreases platelet aggregation which may precipitate bleeding.	Caps: 25, 50 mg Sustained Release Cap: 75 mg Liquid: 25 mg/5 ml Suppository: 50 mg Inj: 1 mg/vial

Continued

APPENDIX III. Drug Table—cont'd

Drug	Dose	Comments	Dosage Forms
Indomethacin—cont'd		Injection used for PDA closure in neonates.	
Ketamine (Ketalar)	IV: 0.5-2 mg/kg IM: 3-7 mg/kg Infusion: 5-20 μg/kg/minute	Contraindicated in patients with increased ICP. Emergence reactions occur in greater than 10% of patients and are most frequent in patients greater than 15 years old. Psychological manifestations may vary between pleasant dream-like states to hallucinations and delirium. Manage emergence reactions with small doses of midazolam, lorazepam, or diazepam.	Inj: 10 mg/ml 50 mg/ml 100 mg/ml
Ketoprofen (Orudis)	PO: 25-50 mg q 6-8 hrs Max dose: 300 mg/day (0.5 mg-1 mg/kg per dose)	NSAID. Prominent adverse reactions are gastrointestinal in	Caps: 25, 50, 75 mg Extended Release Cap: 200 mg

	Antiinflammatory: PO: 50-75 mg q 6-8 hrs Max dose: 300 mg/day (1.0-1.5 mg/kg per dose)	nature.	
Ketorolac (Toradol)	PO: 0.5 mg/kg dose q 6 hrs Max dose: 40 mg/day IV/IM: 0.5 mg/kg dose q 6 hrs Max dose: 120 mg/day	Should not be given for more than 5 days. Use cautiously in patients with hypersensitivity to aspirin or other NSAIDs.	Tab: 10 mg Inj: 15 mg/ml 30 mg/ml 60 mg/2 ml (IM Only)
Levorphanol (Levo-Dromoran)	Children >18 yrs old: PO: 1.5-4.5 mg/dose q 12-24 hrs IM: 2-4 mg/dose IV: 250-500 µg (1.5-2 mg max total dose)	For control of moderate to severe pain. Long half-life of 12-24 hours. Adjunct to nitrous oxide and oxygen anesthesia	Tab: 2 mg Inj: 2 mg/ml
Lidocaine (Xylocaine)	Inj: 0.5% (1 ml/kg) 1% (0.2-0.4 ml/kg) 2% (0.1-0.2 ml/kg) Infiltration: 0.5%-1% Intercostal, paravertebral, pudendal, paracervical,	Lidocaine solution containing epinephrine should not be used in the digits, nose, ears, or penis. Avoid large doses in patients with conduction	Inj: 0.5, 1, 1.5, 2, 4, 10, 20% 0.5% (with epinephrine 1:200,000) 1% (with epinephrine 1:100,000)

Continued

APPENDIX III. Drug Table—cont'd

Drug	Dose	Comments	Dosage Forms
Lidocaine—cont'd	cervical, lumbar, thoracic epidural, lumbar analgesia, obstetrical analgesia: 1%-2% Brachial, lumbar epidural anesthesia: 1.5%-2% Max dose: 5 mg/kg	defects.	1% (with epinephrine 1:200,000) 1.5% (with epinephrine 1:200,000) 1.5% (with 7.5% Dextrose) 5% (with 7.5% Dextrose)
Lorazepam (Ativan)	PO, IV: 0.025-0.05 mg/kg Infusion: 0.025-0.1 mg/kg/hr Max starting dose: 4 mg	Maximum dilution 0.25 mg/ml. Observe for precipitation.	Tabs: 0.5, 1, 2 mg Liquid: 2 mg/ml Inj: 2 mg/ml 4 mg/ml
Meperidine (Demerol)	PO, IV: 1-1.5 mg/kg/dose Infusion: 0.5-0.7 mg/kg/hr	Use with caution in patients with cardiac arrhythmias, asthma, and increased ICP. Normeperidine may accumulate in patients with renal failure.	Tabs: 50, 100 mg Liquid: 50 mg/5 ml Inj: 10 mg/ml 25 mg/ml 50 mg/ml 100 mg/ml
Mepivacaine (Carbocaine)	Brachial, cervical, intercostal, pudendal nerve block: 1% or 2%	Central nervous system and cardiovascular toxicity is primarily due to excessive	Inj: 1%, 1.5%, 2%

	solution Caudal or epidural block: 1%, 1.5%, 2% Therapeutic block: 1% or 2%	doses, inadvertent intravascular injection, and too rapid administration.	
Methadone (Dolophine)	IV, PO: 0.025 to 0.2 mg/kg/dose q 12 hrs	Drug may accumulate with repeated dosing. The effects on respiration appear to last longer than the analgesic effects equipotent with morphine.	Tabs: 5, 10, 40 mg Liquid: 5 mg/5 ml 10 mg/5 ml 10 mg/10 ml 10 mg/ml
Methohexital (Brevital)	IV: 2-3 mg/kg PR: 20-30 mg/kg	Administer IV in concentration no greater than 1%. Use with caution in patients with liver impairment, asthma, or cardiovascular instability.	Inj: 500 mg 2.5 g 5 g
Metoclopramide (Reglan)	IV, PO: 0.1-0.2 mg/kg/dose q 6 hrs	May cause extrapyramidal symptoms. Use cautiously in patients with seizure disorders.	Tabs: 5, 10 mg Liquid: 5 mg/5 ml Inj: 5 mg/ml

Continued

APPENDIX III. Drug Table—cont'd

Drug	Dose	Comments	Dosage Forms
Midazolam (Versed)	PO: 0.5-0.7 mg/kg IV: 0.05-0.2 mg/kg Infusion 0.05-0.2 mg/kg/hr Intranasal 0.3-0.4 mg/kg	Has been associated with respiratory depression—especially when administered with opioids.	Liquid: 2.5 mg/ml (Formulation on file) Inj: 1 mg/ml 5 mg/ml
Milk of magnesia (MOM) (Various manufacturers)	PO: 0.5 ml/kg/dose p.r.n. Children 2-5 yrs old: 5-15 ml/day p.r.n. Children 6-12 yrs old: 15-30 ml/day p.r.n. Adults >12 yrs old: 30-60 ml/day p.r.n.	Laxative effect occurs in 4-8 hours. May cause hypermagnesemia.	Tab: 311 mg Liquid: 400 mg/5 ml 800 mg/5 ml
Mivacurium (Mivacron)	IV: 0.2 mg/kg Infusion: 5-30 μg/kg/min	Short-acting, nondepolarizing skeletal muscle relaxant. Duration of action 5-10 minutes.	Inj: 0.5 mg/ml 2 mg/ml
Morphine (Roxanol, Duramorph, Astramorph)	PO: 0.2-0.5 mg/kg/dose q 4-6 hrs p.r.n. (immediate release)	Metabolized hepatically to M6G. M6G is renally excreted. May accumulate	Tabs: 10, 15, 30 mg 30, 60 mg sustained release

	IV: 0.05-0.1 mg/kg PCA: Bolus 0.02 mg q 10 mins Infusion: 0.005-0.01 mg/kg/hr	and cause respiratory depression in renal failure.	Liquid: 10 mg/5 ml 20 mg/5 ml 20 mg/ml 100 mg/5 ml Suppositories: 5, 10, 20, 30 mg Inj: 0.5 mg/ml 1 mg/ml 2 mg/ml 3 mg/ml 4 mg/ml 5 mg/ml 8 mg/ml 10 mg/ml 15 mg/ml
Nalbuphine (Nubain)	IV: 0.05-0.2 mg/kg	Opioid agonist/antagonist. Structurally similar to oxymorphone and naloxone. Equipotent to morphine.	Inj: 10 mg/ml 20 mg/ml
Nalmefene (Revex)	Safety and efficacy not established in children	Pure opioid antagonist. Structurally similar to naloxone but with a	Inj: 100 μg/ml 1 mg/ml

Continued

APPENDIX III. Drug Table—cont'd

Drug	Dose	Comments	Dosage Forms
Nalmefene—cont'd		longer half-life and duration of activity (4-8 hrs with IV administration).	
Naloxone (Narcan)	IV: 1-2 μg/kg (up to 0.2 mg) q 2-3 minutes	Can precipitate withdrawal in patients chronically receiving opioids. Repeated doses may be necessary if the duration of action of the opioid exceeds that of naloxone. Use with caution in patients with preexisting cardiac disease.	Inj: 0.4 mg/ml 1 mg/ml 0.02 mg/ml
Naltrexone (Trexan)	Limited information for use in children.	Semisynthetic opioid antagonist similar in structure to naloxone. Administered orally.	Tab: 50 mg
Naproxen (Naprosyn,	>2 yrs old	Use with caution in patients	Tabs: 200, 250, 375,

Anaprox)	PO: 5-7 mg/kg/dose q 8-12 hrs Max dose: 1.25 gm/day	with gastrointestinal disease, cardiac disease, or renal-hepatic dysfunction.	500 mg Liquid: 125 mg/5 ml
Nortriptyline (Aventyl, Pamelor)	5-9 yrs old PO: 0.1 mg/kg qhs 10-16 yrs PO: 25-50 mg	Tricyclics lower the seizure threshold. May cause tardive dyskinesia. Use with caution in patients with seizure disorders, cardiovascular disorders, glaucoma, or hyperthyroidism.	Caps: 10, 25, 50, 75 mg Liquid: 10 mg/5 ml
Ondansetron (Zofran)	4-11 yrs old PO: 4 mg >11 yrs old PO: 8 mg IV: 0.15 mg/kg/dose Max dose IV: 4 mg	IV formulation may be given orally. Has been reported to cause bronchospasm, tachycardia, angina, seizures, and hyperkalemia.	Tabs: 4, 8 mg Inj: 2 mg/ml
Oxycodone (Various manufacturers)	PO: 0.05-0.15 mg/kg/dose q 4-6 hrs p.r.n. (up to 5 mg/dose)	Opioid analgesic that may cause respiratory depression.	Tabs: 5 mg Liquid: 5 mg/5 ml 20 mg/ml

Continued

APPENDIX III. Drug Table—cont'd

Drug	Dose	Comments	Dosage Forms
Oxycodone with acetaminophen (Percocet, Tylox)	PO: 0.05-0.15 mg/kg/dose q 4-6 hrs p.r.n. (up to 5 mg/dose) (Based on oxycodone component)	Opioid analgesic that may cause respiratory depression.	Caps/Tabs: 5 mg oxycodone/500 mg acetaminophen 5 mg oxycodone/325 mg acetaminophen Liquid: 5 mg oxycodone/325 mg acetaminophen in 5 ml
Oxymorphone (Numorphan)	Dosing in children <12 yrs old not established >12 yrs old IV: 0.5 mg initially SQ, IM: 1-1.5 mg q 4-6 hrs p.r.n. PR: 5 mg q 4-6 hrs p.r.n.	Opioid agonist with a significant potential to cause respiratory depression, emesis, and physical dependence.	Inj: 1 mg/ml 1.5 mg/ml Suppository: 5 mg
Pancuronium (Pavulon)	IV: 0.05-0.1 mg/kg/dose Infusion: 0.05-0.1 mg/kg/hr	Use with caution in patients with preexisting tachycardia or renal dysfunction.	Inj: 1 mg/ml 2 mg/ml

Pentazocine (Talwin)	IV: 0.1-0.3 mg/kg/dose q 3-4 hrs	Opioid agonist/antagonist. Withdrawal has been reported in some patients previously receiving opioids. May produce euphoria and hallucinations. Elevates systemic and pulmonary arterial pressure, systemic vascular resistance, and left ventricular end diastolic pressure.	Tabs: 50 mg pentazocine/0.5 mg naloxone Inj: 30 mg/ml
Pentobarbital (Nembutal)	IV: Bolus: 1-4 mg/kg Infusion: 1-4 mg/kg/hr IM: 5-7 mg/kg PO: 2-4 mg/kg	Useful in the treatment of patients with increased ICP. Serum concentrations: Sedation: 1-5 mg/L Hypnosis: 5-15 mg/L Coma: 20-40 mg/L	Inj: 10 mg/ml
Phenytoin (Dilantin)	IV, PO: Bolus: 10-20 mg/kg up to 1 g Maintenance dose: 6-10 mg/kg/day q 8-12 hrs	Contraindicated in patients with heart block or sinus bradycardia. Therapeutic concentration 10-20 mg/L.	Tab: 50 mg Caps: 30, 100 mg Liquid: 30 mg/5 ml 125 mg/5 ml Inj: 50 mg/ml

Continued

APPENDIX III. Drug Table—cont'd

Drug	Dose	Comments	Dosage Forms
Piroxicam (Feldene)	Dosage not established in children. Adults: PO: 20 mg daily	Use cautiously in patients with impaired cardiac or renal function, gastrointestinal disease, and patients receiving anticoagulants.	Caps: 10, 20 mg
Prilocaine (Citanest)	Dosage not established in children. Regional anesthesia 0.5% solution (Max dose 5 mg/kg)	Metabolite can induce methemoglobinemia.	Inj: 4% 4% (with epinephrine 1:200,000)
Procaine (Novocain)	Infiltration anesthesia: 0.25%-1% Peripheral nerve block: 0.5%-2% Spinal anesthesia: 10% (diluted in appropriate amount of fluid)	CNS and cardiovascular effects are due to excessive dosage, rapid absorption, or inadvertent intravascular injection.	Inj: 1%, 2%, 10%
Promethazine (Phenergan)	Antihistamine: PO: 0.1 mg/kg/dose q 6 hrs Antiemetic:	Use cautiously in patients with cardiac disease or seizures. May cause	Tabs: 12.5, 25, 50 mg Liquid: 6.25 mg/5 ml 25 mg/5 ml

	PO, IM, IV, PR: 0.25-1 mg/kg/dose q 4-6 hrs Sedation: PO, IV, IM, PR: 0.5-1 mg/kg/dose q 6 hrs	extrapyramidal and anticholinergic symptoms.	Suppositories: 12.5, 25, 50 mg Inj: 25, 50 mg/ml
Propofol (Diprivan)	IV: Bolus: 0.5-3 mg/kg Infusion: 25-200 µg/kg/min	Local pain upon injection. Formulation is an oil-in-water emulsion and may result in elevated serum triglycerides when administered for extended periods of time.	Inj: 10 mg/ml
Ranitidine (Zantac)	PO: 1-2 mg/kg/dose q 12 hrs Max dose: 300 mg/day IM/IV: 1 mg/kg/dose q 8 hrs Infusion: 0.1-0.25 mg/kg/hr	Adjust dose in renal failure.	Tabs: 150, 300 mg Liquid: 15 mg/ml Inj: 25 mg/ml
Rocuronium (Zemuron)	IV: Bolus: 0.6-1 mg/kg Infusion: 0.6 mg/kg/hr	Nondepolarizing neuromuscular blocking agent. Similar pharmacokinetic profile to vecuronium. Onset is 60 seconds.	Inj: 10 mg/ml

Continued

APPENDIX III. Drug Table—cont'd

Drug	Dose	Comments	Dosage Forms
Sodium bicarbonate (Various manufacturers)	Cardiac Arrest: IV: 1 mEq/kg slow IVP, repeat 0.5 mEq/kg in 10 min p.r.n. for acid-base status	Rate of administration not greater than 10 mEq/min.	Tabs: 300, 325, 520, 600, 650 mg Inj: 4, 4.2, 7.5, 8.4%
Succinylcholine (Anectine)	IV: 1-2 mg/kg IM: 2.5-4 mgkg	May be given by rapid IV injection. Onset 30-45 seconds. May increase serum potassium.	Inj: 20, 50, 100 mg/ml Powder for Inj: 100, 500, 1000 mg
Sufentanil (Sufenta)	Induction: (For cardiovascular surgery) IV: 10-25 μg/kg	Has a quicker onset and shorter duration of action than fentanyl. Approximately 10 times more potent than fentanyl.	Inj: 50 μg/ml
Tetracaine (Pontocaine)	Spinal anesthesia: (Adults) Perineum and lower extremities: 10 mg Up to costal margin: 15-20 mg	Duration of anesthesia is age dependent. High block may compromise cardiorespiratory function.	Inj: 1% 0.2% with 6% Dextrose 0.3% with 6% Dextrose

	Saddle block: 2-5 mg in dextrose 6% Dosing in children is based on age and desired level of block.		Powder for reconstitution: 20 mg
Thiamylal (Surital)	Test dose: Inject a very small amount of 2.5% solution and observe patient for unusual sensitivities. Titrate dose to patient response (3-4 mg/kg)	Sterile water for injection, USP is the preferred diluent. Do not reconstitute with lactated ringers or solutions containing bacteriostatic compounds, since precipitation has occurred.	Inj: 1, 5, 10 g
Thiopental (Pentothal)	IV (induction of anesthesia): Neonates: 3-4 mg/kg/dose Children: 5-8 mg/kg/dose Adults: 3-5 mg/kg/dose PR (sedation): 20-30 mg/kg/dose	Use with caution in patients with asthma, since it may cause bronchospasm. Has a shorter half-life in children than adults. Lipid soluble; therefore, may accumulate in chronic dosing.	Inj: 250, 400, 500 mg 1, 2.5, 5 g Rectal suspension: 400 mg/ml

Continued

APPENDIX III. Drug Table—cont'd

Drug	Dose	Comments	Dosage Forms
Tolmetin (Tolectin)	Not recommended for use in children <2 yrs old Antiinflammatory dose: Initial: 15-20 mg/kg/day q 8 hrs Acute Pain: 5-7 mg/kg/dose q 6-8 hrs Adult dose: Starting: 400 mg q 8 hrs Max dose: 2000 mg/day	NSAID with gastrointestinal side effects. (Bleeding, nausea, diarrhea, constipation, ulcers). Take with food, milk, or antacids to reduce gastrointestinal adversities.	Cap: 400 mg Tabs: 200, 600 mg
Tramadol (Ultram)	Dosing not established in children <16 yrs old Children >16 yrs old: PO: 50-100 mg q 4-6 hrs Note: several factors affect patient specific dosing, including renal function, hepatic function, and concomitant drug administration.	Synthetic analog of codeine with a low affinity for opioid receptors. Most common adverse side effects are dizziness, nausea, sedation, constipation, headache, and drowsiness.	Tab: 50 mg

Vecuronium (Norcuron)	IV: Bolus: 0.08-0.1 mg/kg/dose Infusion: 0.1 mg/kg/hr	Neuromuscular blockade may be potentiated by the following drugs: enflurane, isoflurane, aminoglycosides, tetracyclines, metronidazole, clindamycin, quinidine, piperacillin, mezlocillin, and verapamil. Children between the ages of 1 and 10 yrs may require more frequent dosing than adults.	Inj: 10 mg vial

APPENDIX IV
Generic and Trade Names

Generic Name	Trade Name
Acetaminophen	Tylenol, Panadol
Acetaminophen with codeine	Tylenol with codeine
Alfentanil	Alfenta
Amitriptyline	Elavil
Aspirin	various manufacturers
Atropine	various manufacturers
Atracurium	Tracrium
Bethanecol	Urecholine
Bisacodyl	Dulcolax
Bretylium	Bretylol
Bupivacaine	Marcaine, Sensorcaine
Buprenophine	Buprenex
Butorphanol	Stadol
Cascara sagrada	various manufacturers
Chloral hydrate	Noctec, Aquachloral
Chloroprocaine	Nesacaine
Chlorpromazine	Thorazine
Choline magnesium trisalicylate	Trilisate
Cimetidine	Tagamet
Cisapride	Propulsid
Clomipramine	Anafranil
Clonidine	Catapres
Cocaine	Cocaine
Codeine	various manufacturers
Dezocine	Dalgan
Diazepam	Valium
Diclofenac	Voltaren
Diphenhydramine	Benadryl
Doxacurium	Nuromax
Doxepin	Adapin, Sinequan
Droperidol	Inapsine
Etidocaine	Duranest
Etomidate	Amidate
Eutectic mixture of local anesthetics	EMLA cream
Fentanyl	Sublimaze
Flumazenil	Romazicon
Fluoxetine	Prozac
Glucose	various manufacturers

APPENDIX IV
Generic and Trade Names—cont'd

Generic Name	Trade Name
Glycopyrrolate	Robinul
Haloperidol	Haldol
Hydrocodone	Hydrocet
Hydrocodone with acetaminophen	Vicodin, Lortab
Hydromorphone	Dilaudid
Hydroxyzine	Atarax, Vistaril
Ibuprofen	Motrin, Advil
Imipramine	Tofranil
Indomethacin	Indocin
Ketamine	Ketalar
Ketoprofen	Orudis
Ketorolac	Toradol
Levorphanol	Levo-Dromoran
Lidocaine	Xylocaine
Lorazepam	Ativan
Meperidine	Demerol
Mepivacaine	Carbocaine
Methadone	Dolophine
Methohexital	Brevital
Metoclopramide	Reglan
Midazolam	Versed
Milk of magnesia (MOM)	various manufacturers
Mivacurium	Mivacron
Morphine	Roxanol, Duramorph, Astramorph
Nalbuphine	Nubain
Naloxone	Narcan
Naltrexone	Trexan
Naproxen	Naprosyn, Anaprox
Nortriptyline	Aventyl, Pamelor
Ondansetron	Zofran
Oxycodone	various manufacturers
Oxycodone with acetaminophen	Percocet, Tylox
Oxymorphone	Numorphan
Pancuronium	Pavulon
Pentazocine	Talwin
Pentobarbital	Nembutal
Phenylephrine	Neo-Synephrine
Phenytoin	Dilantin

APPENDIX IV
Generic and Trade Names—cont'd

Generic Name	Trade Name
Piroxicam	Feldene
Prilocaine	Citanest
Procaine	Novocain
Promethazine	Phenergan
Propofol	Diprivan
Ranitidine	Zantac
Rocuronium	Zemuron
Sodium bicarbonate	various manufacturers
Sodium citrate	Bicitra, Polycitra
Succinylcholine	Anectine
Sufentanil	Sufenta
Tetracaine	Pontocaine
Thiamylal	Surital
Thiopental	Pentothal
Tolmetin	Tolectin
Tramadol	Ultram
Vecuronium	Norcuron

INDEX

A

Abdominal pain, 178
traumatic injury causing, 189-190
Abdominal surgery, pain after, 51
Ablation, radiofrequency, 294-296
Abstinence syndrome, neonatal, 250, 251
Accidents, pain caused by, 187-192
Acetaminophen, 13, 15, 329-330
for burn pain, 184-185
for chest pain, 180
dosage of, 14
for mild postoperative pain, 52-55
for moderate to severe postoperative pain, 55
after myringotomy, 176
oral preparations of, 181
for otitis media pain, 161, 175
for trauma-related pain, 191
Acetylsalicylic acid, 13, 15
for mild postoperative pain, 52
Adapin; *see* Doxepin
Addiction, opioid, 73-74, 227-228, 250-252
Adenosine for emergency, dose of, 320
Adjunctive techniques for management of sickle cell anemia pain, 164-165
Adjuvant medications, psychotropic agents as, 36
Adrenalin; *see* Epinephrine
Advil; *see* Ibuprofen
Agonist/antagonists, opioid, 59, 60
mixed, 22-23
actions of, 16
Airway
difficult, algorithm for, 272-273
laryngeal mask, 276, 278
sizes of, 279
problems with, physical examination focused on, 43
Albuterol for anaphylaxis, 87
Alfenta; *see* Alfentanil
Alfentanil, 16, 17, 20, 330
for endotracheal intubation, 205-206
for moderate to severe postoperative pain, 58
in PICU, 248
potency and half-life of, 59
for radiofrequency ablation, 296
for surgical pain in neonates, 216
Algorithm, difficult airway, 272-273
American Society of Anesthesiologists, physical status classification of, 44, 268, 269
Amidate; *see* Etomidate
Amides, 30, 82
for regional anesthesia, 31
dosing guidelines for, 115
Amitriptyline, 34, 330
for cancer pain, 173
dosage of, 35
Amrinone, pediatric drip for, dosage of, 321
Anafranil; *see* Clomipramine
Analgesia
epidural; *see* Epidural analgesia
interpleural; *see* Interpleural analgesia
intrathecal, opioids for, 89, 90
patient-controlled; *see* Patient-controlled analgesia

Analgesia—cont'd
postoperative, opioids for, 109-110
during procedures, agents for, 269
Analgesics
for endotracheal intubation, 274
during mechanical ventilation, starting doses of, 254
nonopioid, classification of, 53
oral preparations of, formulation of, 181
selection of, 269-270
use of, in PICUs and NICUs, 200
Anaprox; *see* Naproxen
Anectine; *see* Succinylcholine
Anemia, hemolytic, chronic, with sickle cell disease, 158
Anesthesia
caudal, 98-106
advantages and disadvantages of, 103
spinal anesthesia versus, 103
epidural, 92-108
adverse effects of, 106-108
for management of sickle cell anemia pain, 166-167
for trauma-related pain, 192
general, 42
spinal anesthesia combined with, 110
local; *see* Local anesthesia
regional; *see* Local anesthesia; Regional nerve blocks
spinal; *see* Spinal anesthesia
Anesthetic agents
inhalational, 40-41
in PICU, 236-238
systemic effects of, 41
intravenous, 23-26
local; *see* Local anesthetics
Ankle block, 149, 150
dosing guidelines for, 121
Antibiotics for otitis media pain, 174, 175
Anticonvulsants
for burn pain, 185
for cancer pain, 173-174
Antidepressants, 34-35
side effects of, 34-35
tricyclic
for burn pain, 185
for cancer pain, 173
Antihistamines, 35-36
for anaphylaxis, 87
dosage of, 35
for opioid-induced pruritus, 75
Antiinflammatory drugs, nonsteroidal; *see* Nonsteroidal antiinflammatory drugs
Aquachloral; *see* Chloral hydrate
Arrow Theracath
for epidural anesthesia, 94, 95
for interpleural analgesia, 118
ASA; *see* American Society of Anesthesiologists
Aspiration, prophylaxis for, agents for, 266
Aspiration pneumonitis, 265, 266
Aspirin, 330-331
dosage of, 14
Assessment, pain, in neonate, 198, 199
Astramorph; *see* Morphine
Atarax; *see* Hydroxyzine
Ativan; *see* Lorazepam
Atracurium, 39
dosage of, 37
for endotracheal intubation, 277
Atropine, 331
for emergency, dose of, 320
for endotracheal intubation, 205, 274
Aventyl; *see* Nortriptyline
Axillary block, 140-142
interscalene, dosing guidelines

Axillary block—cont'd
for, 121

B

Barbiturates
for CT scanning sedation, 284
for mechanical ventilation, starting doses of, 254
for painful procedures, 307-308
in PICU, 244-246
for sedation, 26-27
Behavioral assessment of pain in neonate and infant, 199
Benadryl; *see* Diphenhydramine
Benzodiazepines, 28-29
antagonists for, 29, 311-312
for mechanical ventilation, 206, 207
starting doses of, 254
painful procedures, 301-302
in PICU, 238-241
for radiofrequency ablation, 296
for radiographic/cardiac catheterization procedures, 286
tapering use of, 241
tolerance to and physical dependence on, 241
for trauma-related pain, 191
Bethanechol, 331-332
Bier block, 142-146, 311
dosing guidelines for, 121
Biofeedback for management of sickle cell anemia pain, 164-165
Bisacodyl, 332
Block; *see also* Nerve blocks
ankle, 149, 150
axillary, 140-142
Bier, 142-146, 311
brachial plexus, 137-142
caudal, for circumcision, 210-212
caudal epidural; *see* Caudal epidural block

Block—cont'd
epidural, for neonates, 221-222
interscalene, 138-139
complications of, 139-140
lumbar plexus, 128-129
obturator nerve block combined with, 132-136
ring, for circumcision, 210
sacral plexus, 128-129
upper extremity, 137-142
wrist, 149, 151, 152-153
Blockage; *see* Nerve block
Blood pressure cuff to monitor during sedation, 44
Bone marrow aspiration, 168, 169
Brachial plexus block, 137-142
Bretylium, 332-333
for arrhythmias associated with bupivacaine toxicity, 33
for emergency, dose of, 320
Bretylol; *see* Bretylium
Brevital; *see* Methohexital
Bronchodilators for anaphylaxis, 87
Bupivacaine, 30, 32, 333
for caudal anesthesia, 102, 104, 211, 212
via chest tube, 182-183
continuous regional anesthesia in neonates, 219, 220, 221, 222
for digital blocks, 148-149
for epidural analgesia for neonate, 223
for epidural anesthesia, 94, 96
dosage of, 97
in neonate, 222
for fascia iliaca obturator nerve/lumbar plexus blockade, 133
for femoral cutaneous nerve block, 132
for femoral nerve block, 131
for ilioinguinal and iliohypogas-

Bupivacaine—cont'd
tric block, 147
for intercostal block, 127
for interpleural analgesia, 118-119
for interscalene block, 138-139
maximum duration of action of, 32
maximum recommended dosage of, 32, 84
for psoas compartment approach to obturator nerve/lumbar plexus blockade, 136
for regional anesthesia, 31
dosing guidelines for, 115, 120-121
for sciatic nerve block, 136
for spinal anesthesia, 103, 109
in neonates, 218, 219, 220
for 3-in-1 obturator nerve/lumbar plexus blockade, 132
toxicity of, 33
Buprenex; *see* Buprenorphine
Buprenorphine, 333
Burns, 183-187
Butorphanol, 22-23, 333-334
epidural administration of, dosage for, 89, 90
intranasal administration of, 69-70
for moderate to severe postoperative pain, 60
potency and half-life of, 59
to prevent side effects of morphine, 90, 91-92
transmucosal administration of, 68
Butyrophenones, 36
dosage of, 35
for opioid adverse effects, 75
in PICU, 252-253

C

Calcitonin, transmucosal administration of, 68
Calcitonin-gene-related peptide
pain sensitivity in neonates and, 12
transmission of nociceptive impulses and, 8
Calcium chloride for emergency, dose of, 320
Cancer pain management model for management of sickle cell anemia pain, 165-166
Candidiasis, 170
Capnometer, end-tidal carbon dioxide, to monitor during sedation, 44
Capsaicin for mucositis, 170, 171
Carbamazepine
for burn pain, 185
for cancer pain, 174
Carbocaine; *see* Mepivacaine
Carbon dioxide monitoring during sedation, 44-45
Cardiac catheterization, sedation for, 292-296
drug strategies for, 286
Cardiac causes of chest pain, 176, 177, 176, 179
related to traumatic injury, 189
Cascara sagrada, 334
Catapres; *see* Clonidine
Catecholamine responses to surgery, neonatal, 13
Catheter
central venous, placement of, sedation during, 200-204
interpleural, placement of, for interpleural anesthesia, 116, 117
Catheterization, cardiac, sedation for, 292-296
drug strategies for, 286
Caudal anesthesia, 98-106; *see also* Caudal epidural block
advantages and disadvantages of, 103
continuous, 104-105

Caudal anesthesia—cont'd
spinal anesthesia versus, 103
Caudal epidural block, 98-99; *see also* Caudal anesthesia
for circumcision, 210-212
needle placement for, 100, 101
no-touch technique for, 101
"Ceiling effect" of mixed opioid agonist-antagonists, 22
Central venous catheter placement, sedation during, 200-204
CGRP; *see* Calcitonin-gene-related peptide
Chaissaignac's tubercle, identification of, 138, 139
Chest pain, 176-183
common causes of, 177
traumatic injury causing, 189
Chest tubes, anesthetics via, 182-183
Chest wall rigidity, opioid use and, 249
Chloral hydrate, 29-30, 334
for CT scanning sedation, 284, 286
for diagnostic cardiac catheterization, 293
for mechanical ventilation, 209
for painful procedures, 304-305
in PICU, 253
for radiographic/cardiac catheterization procedures, 286
Chlorhexidine gluconate
for candidiasis, 170
for mucositis, 170, 171
Chloroprocaine, 30, 335
advantages and disadvantages of, 107
for caudal anesthesia, 104-106, 212
for continuous caudal anesthesia, 219-220
for epidural block in neonate, 222
Chloroprocaine—cont'd
for femoral nerve block, 131
for interscalene block, 139
maximum dose and duration of action of, 32, 84
for regional anesthesia, 31
dosing guidelines for, 115, 121
for topical anesthesia, 300
Chlorpromazine, 335
dosage of, 35
in DPT, 2, 310
Cholecystectomy, intercostal blockade for, 123
Choline magnesium trisalicylate, 13-14, 15, 335
for mild postoperative pain, 52
Cimetidine, 336
for aspiration prophylaxis, 266
Circumcision
sedation for, 209-215
technique for, 213, 214
Cisapride, 336
for aspiration prophylaxis, 266
Citanest; *see* Prilocaine
Clomipramine, 336-337
dosage of, 35
Clonidine, 337
in PICU, 253
Cocaine, 337
for regional nerve blocks, dosing guidelines for, 115
for topical anesthesia, 299
in TAC, 299
Coccyx, anatomy of, 99
Codeine, 16, 21, 337-338
actions of, 16
for chest pain, 180
dosage of, 21
duration of action and potency of, 18
for mild postoperative pain, 54
for moderate to severe postoperative pain, 58
after myringotomy, 176

Codeine—cont'd
oral administration of, 65
oral preparations of, 181
for otitis media pain, 161, 175
for sickle cell anemia pain, 161
side effects of, 21
Cognitive strategies for management of sickle cell anemia pain, 164-165
Computerized tomography, sedation for, 283-288
Conscious sedation, 42
Continuous regional anesthesia in neonates, 219-222
Cortical function during fetal life, 11-12
Corticosteroids
for anaphylaxis, 87
for cancer pain, 174
for management of sickle cell anemia pain, 165
Cricothyrotomy, needle, 276, 278-279
CT scanning, sedation for, 283-288

D

Dalgan; *see* Dezocine
Deep sedation, 42
Delta receptors, 15-16
Demerol; *see* Meperidine
Dependence, physical; *see* Physical dependence
Depression, respiratory, from opioid administration, 71-73, 90, 91-92
Desflurane, 40
in PICU, 236
Developing pain system, neuroanatomy and neurophysiology of, 4-13
Dexamethasone for cancer pain, 174
Dextrose, 338
for emergency, dose of, 320
Dezocine, 338
Diagnostic cardiac catheterization, sedation for, 293
Diagnostic procedures, invasive
for children, list of, 297
sedation for, 296-300
Diamorphine
epidural administration of, dosage of, 90
intrathecal administration of, dosage of, 90
Diazepam, 28-29, 338
dosage of, 28
for painful procedures, 301
in PICU, 238
Diclofenac, 13, 338
dosage of, 14
Difficult airway algorithm, 272-273
Digital blocks, 147-149
dosing guidelines for, 121
Dilantin; *see* Phenytoin
Dilaudid; *see* Hydromorphone
Diphenhydramine, 35-36, 338-339
for anaphylaxis, 87
dosage of, 35
for mucositis, 171
for opioid-induced pruritus, 75-76
for pruritus, 90
Diprivan; *see* Propofol
Disease, pain associated with, management of, 157-195
Dobutamine, pediatric drip for, dosage of, 321
Dolobid; *see* Methadone
Dolophine; *see* Methadone
Dopamine, pediatric drip for, dosage of, 321
Dorsal horn of spinal cord
components and functions of, 7
development of, 8-12
Doxacurium, 39, 339
dosage of, 37

Doxepin, 339
dosage of, 35
DPT (pedi cocktail), 2, 310
Droperidol, 339-340
for opioid adverse effects, 75
Drugs; *see* specific action; specific drug
Dulcolax; *see* Bisacodyl
Duramorph; *see* Morphine
Durarest; *see* Etidocaine
Dyclonine for mucositis, 170, 171

E

Elavil; *see* Amitriptyline
Electrocardiograph to monitor during sedation, 45
Emergency medications, 320-321
EMLA; *see* Eutectic mixture of local anesthetics
End-tidal carbon dioxide capnometer to monitor during sedation, 44
Endotracheal intubation
in awake patient, 273
elective, 273-279
equipment and monitors for, 271
medications to facilitate, 274
sedation for, 270-279
in neonate, 204-209
Enflurane, 40
in PICU, 236-237
Enkephalin, actions of, 16
Epidural analgesia
for burn pain, 185
for chest pain, 182
for neonates, 218-219, 223-225
opioids for, 89, 90
for sickle cell anemia pain, 166-167
and spinal anesthesia/analgesia, 81-112
for trauma-related pain, 192
Epidural anesthesia, 92-108
adverse effects of, 106-108
Epidural anesthesia—cont'd
caudal, 98-106
for neonates, 221-222
Epidural block, caudal; *see* Caudal epidural block
Epidural space, 92, 93
Epinephrine
addition of, to local anesthetic injection, 32
for anaphylaxis, 87
for caudal block, 211
for emergency, dose of, 320
pediatric drip for, dosage of, 321
in TAC, 299
for topical anesthesia, 299
Equipment for sedation, minimal, 46
Equipment cart, pediatric, mobile, suggested items for, 281
Esters, 30, 82
for regional anesthesia, 31
dosing guidelines for, 115
Etidocaine, 30, 340
for regional anesthesia, 31
Etomidate, 25-26, 340
for endotracheal intubation, 205, 274
Eutectic mixture of local anesthetics, 33-34, 298-299, 340-341
for central venous catheter placement, 201
before chest tube removal, 183
for circumcision, 212, 214
for procedural pain, 168-169
Examination, physical, 267-268
Excitatory neurotransmitters, 8-9
Extracorporeal membrane oxygenation, sedation during, 225-227
Extremity pain, traumatic injury causing, 189, 190

F

Fascia iliaca block of lumbar

plexus, 128, 132-133
dosing guidelines for, 120
Fasting guidelines for sedation, 45, 47
Feldene; *see* Piroxicam
Femoral cutaneous nerve, cutaneous sensory innervation of, 129
Femoral cutaneous nerve block, 131-132
dosing guidelines for, 120
Femoral nerve
cutaneous sensory innervation of, 129
location of, 130
Femoral nerve block, 129-131
dosing guidelines for, 120
Fentanyl Oralet, 20
for painful procedures, 303-304
Fentanyl, 16, 17, 20, 341
actions of, 16
for Bier block, 145
for burn pain, 186
for cancer pain, 173
for central venous catheter placement, 202-203
for diagnostic cardiac catheterization, 293
dosage of, 17, 20
duration of action and potency of, 18
for emergency, dose of, 320
for endotracheal intubation, 205-206, 274
epidural administration of, dosage for, 89, 90
for epidural anesthesia, 96, 97
in neonate, 222, 223, 224
for extracorporeal membrane oxygenation cannula placement, 225-226
intranasal administration of, 68-69
intrathecal administration of, dosage of, 89, 90
Fentanyl—cont'd
for local anesthesia, 88-89
for mechanical ventilation, 206, 207, 208-209
starting doses of, 254
for mild postoperative pain, 54
for moderate to severe postoperative pain, 58
for painful procedures, 303
in PICU, 248
potency and half-life of, 59
for radiofrequency ablation, 296
for radiographic/cardiac catheterization procedures, 286
side effects of, 17
subcutaneous administration of, 68
subcutaneous infusion of, 248
for surgical pain in neonates, 215, 216-217
transdermal administration of, 66-67, 246-247
transmucosal administration of, 68, 71
for painful procedures, 303-304
Fetal life, cortical function during, 11-12
Field infiltration in neonates, local anesthetics for, 202
Finger, nerve blocks for, 147-149
Flumazenil, 29, 341-342
as benzodiazepine antagonist, 312
in PICU, 240
Fluoxetine, 34, 341
dosage of, 35
Fluvoximine, 34

G

Gadolinium, 292
Gastrointestinal causes of abdominal pain related to traumatic injury, 190

Gastrointestinal causes of chest pain, 177, 178, 179
related to traumatic injury, 189
Gate-control theory of pain, physiologic basis for, 9
General anesthesia, 42
spinal anesthesia combined with, 110
Generic and trade name index, 358-360
Genitourinary causes of abdominal pain related to traumatic injury, 190
Global assessment of pain in neonate and infant, 199
Glucose, 342
Glutamate
pain sensitivity in neonates and, 12
transmission of nociceptive impulses and, 8
Glycopyrrolate, 342
for endotracheal intubation, 274
for painful procedures, 306-307
Granisetron for opioid adverse effects, 75
Gynecologic causes of abdominal pain related to traumatic injury, 190

H

Haldol; *see* Haloperidol
Haloperidol, 36, 342
dosage of, 35
in PICU, 252
Halothane, 40
for myringotomy, 176
in PICU, 236
Head injury, 187
traumatic, 187-188
Head pain, traumatic injury causing, 188
Headache, causes of, related to traumatic injury, 188
Hemoglobinopathies, sickle cell disease and associated, 158-168
Hemolytic anemia, chronic, with sickle cell disease, 158
Herniorrhaphy
caudal anesthesia for, 102
ilioinguinal and iliohypogastric blocks for, 146
spinal anesthesia for, 218
History, patient, 267-268
Hydrocodone, 342-343
for cancer pain, 173
for chest pain, 180
for mild postoperative pain, 54
oral preparations of, 181
Hydrocoelectomy, ilioinguinal and iliohypogastric blocks for, 146
Hydromorphone, 16, 22, 343
for cancer pain, 173
duration of action and potency of, 18
epidural administration of, dosage of, 90
for moderate to severe postoperative pain, 58, 61
oral administration of, 65, 66
oral preparations of, 181
in PICU, 249-250
potency and half-life of, 59
for sickle cell anemia pain, 162
subcutaneous administration of, 68
subcutaneous infusion of, 248
Hydroxyzine, 35-36, 343
dosage of, 35
Hypnosis for management of sickle cell anemia pain, 164-165

I

Ibuprofen, 13, 15, 343
for chest pain, 180
dosage of, 14
for mild postoperative pain, 52-55

Ibuprofen—cont'd
for moderate to severe postoperative pain, 55
after myringotomy, 176
oral preparations of, 181
for otitis media pain, 161, 175
for sickle cell anemia pain, 161
for trauma-related pain, 191
Iliohypogastric block, 146-147
dosing guidelines for, 121
Ilioinguinal block, 146-147
dosing guidelines for, 121
Imaging
and invasive procedures, sedation for, 263-318
magnetic resonance
exclusion from, criteria for, 288
sedation for, 288-292
Imagnabix, 292
Imipramine, 343-344
dosage of, 35
Inapsine; *see* Droperidol
Indocin; *see* Indomethacin
Indoles, 13
Indomethacin, 13, 344
for central venous catheter placement, 204
dosage of, 14
for moderate to severe postoperative pain, 55-57
Inhalational anesthetic agents, 40-41
in PICU, 236-238
systemic effects of, 41
Injury, thermal, 183-187
Insulin, transmucosal administration of, 68
Intensive care unit
neonatal, use of analgesics in, 200
pediatric; *see* Pediatric intensive care unit
Intercostal blockade, 123-128
adverse effects of, 127-128
Intercostal blockade—cont'd
for chest pain, 183
dosing guidelines for, 120
positioning of child for, 125, 126
technique for, 123-127
Intercostal space, needle placement in, for intercostal blockade, 124, 125
Interpleural analgesia, 116-123
additional uses of, 123
adverse effects of, 119, 122
regional nerve blocks and, 113-156
technique for, 116-119
Interpleural block, dosing guidelines for, 120
Interpleural catheter, placement of, for interpleural anesthesia, 116, 117
Interscalene axillary block, dosing guidelines for, 121
Interscalene block, 138-140
complications of, 139-140
Interventional cardiac catheterization, sedation for, 293-294
Intracranial pressure, increased, opioid use and, 248-249
Intrathecal analgesia, opioids for, 89, 90
Intravenous anesthetic agents, 23-26
Intubation, endotracheal; *see* Endotracheal intubation
Invasive procedures
in neonate
list of, 200
sedation during, 198-215
sedation for, 263-318
therapeutic and diagnostic, sedation for, 296-300
Isoflurane, 40
in PICU, 236-238
Isoproterenol
for anaphylaxis, 87

Isoproterenol—cont'd
pediatric drip for, dosage of, 321

J

Jet injection devices, 300

K

Kappa receptors, 16
Ketalar; *see* Ketamine
Ketamine, 24-25, 344-345
actions of, 16
for Bier block, 145-146
for burn pain, 186
for central venous catheter placement, 203
for CT scanning sedation, 286
for diagnostic cardiac catheterization, 293
dosing of, based on route of delivery, 305
for endotracheal intubation, 206, 274
for interventional cardiac catheterization, 294
for mechanical ventilation, starting doses of, 254
for painful procedures, 305-307
in PICU, 241-243
for radiographic/cardiac catheterization procedures, 286
Ketoprofen, 13, 345
dosage of, 14
Ketorolac, 13, 15, 345
adverse effects of, 57
for chest pain, 180
dosage of, 14, 15
for moderate to severe postoperative pain, 55-57
nephrotoxicity of, 14
oral preparations of, 181
for trauma-related pain, 191
Knee surgery
obturator nerve blockade for, 132
sciatic nerve block for, 136

L

Laparotomy, caudal anesthesia for, 102
Laryngeal mask airway, 276, 278
sizes of, 279
Levo-Dromoran; *see* Levorphanol
Levorphanol, 16, 345
for moderate to severe postoperative pain, 58
Lidocaine, 30, 32, 346
for Bier block, 145
for burn pain, 185
for central venous catheter placement, 201, 202
for circumcision, 212
for digital blocks, 148
for emergency, dose of, 320
for endotracheal intubation, 274
for epidural analgesia for neonate, 223
maximum dose and duration of action of, 32, 84
for mucositis, 170, 171
pediatric drip for, dosage of, 321
for penile block, 210
for regional anesthesia, 31, 311
dosing guidelines for, 115, 121
for ring block, 210
for spinal anesthesia, 103, 109
topical anesthesia, 300
Local anesthesia, 82-92; *see also* Regional nerve blocks
for circumcision, 209-211
continuous, in neonates, 219-222
contraindications to, 82
for invasive procedures, 298-300
opioids for, 87-92
techniques for, 311
Local anesthetics, 30-34
absorption of
rate of, according to site of injection, 84
from regional blocks, 115
classification of, 83

Local anesthetics—cont'd
dosage of, 84
maximum recommended, 84
for regional nerve blocks, 115
for epidural anesthesia, 92-94
eutectic mixture of; *see* Eutectic mixture of local anesthetics
mechanism of action of, 82-83
rate of absorption of, 31
for skin and field infiltration in neonates, 202
for spinal anesthesia, 103
toxicity of, 32-33, 83, 85-87
determinants of, 83
management of, 85
Lorazepam, 28-29, 346
for burn pain, 186
dosage of, 28
for mechanical ventilation, 206, 207-208
starting doses of, 254
for painful procedures, 301
in PICU, 238, 240, 241
Lorcet HD; *see* Hydrocodone
Lorcet Plus; *see* Hydrocodone
Lortab; *see* Hydrocodone
Lower extremity block, 128-137
Lower extremity pain, traumatic injury causing, 189, 190
Lumbar plexus block, 128-129
obturator nerve block combined with, 132-136
Lumbar puncture, 168, 169

M

Magnesium for arrhythmias associated with bupivacaine toxicity, 33
Magnetic resonance imaging
exclusion from, criteria for, 288
sedation for, 288-292
Magnetic resonance imaging suite, diagram of, 282
Major tranquilizers, 36
Mallampati classification of upper airway, 43, 268
Marcaine; *see* Bupivacaine
Mature pain system, 4-5
Mechanical ventilation
sedation for, 204-209
sedative and analgesic agents for, starting doses of, 254
Median nerve, anesthesia of, 149, 151, 152-153
Meperidine, 16, 346
in DPT, 2, 310
duration of action and potency of, 18
epidural administration of, dosage of, 90
intrathecal administration of, dosage of, 90
metabolism of, 17
for moderate to severe postoperative pain, 58, 61-62
for painful procedures, 303
in "pedi cocktail," 2, 310
in PICU, 249, 250
potency and half-life of, 59
for sickle cell anemia pain, 162-163
for surgical pain in neonates, 217
Mepivacaine, 30, 347
for regional anesthesia, 31
dosing guidelines for, 115
maximum dose and duration of action of, 32, 84
Metabolic responses to surgery, neonatal, 13
Methadone, 16, 21-22, 347
dosage of, 21-22
duration of action and potency of, 18
epidural administration of, dosage of, 90
for moderate to severe postoperative pain, 58, 61, 62-63
for opioid withdrawal, 252

Methadone—cont'd
oral administration of, 65, 66
in PICU, 249
potency and half-life of, 59
for sickle cell anemia pain, 162, 173
Methadone sliding scale, 227-228
Methohexital, 27, 347
for painful procedures, 307
in PICU, 245
for radiographic/cardiac catheterization procedures, 286
Methylprednisolone for sickle cell anemia pain, 165
Metoclopramide, 347-348
for aspiration prophylaxis, 266
for opioid adverse effects, 75
Midazolam, 28-29, 348
for burn pain, 186
for CT scanning sedation, 286
for diagnostic cardiac catheterization, 293
dosage of, 28
based on route of delivery, 301
for emergency, dose of, 320
for endotracheal intubation, 205, 274
for extracorporeal membrane oxygenation cannula placement, 225
for mechanical ventilation, 206, 207
starting doses of, 254
for painful procedures, 301-302, 306-307
in PICU, 238-240, 241
for preoperative premedication, 53
for radiographic/cardiac catheterization procedures, 286
transmucosal administration of, 68
Milk of magnesia, 348
Mivacron; *see* Mivacurium
Mivacurium, 39-40, 348
for endotracheal intubation, 277
Mobile pediatric equipment cart, suggested items for, 281
Monitoring
after opioid administration, 90-91
of sedation, 44-45
Morphine, 16, 17, 348-349
actions of, 16
for cancer pain, 173
for caudal anesthesia, 102
for diagnostic cardiac catheterization, 293
dosing guidelines for, 61
duration of action and potency of, 18
epidural administration of, dosage for, 89, 90
for epidural analgesia for neonate, 224
intrathecal administration of, dosage of, 89, 90
for local anesthesia, 88, 89
for mechanical ventilation, 206, 208-209
starting doses of, 254
metabolism of, 17
for mild postoperative pain, 54
for moderate to severe postoperative pain, 58, 60-65
nebulized, 70
oral administration of, 65-66
for painful procedures, 303
in PICU, 249
for postoperative analgesia, 110
potency and half-life of, 59
pruritus caused by, 90
for sickle cell anemia pain, 162, 165-166
subcutaneous administration of, 68
subcutaneous infusion of, 248
for surgical pain in neonates, 216, 217

Morphine-6-glucuronide, 17
Motrin; *see* Ibuprofen
MS-Contin; *see* Morphine
Mu receptors, 15-16
Mucositis, 169-172
 agents used in treatment of, 171
 prevention/treatment of, 172
Multidisciplinary approach to management of sickle cell anemia pain, 164
Muscle relaxants, for radiographic/cardiac catheterization procedures, 286
Musculoskeletal causes of chest pain, 177, 178, 179-180
 related to traumatic injury, 189
Mylanta for mucositis, 171
Myringotomy, 174, 175-176

N

Nalbuphine, 22-23, 349
 potency and half-life of, 59
Naloxone, 23, 349-350
 actions of, 16
 dosage of, 23
 for emergency, dose of, 320
 as opioid antagonist, 311
 for pruritus, 90
 for respiratory depression from opioids, 73
 to reverse respiratory depression, 90
Naltrexone, 350
Naprosyn; *see* Naproxen
Naproxen, 13, 15, 350
 dosage of, 14
 for mild postoperative pain, 52
Narcan; *see* Naloxone
Neck pain, traumatic injury causing, 188
Needle, placement of, for caudal epidural block, 100, 101
Needle cricothyrotomy, 276, 278-279
Nembutal; *see* Pentobarbital
Neonatal abstinence syndrome, 250, 251
Neonatal intensive care unit, use of analgesics in, 200
Neonate
 continuous regional anesthesia in, 219-222
 epidural analgesia for, 223-225
 epidural anesthesia in, 218-219
 extracorporeal membrane oxygenation in, sedation during, 225-227
 increased pain sensitivity in, evidence for, 12-13
 invasive procedures in
  list of, 200
  sedation during, 198-215
 opioid tolerance and physical dependence in, 227-228
 pain assessment in, 198, 199
 pain management for, 197-234
 pain perception by, 4, 6
 postoperative pain in, 215-225
 skin and field infiltration in, local anesthetics for, 202
 spinal anesthesia in, 218-219
 surgical pain in, 215-225
Nerve
 femoral
  cutaneous sensory innervation of, 129
  location of, 130
 femoral cutaneous, cutaneous sensory innervation of, 129
 median, anesthesia of, 149, 151, 152-153
 obturator, cutaneous sensory innervation of, 129
 peroneal, anesthesia of, 149, 150
 radial, anesthesia of, 151, 152-153
 saphenous, anesthesia of, 149, 150

Nerve—cont'd
sural, anesthesia of, 149, 150
tibial, posterior, anesthesia of, 149, 150
ulnar, anesthesia of, 149, 151, 152-153
Nerve block; *see also* Blocks
digital, 147-149
fascia iliaca, of lumbar plexus, 128, 132-133
femoral, 129-131
femoral cutaneous, 131-132
iliohypogastric, 146-147
ilioinguinal, 146-147
intercostal; *see* Intercostal blockade
lower extremity, 128-137
obturator, 132-136
penile, technique for, 210, 211
peripheral, 146-151
psoas compartment, of lumbar plexus, 128, 132, 134-136
sciatic, 136
needle entry for, 137
3-in-1, of lumbar plexus, 128, 129, 132, 133, 134
Nervous system, development of, pain perception and, 8-12
Nesacaine; *see* Chloroprocaine
Neuraxial opioids, 88, 89
adverse effects of, 89-90
Neuroanatomy and neurophysiology of developing pain system, 4-13
Neuromuscular blocking agents, 36-40
for endotracheal intubation, 274, 275-276
nondepolarizing, 277
for endotracheal intubation, 276
Neuropeptide Y, transmission of nociceptive impulses and, 8
Neurophysiology and neuroanatomy of developing pain system, 4-13
Neurotransmitters, excitatory, 8-9
Nitroglycerin, pediatric drip for, dosage of, 321
Nitroprusside, pediatric drip for, dosage of, 321
Nitrous oxide, 40
for myringotomy, 175
for painful procedures, 309-310
No-touch technique for caudal epidural block, 101
Nociceptors, development of, 6, 8
Noctec; *see* Chloral hydrate
Nondepolarizing neuromuscular blocking agents, 277
for endotracheal intubation, 276
Nonintravenous routes of opioid administration, 65-71
Nonopioid analgesics, classification of, 53
Nonpharmacologic methods of sedation, 312
Nonsteroidal antiinflammatory drugs, 13-15, 53
adverse effects of, 57-58
for burn pain, 185
for cancer pain, 173
for central venous catheter placement, 204
for chest pain, 178, 180
for mild postoperative pain, 52-55
for moderate to severe postoperative pain, 55-58
nephrotoxicity of, 14
pharmacology of, 14
for sickle cell anemia pain, 161, 164
side effects of, 14-15
for trauma-related pain, 191
Norcuron; *see* Vecuronium
Norepinephrine
for anaphylaxis, 87

Norepinephrine—cont'd
pediatric drip for, dosage of, 321
Normeperidine, 17
for moderate to severe postoperative pain, 62
Nortriptyline, 350
for cancer pain, 173
dosage of, 35
Novel antidepressants, dosage of, 35
Novocain; *see* Procaine
NPO guidelines for children, 47, 265
NPO status before sedation, 264, 265-266
NSAIDs; *see* Nonsteroidal antiinflammatory drugs
Nubain; *see* Nalbuphine
Numorphan; *see* Oxymorphone
Nuromax; *see* Doxacurium
Nystatin, for candidiasis, 170

O

Obturator nerve, cutaneous sensory innervation of, 129
Obturator nerve block, 132-136
Oncologic diseases, 168-174
Ondansetron, 350-351
for opioid adverse effects, 75
Opioid agonist/antagonists, mixed, 22-23
actions of, 16
Opioid antagonist, 23
Opioid receptors and brain development in neonates, 12
Opioids, 58-76
addiction from, 73-74
adverse effects of, 71-76
patients at risk for, 73
of agonist/antagonist class, 59, 60
and analogs, 15-23
antagonists for, 311-312
for burn pain, 184, 185-187

Opioids—cont'd
for central venous catheter placement, 204
for chest pain, 180
classification of, 16, 58
for mechanical ventilation, 206, 208-209
starting doses of, 254
for mucositis, 170, 172-173
naturally occurring, 16, 58
nebulized forms of, 70
neuraxial, 88, 89
adverse effects of, 89-90
nonintravenous routes of administration of, 65-71
oral administration of, 65-66
for painful procedures, 302-303
for patient-controlled analgesia, 63-65, 67-68
in PICU, 246-252
for postoperative analgesia, 109-110
potency and half-life of, 59
for radiographic/cardiac catheterization procedures, 286
for regional anesthesia, 87-92
monitoring after, 90-91
semisynthetic, 58
for sickle cell anemia pain, 161-166
subcutaneous administration of, 67-69
subcutaneous infusion of, 247-248
sublingual administration of, 70-71
for surgical pain in neonates, 215-216
synthetic, 58, 60-61
for radiofrequency ablation, 296
tapering use of, 227, 250-252
tolerance to and physical dependence on, 227-228, 250-252

Opioids—cont'd
transdermal administration of, 66-67
transmucosal administration of, 68-69
for trauma-related pain, 191
Orchiopexy, ilioinguinal and iliohypogastric blocks for, 146
Orudis; *see* Ketoprofen
Otitis media, pain caused by, 174-176
treatment of, 161
Oxicam, 13
Oximeter, pulse, to monitor during sedation, 44
Oxycodone, 16, 351
for cancer pain, 173
for chest pain, 180
duration of action and potency of, 18
for mild postoperative pain, 54-55
for moderate to severe postoperative pain, 58
oral administration of, 65
oral preparations of, 181
for sickle cell anemia pain, 161
Oxygenation, extracorporeal membrane, sedation during, 225-227
Oxymorphone, 16, 351
for moderate to severe postoperative pain, 58
potency and half-life of, 59

P

Pain
abdominal, 178
assessment of, in neonate, 198, 199
basic aspects of, 1-48
burns and thermal injury causing, 183-187
chest, 176-183

Pain—cont'd
chest—cont'd
common causes of, 177
gate-control theory of, physiologic basis for, 9
increased sensitivity to, in neonates, evidence for, 12-13
management of
nonpharmacologic approaches to, 206
rational approach to, 3
medical disease causing, management of, 157-195
neonatal, management of, 197-234
oncologic diseases causing, 168-174
otitis media causing, 174-176
treatment of, 161
perception of, 3
by neonates, 4, 6
nervous system development and, 8-12
postoperative; *see* Postoperative pain
procedural, 168-169
rating scales for, 199
surgical, in neonate, 215-225
theories on, 8-11
trauma-related, 187-192
Pain system
developing, neuroanatomy and neurophysiology of, 4-13
mature, 4-5
peripheral, components and functions of, 7
Pain threshold, decreases in, 13
Painful crises with sickle cell disease, 158
Pamelor; *see* Nortriptyline
Panadol; *see* Acetaminophen
Pancuronium, 38, 351-352
dosage of, 37
for emergency, dose of, 320

Pancuronium—cont'd
for endotracheal intubation, 274, 275, 277
Papaverine, 16
for moderate to severe postoperative pain, 58
Paraaminophenol derivatives, 13, 53
for mild postoperative pain, 52
Patient assessment before surgical procedure, 42-43
Patient history, 267-268
Patient-controlled analgesia
for burn pain, 186-187
for moderate to severe postoperative pain, 55, 63-65
for sickle cell anemia pain, 163-164
for trauma-related pain, 191
Pavulon; *see* Pancuronium
"Pedi cocktail," 2, 310
Pediaprofen; *see* Ibuprofen
Pediatric drips for emergency medications, 321
Pediatric equipment cart, mobile, suggested items for, 281
Pediatric intensive care unit
sedation in, 235-261
agents for, 236-255
use of analgesics in, 200
use of barbiturates in, 244-246
use of benzodiazepines in, 238-241
use of butyrophenones in, 252-253
use of inhalational anesthetic agents in, 236-238
use of ketamine in, 241-243
use of opioids in, 246-252
use of phenothiazines in, 252-253
use of propofol in, 243-244
Pediatric pain; *see* Pain
Penile nerve block, technique for, 210, 211
Pentazocine, 16, 22-23, 352
for moderate to severe postoperative pain, 58
potency and half-life of, 59
Pentobarbital, 27, 352
for extracorporeal membrane oxygenation cannula placement, 226-227
for mechanical ventilation, starting doses of, 254
for painful procedures, 308
in PICU, 245-246
for radiographic/cardiac catheterization procedures, 286
Pentothal; *see* Thiopental
Peptide, calcitonin-gene-related
pain sensitivity in neonates and, 12
transmission of nociceptive impulses and, 8
Percocet; *see* Oxycodone
Percodan; *see* Oxycodone
Peripheral nerve block, 146-151
Peripheral pain system, components and functions of, 7
Peroneal nerve, anesthesia of, 149, 150
Phencyclidine, actions of, 16
Phenergan; *see* Promethazine
Phenobarbital
for moderate to severe postoperative pain, 62
in PICU, 245
Phenothiazines, 36
combination of, 310
dosage of, 35
for opioid adverse effects, 75
in PICU, 252-253
Phenylacetic acid derivatives, 13
Phenylephrine, pediatric drip for, dosage of, 321
Phenytoin, 352-353
for arrhythmias associated with bupivacaine toxicity, 33

Phenytoin—cont'd
for cancer pain, 174
Physical dependence
on benzodiazepines, 241
on opioids, 227-228, 250-252
Physical examination, 267-268
before surgery, 42-43
Physical status classification of American Society of Anesthesiologists, 44, 268, 269
Physiologic assessment of pain in neonate and infant, 199
Piroxicam, 13, 353
dosage of, 14
Platelet disorders, drugs for patients with, 57
Pneumonitis, aspiration, 265, 266
Polypeptide, vasoactive intestinal
pain sensitivity in neonates and, 12
transmission of nociceptive impulses and, 8
Pontocaine; *see* Tetracaine
Postoperative analgesia, opioids for, 109-110
Postoperative pain
management of, 49-50
strategies for, 52
mild, 51-55
moderate to severe, 55-58
in neonate, 215-225
Postsurgical stress response, 49-50
Prilocaine, 30, 353
for Bier block, 145
for central venous catheter placement, 201
for regional anesthesia, 31
dosing guidelines for, 121
Procaine, 30, 353
for regional anesthesia, 31
dosing guidelines for, 115
maximum dose and duration of action of, 32
Procedural pain, 168-169
Promethazine, 353-354
in DPT, 2, 310
for opioid adverse effects, 75
in "pedi cocktail," 2, 310
Propionic acid derivatives, 13
Propofol, 26, 354
for burn pain, 186
for diagnostic cardiac catheterization, 293
for endotracheal intubation, 274
for interventional cardiac catheterization, 294
for mechanical ventilation, starting doses of, 254
for painful procedures, 308-309
in PICU, 243-244
for radiofrequency ablation, 296
for radiographic/cardiac catheterization procedures, 286
Propoxyphene for sickle cell anemia pain, 161
Propulsid; *see* Cisapride
Prostaglandin synthesis inhibitors for mild postoperative pain, 51-55
Prozac; *see* Fluoxetine
Pruritus, opioid-induced, 75-76
Psoas compartment block of lumbar plexus, 128, 132, 134-136
dosing guidelines for, 120
Psychotropic agents, 34-36
Pulmonary causes of chest pain, 177, 179-180
related to traumatic injury, 189
Pulse oximeter to monitor during sedation, 44
Puncture, lumbar, 168, 169
Pyloromyotomy, caudal anesthesia for, 101
Pyrroles, 13

R

Radial nerve, anesthesia of, 151, 152-153

Radiofrequency ablation, 294-296
Radiographic procedures, sedation for, drug strategies for, 286
Radiologic procedures, sedation for, 279-292
Ranitidine, 354
for anaphylaxis, 87
for aspiration prophylaxis, 266
Rectal nonsteroidal antiinflammatory drugs for moderate to severe postoperative pain, 55
Reflexes
sensory, development of, 6, 8
threshold for, in neonates, 12
Regional anesthesia; *see* Local anesthesia
Regional blockade; *see* Local anesthesia
Regional nerve blocks; *see also* Local anesthesia; Local anesthetics
dosing guidelines for, 120-121
and interpleural analgesia, 113-156
local anesthetics for
absorption of, 115
dosing guidelines for, 115
for management of sickle cell anemia pain, 167
therapeutic uses of, 114
Reglan; *see* Metoclopramide
Relaxation training for management of sickle cell anemia pain, 164-165
Remifentanil for moderate to severe postoperative pain, 58
Respiratory depression from opioid administration, 71-73, 90, 91-92
Response, postsurgical stress, 49-50
Reye's syndrome, 14, 52
Ring block for circumcision, 210
Robinul; *see* Glycopyrrolate
Rocuronium, 40, 354
for endotracheal intubation, 274, 277
Romazicon; *see* Flumazemil
Ropivacaine, 30
Roxanol; *see* Morphine

S

Sacral cornu, identification of, for caudal anesthesia, 98, 99
Sacral plexus block, 128-129
Sacrum, anatomy of, 99
Safety of sedation, 41-47
Salicylates, 13, 53
for mild postoperative pain, 52
Saphenous nerve, anesthesia of, 149, 150
Scalp pain, related to traumatic injury, 187
Sciatic nerve block, 136
dosing guidelines for, 121
entry for, 137
Sedation
agents for, for painful procedures, 301-312
for cardiac catheterization, 292-296
drug strategies for, 286
for central venous catheter placement, 200-204
for circumcision, 209-215
for computerized tomography, 283-288
conscious, 42
deep, 42
for endotracheal intubation, 204-209
equipment and drugs for, minimal, 46
during extracorporeal membrane oxygenation, 225-227
fasting guidelines for, 45, 47
for imaging and invasive proce-

Sedation—cont'd
dures, 263-318
for invasive therapeutic and diagnostic procedures, 296-300
in neonate, 198-215
for magnetic resonance imaging, 288-292
for mechanical ventilation, 204-209
monitoring of, 44-45
opioid-induced, prevention of, 74
in pediatric intensive care unit, 235-261
agents for, 236-255
pediatric pain and, basic aspects of, 1-48
during procedures, agents for, 269
for radiologic procedures, 279-292
drug strategies for, 286
rational approach to, 3
safety considerations with, 41-47
Vanderbilt University Medical Center policy on, 321-328
Sedation log, 169
Sedatives, 26-30
during mechanical ventilation, starting doses of, 254
selection of, 269-270
Semisynthetic opioids, 58
Sensitivity to pain, increased, in neonates, evidence for, 12-13
Sensorcaine; *see* Bupivacaine
Sensory receptors, fetal, 6
Sensory reflexes, development of, 6, 8
Sevoflurane in PICU, 236
Sickle cell disease and associated hemoglobinopathies, 158-168
Sigma receptors, 16
Sinequan; *see* Doxepin
Skin infiltration in neonates, local anesthetics for, 202
Skull, traumatic injury to, 187
Sodium bicarbonate, 354-355
for emergency, dose of, 320
for mucositis, 171
Sodium citrate for aspiration prophylaxis, 266
Sodium thiopental for endotracheal intubation, 205
Solu-Medrol for anaphylaxis, 87
Somatostatin, transmission of nociceptive impulses and, 8
Spinal anesthesia, 108-110
advantages and disadvantages of, 103
caudal anesthesia versus, 103
and epidural anesthesia/analgesia, 81-112
general anesthesia combined with, 110
local anesthetics for, 103
in neonates, 218-219
Spinal cord, dorsal horn of
components and functions of, 7
development of, 8-12
Stadol; *see* Butorphanol
Steroids for central venous catheter placement, 204
Stress, postsurgical, response to, 49-50
Subcutaneous infusion of opioids, 247-248
Sublimaze; *see* Fentanyl
Substance P
pain sensitivity in neonates and, 12
transmission of nociceptive impulses and, 8
Succinylcholine, 37-38, 355
contraindications to, 275
dosage of, 37
for emergency, dose of, 320
for endotracheal intubation, 274, 275
Sucralfate for mucositis, 171

Sufenta; *see* Sufentanil
Sufentanil, 16, 17, 20, 355
  dosage of, 20
  epidural administration of, dosage of, 89, 90
  intrathecal administration of, dosage of, 90
  for moderate to severe postoperative pain, 58
  in PICU, 248
  potency and half-life of, 59
  for radiofrequency ablation, 296
Supraspinal centers, components and functions of, 7
Sural nerve, anesthesia of, 149, 150
Surgery
  abdominal, pain after, 51
  catecholamine and metabolic responses to, 13
  pain after, management of, 49-80
  pain from, in neonate, 215-225
  patient assessment before, 42-43
  thoracic, pain after, 51
Surital; *see* Thiamylal
Synthetic opioids, 58, 60-61
  for radiofrequency ablation, 296

T

TAC, 299-300
Tagamet; *see* Cimetidine
Talwin; *see* Pentazocine
Tetracaine, 30, 355
  maximum dose and duration of action of, 32, 84
  for regional anesthesia, 31
    dosing guidelines for, 115
  for spinal anesthesia, 103, 109
    in neonates, 218
  in TAC, 299
  for topical anesthesia, 299
Thebaine, 16
  for moderate to severe postoperative pain, 58
Theracath, Arrow
  for epidural anesthesia, 94, 95
  for interpleural analgesia, 118
Therapeutic procedures, invasive
  for children, list of, 297
  sedation for, 296-300
Thermal injury, 183-187
Thiamylal, 355-356
  in PICU, 245
Thiopental, 27, 356
  for emergency, dose of, 320
  for endotracheal intubation, 274
  for painful procedures, 307-308
  in PICU, 245
Thoracic surgery, pain after, 51
Thoracotomy
  caudal anesthesia for, 102
  intercostal blockade for, 123
  interpleural analgesia for, 117-118
Thorazine; *see* Chlorpromazine
  3-in-1 block
    dosing guidelines for, 120
    of lumbar plexus, 128, 129, 132, 133, 134
    sensory distribution anesthetized by, 134
Tibial nerve, posterior, anesthesia of, 149, 150
Toes, nerve blocks for, 147-149
Tofranil; *see* Imipramine
Tolectin; *see* Tolmetin
Tolerance, 227
  to benzodiazepines, 241
  to opioids, 227-228, 250-252
Tolmetin, 13, 15, 356
  for mild postoperative pain, 52
Tomography, computerized, sedation for, 283-288
Topical anesthesia for invasive procedures, 298-300
Toradol; *see* Ketorolac
Trade name and generic name index, 358-360

Tramadol, 357
for mechanical ventilation, 209
Tranquilizers, major, 36
Transarterial approach to axillary block, 140-141
Transdermal delivery of fentanyl, 246-247
Transmucosal fentanyl for painful procedures, 303-304
Trauma-related pain, 187-192
Trexan; *see* Naltrexone
Tricyclic antidepressants
for burn pain, 185
for cancer pain, 173
dosage of, 35
Trilisate; *see* Choline magnesium trisalicylate
d-Tubocurarine, 38
Tylenol; *see* Acetaminophen
Tylenol #2, 181
for mild postoperative pain, 54
Tylenol #3, 181
for mild postoperative pain, 54
Tylenol #4, 181
for mild postoperative pain, 54
Tylox; *see* Oxycodone

U

Ulnar nerve, anesthesia of, 149, 151, 152-153
Ultram; *see* Tramadol
Upper extremity blockade, 137-142
Upper extremity pain, traumatic injury causing, 189, 190
Urecholine; *see* Bethanechol

V

Valium; *see* Diazepam
Vanderbilt University Medical Center Sedation Policy, 321-328
Vasoactive intestinal polypeptide
pain sensitivity in neonates and, 12
transmission of nociceptive impulses and, 8
Vasoocclusive crisis with sickle cell disease, 158, 159, 160, 161
Vasopressin, transmucosal administration of, 68
Vecuronium, 38-39, 357
dosage of, 37
for endotracheal intubation, 205, 274, 275, 277
for radiofrequency ablation, 296
Venipuncture, 168
Ventilation, mechanical
sedation for, 204-209
sedative and analgesic agents for, starting doses of, 254
Versed; *see* Midazolam
Vicodin; *see* Hydrocodone
Vicodin ES; *see* Hydrocodone
VIP; *see* Vasoactive intestinal polypeptide
Vistaril; *see* Hydroxyzine
Volatile anesthetic agents, 40
Voltaren; *see* Diclofenac

W

Windup phenomenon, 13
Withdrawal, drug, 227-228
Wrist block, 149, 151, 152-153
dosing guidelines for, 121

X

Xylocaine; *see* Lidocaine

Z

Zantac; *see* Ranitidine
Zemuron; *see* Rocuronium
Zofran; *see* Ondansetron